Williams
Obstetrics

21ST EDITION Study Guide

This study guide includes continuing medical education material, an educational activity sponsored by:

SOUTHWESTERN
THE UNIVERSITY OF TEXAS
SOUTHWESTERN MEDICAL CENTER
AT DALLAS

ACCME Accreditation

The University of Texas Southwestern Medical Center at Dallas is accredited by the Accreditation Council for Continuing Medical Education to sponsor continuing medical education for physicians.

AMA/PRA Credit Designation

The University of Texas Southwestern Medical Center at Dallas designates this educational activity for a maximum of 50 hours in Category I credit towards the AMA Physician's Recognition Award. Each physician should claim only those hours of credit that he/she actually spent in the educational activity.

This continuing medical education activity was planned and produced in accordance with the Essential Areas and Policies of the ACCME.

Date of original release: June 2001. Term of approval: 3 years

See page 283 for additional CME instructions.

The University of Texas Southwestern Medical Center at Dallas Office of Continuing Education

DISCLOSURE OF SIGNIFICANT RELATIONSHIPS WITH RELEVANT COMMERCIAL COMPANIES/ORGANIZATIONS

Williams Obstetrics 21st Edition Study Guide
June 2001

According to the University of Texas Southwestern "Disclosure Policy," faculty involved in continuing medical education activities are required to complete a "Conflict of Interest Disclosure" to disclose any real or apparent conflict(s) of interest related directly or indirectly to the program. This information is acknowledged solely for the information of the participant.

The faculty listed below have disclosed a financial interest or other relationship with a commercial concern related directly or indirectly to the activity (names of companies are listed after each presenter's name). Those presenters not listed have disclosed no financial interest or relationship.

UT Southwestern does not view the existence of these interests or relationships as implying bias or decreasing the value of the presentation.

This educational activity has been planned to be well balanced and objective in discussion of comparative treatment regimens. Information and opinions offered by the authors represent their viewpoints. Conclusions drawn by the reader should be derived from careful consideration of all available scientific information. Products may be discussed in treatment of indications outside current approved labeling.

Faculty

Susan M. Cox, MD	*Williams Obstetrics 21st Edition Study Guide*, June 2001
Claudia L. Werner, MD	*Williams Obstetrics 21st Edition Study Guide*, June 2001
Larry C. Gilstrap III, MD	*Williams Obstetrics 21st Edition Study Guide*, June 2001
F. Gary Cunningham, MD	*Williams Obstetrics 21st Edition Study Guide*, June 2001

Williams Obstetrics

21ST EDITION Study Guide

Susan M. Cox, MD
Professor
Department of Obstetrics and Gynecology
University of Texas Southwestern Medical Center at Dallas
Dallas, Texas

Claudia L. Werner, MD
Assistant Professor
Department of Obstetrics and Gynecology
University of Texas Southwestern Medical Center at Dallas
Dallas, Texas

Larry C. Gilstrap III, MD
Professor and Chairman
Department of Obstetrics and Gynecology
University of Texas Medical School at Houston
Houston, Texas

F. Gary Cunningham, MD
Professor and Chairman
Department of Obstetrics and Gynecology
Jack A. Pritchard Professor of Obstetrics and Gynecology
Beatrice & Miguel Elias Distinguished Chair in Ob/Gyn
University of Texas Southwestern Medical Center at Dallas
Chief of Obstetrics and Gynecology
Parkland Memorial Hospital
Dallas, Texas

McGRAW-HILL
Medical Publishing Division

New York   Chicago   San Francisco   Lisbon   London   Madrid   Mexico City
Milan   New Delhi   San Juan   Seoul   Singapore   Sydney   Toronto

McGraw-Hill

A Division of The McGraw·Hill Companies

NOTICE

Medicine is an ever-changing science. As new research and clinical experience broaden our knowledge, changes in treatment and drug therapy are required. The authors and the publisher of this work have checked with sources believed to be reliable in their efforts to provide information that is complete and generally in accord with the standards accepted at the time of publication. However, in view of the possibility of human error or changes in medical sciences, neither the authors nor the publisher nor any other party who has been involved in the preparation or publication of this work warrants that the information contained herein is in every respect accurate or complete, and they disclaim all responsibility for any errors or omissions or for the results obtained from use of the information contained in this work. Readers are encouraged to confirm the information contained herein with other sources. For example and in particular, readers are advised to check the product information sheet included in the package of each drug they plan to administer to be certain that the information contained in this work is accurate and that changes have not been made in the recommended dose or in the contraindications for administration. This recommendation is of particular importance in connection with new or infrequently used drugs.

This book was set in Garamond by TechBooks.
The editors were Andrea Seils, Susan Noujaim, and Karen Davis.
The production supervisor was Lisa Mendez.
The cover designer was Mary McKeon.
The index was prepared by Coughlin Indexing Services, Inc.
Courier Stoughton was printer and binder.

This book is printed on acid-free paper.

Contents

Preface

This *Williams Obstetrics 21st Edition Study Guide* is designed to assess comprehension and retention of materials covered in the 21st edition of *Williams Obstetrics.* A feature of this study guide is the provision for earning continuing medical education (CME) credit.

The questions for each section are based on the key points from each chapter and are in the same order as the text. There are a total of 2524 questions from the 59 chapters. The questions are in multiple choice format with one single best answer. It is suggested that the user first read the question and think of the answer prior to choosing the correct answer from the four choices given. The questions are followed by a section that contains the answers and page numbers in the textbook where answers can be found.

We hope that the simplified format used in this study guide will make the task of assimilating the information from the 21st edition of *Williams Obstetrics* less formidable. It is also hoped that the provision for earning CME credit will lend itself to the extremely busy, everyday practice of clinical medicine.

Susan M. Cox, MD
Claudia L. Werner, MD
Larry C. Gilstrap III, MD
F. Gary Cunningham, MD

Williams Obstetrics

21ST EDITION Study Guide

1

Obstetrics in Broad Perspective

1–1. At the beginning of the 1900s, what proportion of women giving birth died of pregnancy-related complications?

   a. 1 in 10
   b. 1 in 50
   c. 1 in 100
   d. 1 in 1000

1–2. What is the infant mortality rate per 1000 livebirths in the United States as of 1997?

   a. 1
   b. 7
   c. 15
   d. 27

1–3. What is the maternal mortality rate per 100,000 livebirths in the United States as of 1997?

   a. 2
   b. 8
   c. 12
   d. 28

1–4. What year was the Bureau of the Census established?

   a. 1858
   b. 1902
   c. 1928
   d. 1952

1–5. Which of one of the following gestations corresponds to the perinatal period?

   a. 22 to 28 weeks
   b. 22 to 34 weeks
   c. 20 to 40 weeks
   d. 20 weeks to 4 weeks postpartum

1–6. The term *birth* usually refers to fetuses born weighing at least what amount?

   a. 250 g
   b. 500 g
   c. 1000 g
   d. 1500 g

1–7. Which of the following describes the number of livebirths per 1000 population?

   a. fertility rate
   b. birth rate
   c. perinatal birth rate
   d. delivery rate

1–8. What is the term for the number of deaths per 1000 births occurring during the first 28 days of life?

   a. stillbirth rate
   b. fetal death rate
   c. perinatal mortality rate
   d. neonatal mortality rate

1–9. How is low birthweight defined?

   a. <1000 g
   b. <1500 g
   c. <2000 g
   d. <2500 g

1–10. What is the gestational age cutoff for defining the birth of a preterm infant?

   a. <29 weeks
   b. <33 weeks
   c. <35 weeks
   d. <37 weeks

1–11. How is an infant classified that is born between 260 and 294 days of gestation?

   a. preterm
   b. term
   c. postterm
   d. postmature

1–12. How would a maternal death secondary to mitral stenosis be classified?

   a. direct maternal death
   b. indirect maternal death
   c. nonmaternal death
   d. nonobstetrical death

1–13. Currently, how many pregnancies do American women average over their lifetimes?

   a. 1.6
   b. 2.5
   c. 3.2
   d. 4.8

1–14. Approximately what percentage of pregnancies in the United States are wanted or planned?

   a. 25
   b. 50
   c. 75
   d. 95

1–15. In 1995, what percentage of babies born to never-married women were placed for adoption?

   a. 1
   b. 10
   c. 20
   d. 40

1–16. What is the average number of livebirths per woman in the United States?

   a. 1
   b. 2
   c. 3
   d. 4

1–17. Approximately what percentage of pregnancies in the United States result in livebirths?

   a. 50
   b. 60
   c. 70
   d. 90

1–18. Approximately what percentage of pregnancies in the United States end by induced termination?

   a. 5
   b. 10
   c. 15
   d. 20

1–19. Approximately what percentage of pregnancies in the United States end as spontaneous miscarriages?

   a. 5
   b. 10
   c. 15
   d. 20

1–20. What is the most common cause of non-delivery-related hospitalization during pregnancy?

   a. preterm labor
   b. preeclampsia
   c. gestational diabetes
   d. pyelonephritis

1–21. What percentage of infant deaths involve low birthweight infants?

   a. 25
   b. 33
   c. 50
   d. 66

1–22. Although thought to be an underestimation, approximately how many maternal deaths in the United States in 1997 were identified by vital statistics?

   a. 327
   b. 3270
   c. 32,700
   d. 327,000

1–23. How does the maternal mortality rate of African-American women compare to that of Caucasian women?

   a. equal
   b. slightly less
   c. twice as high
   d. four times as high

1–24. What percentage of births in the United States occur in 15- to17-year-old teenagers?

    a. 1.5
    b. 4.5
    c. 8.5
    d. 16.5

1–25. How many of the 270 million people living in the United States are medically uninsured?

    a. 2 million
    b. 11 million
    c. 22 million
    d. 44 million

2

Pregnancy: Overview, Organization, and Diagnosis

2–1. In a woman who does not use contraception, how many lifetime opportunities are there for pregnancy?

    a. 100
    b. 250
    c. 500
    d. 1000

2–2. What percentage of married couples have relative or absolute infertility?

    a. 1
    b. 5
    c. 10
    d. 20

2–3. What is the approximate success of in vitro fertilization and embryo transfer in producing a live-born fetus?

    a. <12 percent
    b. <25 percent
    c. <41 percent
    d. <65 percent

2–4. Which of the following mammals menstruates?

    a. chimpanzees
    b. cows
    c. dolphins
    d. rabbits

2–5. What is the average age of menarche for women in the United States?

    a. $11\frac{1}{2}$ years
    b. $12\frac{1}{2}$ years
    c. $13\frac{1}{2}$ years
    d. $14\frac{1}{2}$ years

2–6. Modern cultural and nutritional influences have led to all EXCEPT which of the following?

    a. choice of infertility or delayed childbearing
    b. earlier menarche
    c. improved infant survival
    d. increased lactational amenorrhea

2–7. What is the site of synthesis of follicular estrogen?

    a. granulosa cells
    b. theca cells
    c. stroma cells
    d. endometrium

2–8. The wide fluctuations in estrogen levels during the ovarian cycle are most important to the functioning of which of the following?

    a. bone
    b. brain or pituitary gland
    c. liver
    d. skin

2–9. Compared with primitive human tribes and apes, modern women experience more of which of the following?

    a. amenorrhea due to lactation
    b. episodes of menstruation
    c. lean body mass
    d. live births

2–10. Which of the following is NOT a component of the paracrine arm of the fetal-maternal communication system?

    a. amnion or amniotic fluid
    b. chorion laeve
    c. maternal decidua
    d. spiral arteries

2–11. Anatomically, the placental arm of the fetal-maternal communication system consists of all EXCEPT which of the following?

    a. decidua parietalis
    b. fetal blood cells
    c. maternal blood cells
    d. syncytium

2–12. What lies in direct contact with fetal membranes but NOT underlying the placenta?

    a. decidua basalis
    b. decidua fetalis
    c. decidua maternalis
    d. decidua parietalis

2–13. Which of the following decidual hormones preferentially enters the amniotic fluid?

    a. estrogen
    b. progesterone
    c. prolactin
    d. prostaglandin F_2

2–14. In what anatomical location does fertilization take place?

    a. fallopian tube
    b. ovarian surface
    c. peritoneal cavity
    d. uterine cavity

2–15. How long after fertilization does implantation begin?

    a. 1 day
    b. 3 days
    c. 6 days
    d. 9 days

2–16. What does modulation of expression of major human leukocyte, locus A (HLA) antigens by trophoblasts facilitate?

    a. decidualization of endometrium
    b. degradation of extracellular proteins
    c. immunological acceptance of fetal tissues
    d. maintenance of corpus luteum

2–17. What hormone is responsible for maintenance of the corpus luteum if implantation of the fertilized ovum takes place?

    a. estrogen
    b. progesterone
    c. human chorionic gonadotropin (hCG)
    d. human placental lactogen (hPL)

2–18. The corpus luteum, in the absence of conception, shows a decline in progesterone secretion after how many days?

    a. 3
    b. 7
    c. 10
    d. 15

2–19. After what menstrual age (weeks) does the syncytiotrophoblast become the dominant source of progesterone?

    a. 2
    b. 4
    c. 6
    d. 8

2–20. If the corpus luteum is surgically removed prior to 9 weeks gestation, what is the drug of choice to maintain the pregnancy?

    a. ethinyl estradiol
    b. 17α-hydroxprogesterone caproate
    c. medroxyprogesterone acetate
    d. mestranol

2–21. Where are the C_{19}-steroid precursors used for placental formation of estrogens derived from?

    a. fetal adrenals
    b. maternal adrenals
    c. fetal pituitary gland
    d. maternal ovaries

2–22. Use of maternal low-density lipoprotein cholesterol, as well as its esters and apoproteins, leads to the availability of which of the following?

    a. amino acids
    b. essential fatty acids
    c. progesterone
    d. all of the above

2–23. What hormone plays a key role in maternal blood volume expansion by its conversion to deoxycorticosterone and by stimulating secretion of maternal angiotensin II or aldosterone?

    a. estriol
    b. hCG
    c. progesterone
    d. prolactin

2–24. What happens to fetal iron stores in pregnant women with severe iron-deficiency anemia?

    a. decreases
    b. increases
    c. remains normal
    d. varies tremendously

2–25. Which of the following hormones acts to prevent lactogenesis?

    a. cortisol
    b. hPL
    c. progesterone
    d. prolactin

2–26. Milk let-down, or constriction of myoepithelial cells of the breast ducts, is controlled by the release of which hormone in response to suckling?

    a. cortisol
    b. estradiol
    c. oxytocin
    d. progesterone

2–27. Which of the following is NOT a presumptive symptom of pregnancy?

    a. nausea
    b. fatigue
    c. mastalgia
    d. urinary frequency

2–28. Which of the following is NOT a presumptive sign of pregnancy?

    a. acne
    b. breast changes
    c. Chadwick sign
    d. melasma

2–29. What percentage of pregnancies that do not abort are associated with macroscopic vaginal bleeding?

    a. <5
    b. 20 to 25
    c. 50 to 60
    d. 80 to 90

2–30. Ferning on an air-dried slide of cervical mucus is attributed to an increased concentration of which component?

    a. collagen
    b. glucose
    c. mucopolysaccharide
    d. sodium chloride

2–31. What is the Chadwick sign?

    a. discoloration of the vaginal mucosa
    b. pigmentation of the skin
    c. change in consistency of uterus
    d. implantation bleeding

2–32. Which of the following is NOT considered a probable sign of pregnancy?

    a. enlargement of the abdomen
    b. changes in shape, size, and consistency of uterus
    c. cessation of menses
    d. hCG present in urine

2–33. When does the pregnant uterus first become palpable abdominally?

    a. 8 weeks
    b. 12 weeks
    c. 16 weeks
    d. 20 weeks

2–34. How long after onset of last menstruation until Hegar sign becomes evident?

    a. 1 to 2 weeks
    b. 2 to 4 weeks
    c. 6 to 8 weeks
    d. 10 to 12 weeks

2–35. What is a positive Hegar sign?

    a. ballottement of the fetus
    b. cervical mucous ferning
    c. softening of the uterine isthmus
    d. vasocongestion of the vaginal mucosa

2–36. Chorionic gonadotropin exerts hormonal effects by stimulation of which receptors?

    a. estrogen
    b. follicle-stimulating hormone
    c. luteinizing hormone
    c. progesterone

2–37. What is the earliest time following ovulation that hCG can be detected in maternal urine or plasma?

    a. 5 to 6 days
    b. 8 to 9 days
    c. 10 to 12 days
    d. 14 to 16 days

2–38. What is the doubling time for hCG in early pregnancy?

  a. 1.4 to 2.0 days
  b. 2.4 to 3.0 days
  c. 4.4 to 5.0 days
  d. >5.0 days

2–39. What is the sensitivity of the enzyme-linked immunosorbent assay (ELISA) test for hCG?

  a. 10 mIU/mL
  b. 20 mIU/mL
  c. 50 mIU/mL
  d. 250 mIU/mL

2–40. What is the false-negative rate of home pregnancy tests?

  a. 10 percent
  b. 25 percent
  c. 50 percent
  d. 75 percent

2–41. Fetal heart tones are first heard by auscultation in nonobese women at what week of gestational age?

  a. 9 to 11
  b. 13 to 15

  c. 17 to 19
  d. 21 to 23

2–42. Vaginal probe sonography can detect fetal heart motion as early as what gestational age?

  a. 5 weeks
  b. 7 weeks
  c. 9 weeks
  d. 11 weeks

2–43. Which of the following is NOT a positive sign of pregnancy?

  a. identification of fetal heart tones
  b. positive pregnancy test
  c. perception of fetal movement by examiner
  d. identification of fetus by sonography

2–44. Up to what gestational age is the crown-rump length predictive of gestational age within 4 days?

  a. 8 weeks
  b. 10 weeks
  c. 12 weeks
  d. 14 weeks

3

Anatomy of the Reproductive Tract

3–1. The labia majora are composed largely of what type of tissue?

  a. adipose
  b. corpora cavernosa
  c. smooth muscle
  d. striated muscle

3–2. The labia majora are homologous with which of the following male structures?

  a. glans penis
  b. scrotum
  c. gubernaculum testis
  d. corpora cavernosa

3–3. Which structure becomes more prominent in multiparous women?

    a. fossa navicularis
    b. fourchette
    c. labia majora
    d. labia minora

3–4. By which of the following structures are the labia minora covered?

    a. mucous membrane
    b. hair
    c. transitional epithelium
    d. stratified squamous epithelium

3–5. The clitoris is the homologue of which of the following male structures?

    a. penis
    b. scrotum
    c. gubernaculum testis
    d. corpora cavernosa

3–6. What is the principle erogenous organ or area in women?

    a. vagina
    b. clitoris
    c. labia minora
    d. G-spot

3–7. From which embryonic structure does the vestibule arise?

    a. genital ridge
    b. mesonephric ducts
    c. müllerian ducts
    d. urogenital sinus

3–8. From which embryonic structure does the upper vagina arise?

    a. genital ridge
    b. mesonephric ducts
    c. müllerian ducts
    d. urogenital sinus

3–9. From which embryonic structure does the lower vagina arise?

    a. genital ridge
    b. mesonephric ducts
    c. müllerian ducts
    d. urogenital sinus

3–10. The vagina is lined mostly with what type of epithelium?

    a. cornified squamous epithelium
    b. cuboidal epithelium
    c. glandular epithelium
    d. noncornified squamous epithelium

3–11. Which of the following is the predominant bacteria of the vagina during pregnancy?

    a. *Peptostreptococcus* sp.
    b. *Listeria monocytogenes*
    c. *Lactobacillus* sp.
    d. *Streptococcus agalactiae*

3–12. What is the arterial blood supply to the upper third of the vagina?

    a. cervicovaginal branches of the uterine arteries
    b. inferior vesical arteries
    c. superior vesical arteries
    d. middle rectal and internal pudendal arteries

3–13. What is the arterial blood supply of the middle third of the vagina?

    a. cervicovaginal branches of the uterine arteries
    b. inferior vesical arteries
    c. superior vesical arteries
    d. middle rectal and internal pudendal arteries

3–14. What is the blood supply of the lower third of the vagina?

    a. cervicovaginal branches of the uterine arteries
    b. inferior vesical arteries
    c. superior vesical arteries
    d. middle rectal and internal pudendal arteries

3–15. The major blood supply to the perineum is via which artery and its branches?

    a. cervicovaginal artery
    b. internal pudendal artery
    c. inferior vesical artery
    d. uterine arteries

3–16. What is the origin of the pudendal nerve?

    a. L4-5, S1-2
    b. S1-3
    c. S2-4
    d. S4-5

3–17. Which part of the uterus becomes the lower uterine segment during pregnancy?

    a. cervix
    b. cornua
    c. corpus
    d. isthmus

3–18. What is the average length of a parous uterus?

    a. 2.5 to 3.5 cm
    b. 4 to 6 cm
    c. 6 to 8 cm
    d. 9 to 10 cm

3–19. What is the average weight of a nulliparous adult uterus?

a. 20 to 30 g
b. 50 to 70 g
c. 80 to 90 g
d. 100 to 150 g

3–20. What is the approximate weight of a pregnant uterus at term?

a. 110 g
b. 410 g
c. 610 g
d. 1100 g

3–21. What is the total volume of the uterus at term?

a. 2.5 L
b. 3.5 L
c. 5.0 L
d. 7.0 L

3–22. Approximately what percentage of the normal cervix is composed of muscle?

a. <1
b. 10
c. 25
d. 50

3–23. In utero exposure to what drug can cause structural abnormalities of the uterus and cervix?

a. diethylstilbestrol
b. ethinyl estradiol
c. medroxyprogesterone acetate
d. valproic acid

3–24. Which of the following arteries penetrates the middle third of the uterine wall and runs in a plane parallel to the uterine surface?

a. arcuate artery
b. radial artery
c. basal artery
d. coiled artery

3–25. The uterine artery is a main branch of which of the following arteries?

a. aorta
b. common iliac artery
c. external iliac artery
d. internal iliac artery

3–26. Uterine enlargement in pregnancy is due to what myometrial process?

a. collagen dissociation
b. decidualization

c. hyperplasia
d. hypertrophy

3–27. At which of the following locations does the uterine artery most commonly cross over the ureter?

a. 1 cm lateral to the cervix
b. 2 cm lateral to the cervix
c. 3.5 cm lateral to the cervix
d. 4.5 cm lateral to the cervix

3–28. The ovarian artery is a direct branch of which of the following vessels?

a. aorta
b. common iliac artery
c. external iliac artery
d. internal iliac artery

3–29. The left ovarian vein empties into which of the following veins?

a. external iliac vein
b. internal iliac vein
c. renal vein
d. vena cava

3–30. Which of the following nerve roots provide sensory fibers from the uterus that are associated with the painful stimuli of uterine contractions?

a. T-9 and T-10
b. T-11 and T-12
c. L-1 and L-2
d. S-2, S-3, and S-4

3–31. What portion of the fallopian tube lies within the wall of the uterus?

a. ampulla
b. infundibulum
c. interstitial
d. isthmus

3–32. What type of epithelium lines the oviducts?

a. basaloid epithelium
b. ciliated columnar epithelium
c. cuboidal epithelium
d. stratified columnar epithelium

3–33. The uterus and fallopian tubes arise embryologically from which of the following?

a. mesonephric ducts
b. müllerian ducts
c. urogenital sinus
d. Wolffian ducts

3-34. The blood and nerve supply to the ovaries courses through which of the following ligaments?

    a. broad ligaments
    b. cardinal ligaments
    c. infundibulopelvic ligaments
    d. utero-ovarian ligaments

3-35. What is the single layer of cuboidal epithelium on the surface of the ovary?

    a. tunica albuginea
    b. germinal epithelium of Waldeyer
    c. the primordial layer of Wolffian
    d. tunica cortex

3-36. The primordial germ cells migrate toward the genital ridge from which of the following?

    a. mesonephros
    b. müllerian ducts
    c. urogenital sinus
    d. yolk sac

3-37. What is the estimated number of oocytes at puberty?

    a. 50,000 to 100,000
    b. 200,000 to 400,000
    c. 750,000 to 1 million
    d. 3 to 5 million

3-38. What is the mean number of oocytes in women over age 36?

    a. 340
    b. 34,000
    c. 340,000
    d. 3,400,000

3-39. Gartner duct cysts are remnants of which of the following ducts?

    a. mesonephric ducts
    b. paramesonephric ducts
    c. metanephric ducts
    d. parametanephric ducts

3-40. Which of the following is NOT part of the innominate bone?

    a. ilium
    b. ischium
    c. pubis
    d. sacrum

3-41. Which of the following is NOT part of the superior boundary of the true pelvis?

    a. linea terminalis
    b. ischial spines
    c. promontory of the sacrum
    d. pubic bones

3-42. The true pelvis is bounded below by which of the following structures?

    a. linea terminalis
    b. alae of sacrum
    c. pelvic outlet
    d. upper margins of pelvic bone

3-43. What is the shortest diameter of the pelvic cavity?

    a. diagonal conjugate
    b. interspinous
    c. true conjugate
    d. transverse diameter

3-44. What is the normal angle of the subpubic arch under which the fetal head normally passes?

    a. 40 to 50 degrees
    b. 60 to 70 degrees
    c. 90 to 100 degrees
    d. 120 to 130 degrees

3-45. How does the dorsal lithotomy position for vaginal delivery widen the pelvic outlet?

    a. posterior displacement of the coccyx
    b. anterior rotation of the sacrum
    c. decrease of the interspinous distance
    d. upward movement of the sacroiliac joint

3-46. What are the results of a modified squatting position in the second stage of labor?

    a. a longer than normal second stage
    b. more perineal lacerations
    c. more labial lacerations
    d. less caput and molding

3-47. A gynecoid pelvis is seen in approximately what percentage of white women?

    a. 25
    b. 50
    c. 75
    d. 100

3-48. What does the obstetrical conjugate normally measure?

    a. 9 cm
    b. 10 cm
    c. 11 cm
    d. 12 cm

3-49. What is the shortest distance between the sacral promontory and symphysis pubis?

    a. diagonal conjugate
    b. obstetrical conjugate
    c. true conjugate
    d. sagittal conjugate

3–50. How is the obstetrical conjugate computed?

    a. add 1.5 cm to the diagonal conjugate
    b. subtract 1.5 cm from the diagonal conjugate
    c. average the diagonal and true conjugate
    d. add 1.5 cm to the true conjugate

3–51. What is the narrowest pelvic dimension that must be navigated by the fetal head?

    a. inferior strait
    b. interspinous diameter
    c. obstetrical conjugate
    d. pelvic inlet

3–52. What is the average transverse diameter of the pelvic outlet?

    a. 8 cm
    b. 10 cm
    c. 10.5 cm
    d. 11 cm

3–53. Upon which diameter does the prognosis for vaginal delivery with a narrow midpelvis or pelvic outlet largely depend?

    a. anterior sagittal diameter
    b. transverse diameter
    c. posterior sagittal diameter
    d. anteroposterior diameter

3–54. Which of the following terms best describes a small posterior sagittal diameter, with convergent sidewalls, prominent ischial spines, and a narrow subpubic arch?

    a. gynecoid
    b. android
    c. anthropoid
    d. platypelloid

3–55. What type of pelvis is characterized by a short anterior–posterior diameter and a wide transverse diameter?

    a. gynecoid pelvis
    b. android pelvis
    c. anthropoid pelvis
    d. platypelloid pelvis

3–56. What type of pelvis is associated with an inlet that is round, with straight pelvic sidewalls, spines that are not prominent, and a wide pelvic arch?

    a. gynecoid pelvis
    b. android pelvis
    c. anthropoid pelvis
    d. platypelloid pelvis

3–57. Which type of pelvis is typified by an anteroposterior diameter greater than the transverse and convergent sidewalls?

    a. gynecoid pelvis
    b. android pelvis
    c. anthropoid pelvis
    d. platypelloid pelvis

3–58. In what percentage of white women is the anthropoid pelvis type found?

    a. 3
    b. 10
    c. 25
    d. 33

3–59. What percentage of white women have an android-type pelvis?

    a. 3
    b. 10
    c. 25
    d. 33

3–60. What percentage of nonwhite women have an anthropoid-type pelvis?

    a. 3
    b. 12
    c. 25
    d. 50

3–61. What is the rarest type of pelvis?

    a. gynecoid pelvis
    b. android pelvis
    c. anthropoid pelvis
    d. platypelloid pelvis

3–62. What is considered an adequate pelvic inlet diagonal conjugate?

    a. 10 cm
    b. 10.5 cm
    c. 11 cm
    d. 11.5 cm

3–63. Engagement occurs when the biparietal diameter of the fetal head descends below the level of which of the following?

    a. ischial tuberosities
    b. midpelvis
    c. pelvic floor
    d. pelvic inlet

3–64. What is the approximate distance from the plane of the pelvic inlet to the level of the ischial spines?

   a. 1 cm
   b. 2 cm
   c. 3 cm
   d. 5 cm

3–65. What is the distance from the biparietal plane of the unmolded fetal head to the vertex?

   a. <1 cm
   b. 1 to 2 cm

   c. 3 to 4 cm
   d. 6 to 8 cm

3–66. What is the lower limit of normal transverse (intertuberous) diameter of the pelvic outlet?

   a. 8 cm
   b. 9.5 cm
   c. 11 cm
   d. 12.5 cm

The Endometrium and Decidua: Menstruation and Pregnancy

4–1. At what age does the blastocyst establish cell-to-cell contact with the endometrium?

   a. 3 days post-fertilization
   b. 6 days post-fertilization
   c. 9 days post-fertilization
   d. 12 days post-fertilization

4–2. What is the lifetime cumulative blood loss associated with menstruation?

   a. <5 L
   b. 10 to 20 L
   c. 25 to 35 L
   d. >40 L

4–3. What does the portion of the decidua invaded by the trophoblast become?

   a. decidua basalis
   b. decidua capsularis
   c. decidua vera
   d. decidua parietalis

4–4. Which of the following is NOT produced by the decidua?

   a. 1,25-dihydroxy-vitamin-D_3
   b. corticotropin-releasing hormone
   c. relaxin
   d. thyroid-stimulating hormone

4–5. By which day of the endometrial cycle is restoration of the epithelial surface of the endometrium complete?

   a. 2
   b. 5
   c. 8
   d. 12

4–6. In what phase of the menstrual cycle does infiltration of the stroma by polymorphonuclear and mononuclear leukocytes occur?

   a. late proliferative phase
   b. early secretory phase
   c. midsecretory phase
   d. premenstrual phase

4–7. From what arteries do the spiral arteries arise?

   a. arcuate arteries
   b. uterine arteries
   c. endometrial arteries
   d. decidual arteries

4–8. Which of the following substances is likely to cause the intense vasoconstriction of the spiral arteries 4 to 24 hr before the onset of bleeding?

   a. interleukin-8
   b. monocyte peptide-1
   c. prostaglandin E_2 (PGE_2)
   d. endothelin-1

4–9. During which stage of the menstrual cycle is interleukin-15 preferentially expressed in the endometrium?

   a. menses
   b. proliferative stage
   c. secretory stage
   d. ovulatory stage

4–10. Which of the following cytokines induces proliferation of the decidual natural killer cells?

   a. interleukin-1 (IL-1)
   b. interleukin-6 (IL-6)
   c. interleukin-15 (IL-15)
   d. transforming growth factor-β (TGF-β)

4–11. Which of the following enzymes serves to degrade bioactive peptides such as atrial natriuretic peptide, substance P, and endothelin-1?

   a. enkephalinase
   b. phospholipase A_2
   c. prostaglandin dehydrogenase
   d. phospholipase C

4–12. Which of the following is NOT produced by endometrial stromal cells?

   a. endothelin-1
   b. enkephalinase
   c. parathyroid hormone-related protein (PTH-rP)
   d. 15-hydroxyprostaglandin dehydrogenase (PGDH)

4–13. Approximately what percentage of a woman's cycles will vary more than 2 days from the mean of the length of her cycles?

   a. <1
   b. 5
   c. 33
   d. 50

4–14. What is the average amount of blood lost during a normal menstrual cycle?

   a. 10 to 15 mL
   b. 25 to 60 mL
   c. 85 to 120 mL
   d. 150 mL

4–15. What is the average age of menarche for women living in the United States?

   a. 9 to 10 years
   b. 11 years
   c. 12 to 13 years
   d. 14 to 15 years

4–16. What is the most likely explanation for the premenstrual syndrome (PMS)?

   a. massive estrogen secretion and withdrawal
   b. massive progesterone secretion and withdrawal
   c. massive prostaglandin secretion and withdrawal
   d. massive endothelin secretion and withdrawal

4–17. What is althesin?

   a. prostaglandin inhibitor
   b. cytokine stimulator
   c. menses regulator
   d. steroidal anesthetic

4–18. In what month of gestation is the decidua capsularis most prominent?

   a. first month
   b. second month
   c. fourth month
   d. sixth month

4–19. At what week of gestation is the uterine cavity obliterated by the fusion of the decidua capsularis and parietalis?

   a. week 6 to 8
   b. week 10 to 13
   c. week 14 to 16
   d. week 18 to 20

4–20. Which of the following is defective or absent in the case of placenta accreta?

   a. decidua basalis
   b. Nitabuch's layer
   c. Rohr's stria
   d. decidual stromal cells

4–21. Prolactin levels are highest in which of the following?

   a. fetal plasma
   b. maternal plasma
   c. amniotic fluid
   d. all have equal levels

4–22. Which of the following causes a decrease in decidual prolactin secretion?

   a. IL-1
   b. PGE_2
   c. prostaglandin $F_{2\alpha}$ (PG $F_{2\alpha}$)
   d. thromboxane A (TxA)

5

The Placenta and Fetal Membranes

5–1. What type of placenta characterizes the human?

    a. epitheliochorial placenta
    b. hemochorioendothelial placenta
    c. endotheliochorial placenta
    d. hemoendothelial placenta

5–2. What is the solid ball of cells formed by 16 or more blastomeres?

    a. morula
    b. blastocyst
    c. zygote
    d. embryo

5–3. The fluid-filled cavity that is formed when the morula reaches the uterus converts the morula to which of the following?

    a. zygote
    b. blastomere
    c. blasocyst
    d. embryo

5–4. Up until the end of the 7th week, what term is used to describe the product of conception?

    a. zygote
    b. embryo
    c. fetus
    d. conceptus

5–5. At what stage of development does the conceptus implant?

    a. zygote
    b. morula
    c. blastocyst
    d. embryo

5–6. What is the most common uterine site for implantation in the human?

    a. upper posterior wall
    b. lower posterior wall
    c. upper anterior wall
    d. lower anterior wall

5–7. What is the origin of the syncytiotrophoblast?

    a. inner cell mass
    b. cytotrophoblast
    c. zona pellucida
    d. decidua capsularis

5–8. Which of the following statements is NOT true regarding the hemochorioendothelial placenta?

    a. It is the type of placenta found in most animals.
    b. Maternal blood directly bathes the syncytiotrophoblast.
    c. Fetal blood is separated from maternal blood.
    d. Maternal tissue is juxtaposed to fetal trophoblast and not embryonic cells.

5–9. The term conceptus includes all but which of the following?

    a. embryo
    b. fetal membranes
    c. decidua
    d. placenta

5–10. Pregnancy is least likely to occur if coitus occurs at which time?

    a. at ovulation
    b. 2 days after ovulation
    c. 2 days before ovulation
    d. 1 day before ovulation

5–11. What calcium-dependent adhesion molecule is responsible for cytotrophoblast aggregation?

    a. calmodulin
    b. E-cadherin
    c. desmogin
    d. trophoblastin

5–12. The survival of the conceptus in the uterus is attributable to the immunological peculiarity of which of the following?

    a. decidua
    b. amnion
    c. chorion
    d. trophoblast

5–13. Class II major histocompatibility complex (MHC) antigens are absent from trophoblasts at what stage of gestation?

    a. first trimester
    b. second trimester
    c. third trimester
    d. at all stages

5–14. At what stage of the cycle are uterine large granular lymphocytes present in large numbers?

    a. early follicular stage
    b. midfollicular stage
    c. midluteal stage
    d. late luteal stage

5–15. In what cell type are human leukocyte antigen (HLA-G) antigens expressed?

    a. decidua
    b. villous trophoblasts
    c. cytotrophoblasts
    d. chorion-amnion cells

5–16. What promotes the synthesis of oncofetal fibronectin?

    a. E-cadherin
    b. transforming growth factor-β (TGF-β)
    c. integrins
    d. interleukin-6

5–17. When is a true placental circulation established?

    a. 12th day after fertilization
    b. 14th day after fertilization
    c. 17th day after fertilization
    d. 28th day after fertilization

5–18. What do the villi in contact with the decidua basalis proliferate to form?

    a. chorion frondosum
    b. chorion laeve
    c. chorion basalis
    d. chorion capsularis

5–19. What are a main stem (truncal) villi and its ramifications?

    a. placental cotyledon
    b. maternal cotyledon
    c. stem cotyledon
    d. primary cotyledon

5–20. Leukocytes bearing a Y chromosome have been identified in women for how long after giving birth to a son?

    a. 6 months
    b. 1 year
    c. 2 years
    d. 5 years

5–21. What is the average volume of the term placenta?

    a. 100 mL
    b. 300 mL
    c. 500 mL
    d. 750 mL

5–22. What are fetal macrophages found in the stroma of villi?

    a. Hofbauer cells
    b. Langhan cells
    c. K-cells
    d. septal cells

5–23. Which of the following changes is NOT associated with placental aging?

    a. a decrease in thickness of syncytium
    b. an increase in Langhans cells
    c. a decrease in stroma
    d. an increase in number of capillaries

5–24. How many spiral arterial entries into the intervillous space are present at term?

    a. 30
    b. 60
    c. 90
    d. 120

5–25. Who first described the physiological mechanism of placental circulation?

    a. Ramsey
    b. Benirschke
    c. Bleker
    d. Friedlander

5–26. What is the average length of the umbilical cord?

    a. 25 cm
    b. 55 cm
    c. 95 cm
    d. 125 cm

5–27. What term describes the persistence of the intra-abdominal portion of the duct of the umbilical vessels, which extends from the umbilicus to the intestine?

    a. allantoic remnant
    b. duct of Hoboken
    c. Meckel diverticulum
    d. omphalocele

The Placental Hormones

6–1. Which of the following is NOT true of the chemical characteristics of human chorionic gonadotropin (hCG)?

    a. glycoprotein
    b. highest carbohydrate content of any human hormone
    c. both α- and β-subunits are necessary for bioactivity
    d. the β-subunit is functionally most like the β-subunit of follicle-stimulating hormone (FSH)

6–2. All 8 of the genes for the β-subunit of hCG are located on which of the following chromosomes?

    a. 1
    b. 9
    c. 19
    d. X

6–3. Where is the complete molecule of hCG primarily produced?

    a. syncytiotrophoblast
    b. cytotrophoblast
    c. chorioamnionic membrane
    d. Hofbauer cells

6–4. The hCG molecule is first detectable in maternal serum how long after the midcycle luteinizing hormone (LH) surge?

    a. 3 to 5 days
    b. 7 to 9 days
    c. 11 to 13 days
    d. 15 to 17 days

6–5. The maximum levels of hCG in maternal serum occur at what week of pregnancy?

    a. 4th
    b. 10th
    c. 16th
    d. 20th

6–6. The nadir in the level of hCG in maternal serum is reached at what week of pregnancy?

    a. week 6
    b. week 10
    c. week 16
    d. week 20

6–7. In which of the following are relatively low levels of hCG detected in maternal blood?

    a. Down syndrome
    b. hydatidiform mole
    c. multiple gestation
    d. impending abortion

6–8. The control of hCG synthesis is primarily regulated by what organ?

    a. fetal adrenal gland
    b. fetal pituitary gland
    c. maternal ovaries
    d. not known at present

6–9. The hCG receptor is also the receptor for what other hormone?

    a. estriol
    b. FSH
    c. LH
    d. progesterone

6–10. What is the best known function of HCG?

    a. maintenance of the corpus luteum
    b. protection against paternal antibodies
    c. stimulation of human placental lactogen (hPL) secretion
    d. stimulation of fetal ovaries to produce estrogen

6–11. Other actions of hCG include which of the following?

    a. stimulation of thyroid activity
    b. promotion of relaxin secretion by corpus luteum
    c. promotion of sexual differentiation of the male fetus
    d. all of the above

6–12. Which of the following is NOT true of hPL?

  a. structurally similar to growth hormone and production
  b. levels peak early in gestation, then decline
  c. metabolic role not completely understood
  d. produced mostly by trophoblasts

6–13. What is the half-life of hPL?

  a. 30 min
  b. 4 hr
  c. 24 hr
  d. 36 hr

6–14. During which week of pregnancy does hPL peak in the maternal serum?

  a. week 10 to 12
  b. week 16 to 20
  c. week 28 to 30
  d. week 34 to 36

6–15. Which of the following is NOT derived from the precursor molecule pro-opiomelanocortin (POMC)?

  a. hPL
  b. corticotropin (ACTH)
  c. lipoprotein
  d. β-endorphin

6–16. Which of the following is most likely responsible for the increased thyroid-stimulating activity in women with neoplastic trophoblastic disease?

  a. chorionic thyrotropin
  b. hPL
  c. hCG
  d. corticotropin-releasing hormone (CRH)

6–17. What is the probable role of placental inhibin?

  a. suppresses FSH
  b. suppresses thyroxine-releasing hormone
  c. suppresses gonadtropin-releasing hormone
  d. suppresses CRH

6–18. What is the immediate precursor for estrogen biosynthesis in the human placenta?

  a. acetate
  b. cholesterol
  c. progesterone
  d. dehydroepiandrosterone sulfate

6–19. What is the quantitatively important source of placental estrogen precursor in the human?

  a. maternal adrenal gland
  b. syncytiotrophoblast
  c. cytotrophoblast
  d. fetal adrenal gland

6–20. Markedly decreased levels of maternal urinary estrogens are seen with which fetal condition in particular?

  a. anencephaly
  b. erythroblasts
  c. multiple gestation
  d. renal agenesis

6–21. Which of the following is the enzyme complex responsible for converting precursor substrate to estrogen in the placenta?

  a. aromatase
  b. cyclooxyreductase
  c. hydroxylase
  d. isomerase

6–22. Near term, what percentage of estradiol-17β produced by the placenta is derived from maternal dehydroepiandrosterone sulfate?

  a. 15
  b. 50
  c. 75
  d. 90

6–23. The fetus is the source of approximately what percentage of the precursor of the estriol formed in the placenta?

  a. 5
  b. 25
  c. 50
  d. 90

6–24. Approximately what percentage of the fetal adrenal gland is composed of the fetal zone?

  a. 5
  b. 25
  c. 55
  d. 85

6–25. Relative to body weight, how much larger are the adrenals of the human fetus at term than those of the adult?

  a. 2 times
  b. 10 times
  c. 25 times
  d. 50 times

6–26. What is the precursor used for steroid biosynthesis in the fetal adrenal?

  a. cholesterol
  b. acetate
  c. progesterone
  d. pregnenolone

6–27. What is the major source of fetal plasma low-density-lipoprotein (LDL) cholesterol?

   a. maternal transfer
   b. placental synthesis
   c. fetal liver
   d. fetal adrenal gland

6–28. What is the placental enzyme that "protects" the female fetus from virilization in a pregnant woman with an androgen-secreting ovarian tumor?

   a. aromatase
   b. sulfatase
   c. 17α-hydroxylase
   d. 3β-hydroxysteroid dehydrogenase

6–29. What type of disorder is placental sulfatase deficiency (also associated with ichthyosis)?

   a. multifactorial
   b. X-linked recessive
   c. autosomal dominant
   d. autosomal recessive

6–30. What is the precursor for the biosynthesis of progesterone by the placenta?

   a. placental acetate
   b. maternal cholesterol
   c. fetal pregnenolone
   d. fetal C-19 steroids

6–31. What is the approximate daily production of progesterone in late normal, singleton pregnancies?

   a. 50 mg
   b. 250 mg
   c. 1200 mg
   d. 2400 mg

6–32. Which of the following hormones demonstrates levels that are the most sensitive to the state of fetal well-being?

   a. estriol
   b. hPL
   c. inhibin
   d. progesterone

6–33. Which of the following is true of estrogen and progesterone secretion by the placenta?

   a. over 85 percent secreted into fetal circulation
   b. over 85 percent secreted into amniotic fluid
   c. over 85 percent secreted into maternal circulation
   d. secreted equally into fetal and maternal compartments

6–34. What is the cause of the marked increase in the potent mineralocorticosteroid, deoxycorticosterone, that is seen in pregnancy?

   a. increased fetal adrenal production
   b. increased maternal adrenal production
   c. increased placental production
   d. extra-adrenal conversion of progesterone

6–35. What happens to umbilical cord plasma levels of estrogens and progesterone in infants of women with pregnancy-induced hypertension, chronic hypertension, and severe forms of diabetes mellitus compared with infants of normal women?

   a. increases slightly
   b. increases significantly
   c. decreases slightly
   d. decreases significantly

7

Fetal Growth and Development

7–1. How many days does human pregnancy last, on average, counting from the first day of the last menstrual period?

    a. 260
    b. 270
    c. 280
    d. 290

7–2. Pregnancy is said to consist of 10 lunar months. How long is a real lunar month?

    a. $26\frac{1}{2}$ days
    b. $27\frac{1}{2}$ days
    c. 28 days
    d. $29\frac{1}{2}$ days

7–3. Given the date of a pregnant woman's last menstrual period, what method is used to quickly estimate the due date?

    a. subtract 7 days, subtract 3 months
    b. add 7 days, subtract 3 months
    c. add 7 days, add 3 months
    d. subtract 7 days, add 3 months

7–4. What are the products of conception called prior to implantation?

    a. embryo
    b. fetus
    c. ovum
    d. zygote

7–5. Which of the following best represents the embryonic period?

    a. fertilization to 6 weeks
    b. implantation to 6 weeks
    c. 3rd to 8th week after fertilization
    d. first 11 to 12 weeks of pregnancy

7–6. The embryogenic heart is completely formed by how many weeks after ovulation?

    a. 4
    b. 6
    c. 10
    d. 12

7–7. What is the approximate crown-rump length of the fetus by the end of the 12th week of pregnancy?

    a. 1 to 2 cm
    b. 4 cm
    c. 6 to 7 cm
    d. 10 cm

7–8. In general, spontaneous fetal movements begin at what gestational (weeks) age?

    a. 6
    b. 12
    c. 16
    d. 20

7–9. What is the approximate weight of the fetus at 16 gestational weeks?

    a. 25 g
    b. 50 g
    c. 110 g
    d. 250 g

7–10. Gender of the fetus is first evident by what gestational age (weeks)?

    a. 6
    b. 8
    c. 12
    d. 16

7–11. What is the approximate weight of the fetus at 20 gestational weeks?

    a. 200 g
    b. 300 g
    c. 480 g
    d. 650 g

7–12. At what gestational age (weeks) is the canalicular phase of lung development nearly complete, but terminal air sacs have not yet formed?

    a. 18
    b. 24
    c. 28
    d. 32

7–13. What is the approximate weight of the fetus at 28 gestational weeks?

    a. 750 g
    b. 890 g
    c. 1100 g
    d. 1500 g

7–14. By what gestational age (weeks) has the pupillary membrane disappeared?

    a. 10
    b. 20
    c. 24
    d. 28

7–15. What is the survival rate of an otherwise normal infant born at 28 weeks gestation?

    a. 25%
    b. 50%
    c. 75%
    d. 90%

7–16. What is the average weight of the fetus at 32 gestational weeks?

    a. 1000 g
    b. 1500 g
    c. 1800 g
    d. 2000 g

7–17. What is the average weight of the fetus at 36 gestational weeks?

    a. 1990 g
    b. 2500 g
    c. 2850 g
    d. 3000 g

7–18. What is the average crown-rump length of a term fetus?

    a. 28 cm
    b. 32 cm
    c. 36 cm
    d. 40 cm

7–19. Which of the following is least likely to influence birthweight?

    a. climate
    b. gender
    c. race
    d. socioeconomic status

7–20. What is the largest baby recorded in the medical literature (a stillborn female)?

    a. 14 lb
    b. 16 lb
    c. 18 lb
    d. 25 lb

7–21. In the fetus or neonate, what are the two sutures between the posterior margin of the parietal bones and the upper margin of the occipital bone called?

    a. occipitalis suture
    b. sagittal suture
    c. lambdoid suture
    d. coronal suture

7–22. In the fetus or neonate, what are the two sutures between the frontal and parietal bones?

    a. frontal suture
    b. sagittal suture
    c. lambdoid suture
    d. coronal suture

7–23. Which of the following diameters has the greatest length?

    a. occipitofrontal diameter
    b. biparietal diameter
    c. occipitomental diameter
    d. suboccipitobregmatic diameter

7–24. The plane of which of the following diameters represents the greatest circumference of the head?

    a. occipitofrontal diameter
    b. suboccipitobregmatic diameter
    c. bitemporal diameter
    d. biparietal diameter

7–25. The plane of which of the following diameters represents the smallest circumference of the head?

    a. occipitofrontal diameter
    b. suboccipitobregmatic diameter
    c. bitemporal diameter
    d. biparietal diameter

7-26. Which of these factors corresponds to large fetal infant head size?

    a. white race
    b. male gender
    c. multiparous mother
    d. all of the above

7-27. What is the name of the process by which fetal skull bones shift during labor to accommodate the maternal bony pelvis?

    a. accommodation
    b. conformation
    c. craniosyntosis
    d. molding

7-28. What is the approximate uteroplacental blood flow near term?

    a. 100 to 200 mL/min
    b. 300 to 450 mL/min
    c. 700 to 900 mL/min
    d. 1200 to 1400 mL/min

7-29. What is the estimated total surface area of the chorionic villi at term?

    a. 2 m^2
    b. 10 m^2
    c. 25 m^2
    d. 55 m^2

7-30. Direct transfer of nutrients and oxygen from mother to fetus occurs primarily across which of the following interfaces?

    a. decidua capsularis
    b. fetal membranes
    c. syncytiotrophoblast
    d. yolk sac

7-31. What is the mechanism of transfer of anesthetic gases across the placenta?

    a. simple diffusion
    b. facilitated diffusion
    c. active transport
    d. pinocytosis

7-32. What is the PO_2 (mm Hg) of intervillous space blood?

    a. 10 to 20 mm Hg
    b. 30 to 35 mm Hg
    c. 65 to 75 mm Hg
    d. 90 to 95 mm Hg

7-33. What is the average oxygen saturation of intervillous space blood?

    a. 10 to 15%
    b. 25 to 35%
    c. 65 to 75%
    d. 90 to 95%

7-34. Which of the following fetal attributes compensates for low oxygen tension in the placenta?

    a. high cardiac output
    b. increased fetal hemoglobin
    c. increased hemoglobin concentration
    d. all of the above

7-35. What is the average PO_2 (mm Hg) in the umbilical vein?

    a. 15 mm Hg
    b. 27 mm Hg
    c. 49 mm Hg
    d. 77 mm Hg

7-36. What is the average PO_2 (mm Hg) in the umbilical artery?

    a. 15 mm Hg
    b. 27 mm Hg
    c. 49 mm Hg
    d. 77 mm Hg

7-37. What is the mechanism of iron transport across the placenta?

    a. active transfer
    b. simple diffusion
    c. facilitated diffusion
    d. endocytosis

7-38. How is glucose transferred across the placenta?

    a. active transport
    b. simple diffusion
    c. facilitated diffusion
    d. endocytosis

7-39. After being concentrated in the syncytiotrophoblasts, how are amino acids transferred across the placenta?

    a. active transport
    b. simple diffusion
    c. facilitated diffusion
    d. endocytosis

7-40. Which of the following is an example of a large protein that readily crosses the placenta?

    a. IgG
    b. thyrotropin
    c. insulin
    d. IgM

7–41. How does IgG cross the placenta?

    a. active transport
    b. simple diffusion
    c. facilitated diffusion
    d. endocytosis

7–42. How do calcium and phosphorous cross the placenta?

    a. active transport
    b. simple diffusion
    c. facilitated diffusion
    d. endocytosis

7–43. At what gestational age (weeks) does the fetal kidney begin producing urine?

    a. 8
    b. 12
    c. 16
    d. 20

7–44. Which of the following factors found in amniotic fluid may play a significant role in fetal lung development?

    a. vitamin A
    b. cholecalciferol
    c. prolactin
    d. epidermal growth factors

7–45. Which of the following fetal vessels empties directly into the inferior vena cava?

    a. umbilical vein
    b. portal vein
    c. ductus venosus
    d. hepatic vein

7–46. Which of the following contains the most oxygenated blood in the fetus?

    a. superior vena cava
    b. blood defected by the crista dividens
    c. ductus arteriosus
    d. right ventricle

7–47. What percentage of blood is shunted from the right ventricle to the descending aorta by the ductus arteriosus?

    a. 23
    b. 47
    c. 63
    d. 87

7–48. Which of the following structures represents the intra-abdominal remnants of the umbilical vein?

    a. umbilical ligaments
    b. ligamentum teres

    c. ligamentum venosus
    d. ligamentum portalis

7–49. Which of the following fetal structures is NOT a site of early hematopoiesis?

    a. yolk sac
    b. liver
    c. bone marrow
    d. kidney

7–50. What is the average fetal hemoglobin concentration at term?

    a. 10 g/dL
    b. 13 g/dL
    c. 15 g/dL
    d. 18 g/dL

7–51. Fetal erythropoiesis is primarily controlled by which hormone?

    a. fetal erythropoietin
    b. maternal erythropoietin
    c. fetal thyroxine
    d. maternal thyroxine

7–52. What is the approximate fetoplacental blood volume at term?

    a. 70 mL/kg
    b. 125 mL/kg
    c. 225 mL/kg
    d. 250 mL/kg

7–53. Which of the following hemoglobins contain a pair of alpha chains and a pair of gamma chains?

    a. Gower-1
    b. hemoglobin F
    c. hemoglobin A
    d. hemoglobin A_2

7–54. What percentage of total hemoglobin at birth is hemoglobin F?

    a. 5
    b. 38
    c. 75
    d. 99

7–55. Which of the following vitamins is given prophylactically to infants soon after birth (especially in the breast-feeding newborn)?

    a. vitamin K
    b. vitamin A
    c. vitamin C
    d. vitamin D

7-56. The bulk of IgG acquired by the fetus from its mother occurs during which of the following time periods?

a. 10 to 14 weeks
b. 16 to 20 weeks
c. 24 to 28 weeks
d. last 4 weeks of pregnancy

7-57. Which of the following immunological factors provides protection against enteric infections when ingested in the colostrum?

a. IgG
b. IgM
c. IgA
d. IgE

7-58. At what gestational age (weeks) are fetal respiratory movements first evident?

a. 8 to 10
b. 14 to 16
c. 18 to 20
d. 22 to 24

7-59. How early (weeks) might the fetus hear some sounds in utero?

a. week 12
b. week 18
c. week 24
d. week 30

7-60. Which of the following can lead to intrauterine passage of meconium?

a. cord compression
b. hypoxia
c. normal bowel peristalsis
d. all of the above

7-61. What is the fate of most of the unconjugated bilirubin produced in the fetus?

a. transferred to maternal circulation
b. excreted into and stored in fetal gut
c. conjugated by fetal liver
d. not well understood

7-62. At what gestational age (weeks) is insulin first detectable in fetal plasma?

a. 6
b. 12
c. 16
d. 20

7-63. From what fetal anlage does the mature urinary tact arise?

a. mesonephros
b. metanephros
c. pronephros
d. Wolffian ducts

7-64. What is the approximate daily urine output of a term fetus?

a. 100 mL
b. 350 mL
c. 650 mL
d. 1000 mL

7-65. Where is surfactant primarily produced in the fetal lung?

a. type II pneumocytes
b. alveoli macrophages
c. alveoli basement membrane cells
d. interstitial cells

7-66. Which of the following glycerophospholipids makes up the majority of mature surfactant?

a. phosphatidylinositol
b. phosphatidylethanolamine
c. phosphatidylglycerol
d. phosphatidylcholine

7-67. What percentage of surfactant is composed of specific apoproteins?

a. 10
b. 15
c. 25
d. 30

7-68. What is the major surfactant-associated protein (apoprotein)?

a. SP-A
b. SP-B
c. SP-C
d. SP-D

7-69. Administration of which of the following to the mother has the most significant beneficial effect on surfactant production?

a. betamethasone
b. cyclic adenosine monophosphate
c. prolactin
d. thyroxine

7-70. When can movements of the fetal chest wall first be detected by ultrasound?

a. 11 weeks
b. 18 weeks
c. 24 weeks
d. 26 weeks

7–71. At what gestational age (weeks) does the fetus begin to produce thyroxine?

   a. 7 to 8
   b. 10 to 12
   c. 14 to 16
   d. 22 to 24

7–72. When can corticotropin first be detected in the fetal pituitary gland?

   a. 7 weeks
   b. 11 weeks
   c. 15 weeks
   d. 19 weeks

7–73. What is the most likely explanation for the 46,XX male?

   a. production of müllerian-inhibiting substance by the ovary
   b. Y chromosome was lost from a 47,XXY fetus
   c. translocation of portions of the Y chromosome to the X chromosome
   d. error in karyotyping

7–74. Which of the following statements is correct regarding müllerian-inhibiting substance?

   a. It is an endocrine hormone.
   b. It is produced by the Leydig cells.
   c. It acts locally near its site of formation.
   d. It appears after testosterone.

7–75. The virilizing effect of testosterone on the external genitalia in the male fetus is amplified by its local conversion to which of the following androgens?

   a. 7,21α-epiandrosterone
   b. androstenedione
   c. 5α-dihydrotestosterone
   d. DHEA

7–76. In newborns with either male external genitalia and bilateral cryptorchidism or completely ambiguous external genitalia, what diagnosis should be immediately ruled out?

   a. congenital adrenal hyperplasia
   b. 5α-reductase deficiency
   c. gonadal dysgenesis
   d. maternal androgen-secreting tumor

7–77. Which of the following is NOT characteristic of female pseudohermaphroditism?

   a. Müllerian-inhibiting substance is not produced.
   b. The fetus is exposed to androgen.
   c. The karyotype is 46,XX.
   d. A testis is present on one side.

7–78. Which of the following is NOT characteristic of male pseudohermaphroditism?

   a. Müllerian-inhibiting substance is produced.
   b. Androgenic representation is variable.
   c. Karyotype is 47,XXY.
   d. Testes or no gonads are present.

7–79. Which of the following is NOT characteristic of androgen insensitivity syndrome?

   a. female phenotype
   b. short, blind-ending vagina
   c. no uterus or fallopian tubes
   d. ovarian remnants on one side

7–80. Androgen insensitivity syndrome is characterized by increased testicular secretion of which hormone as compared with a normal male?

   a. androstenedione
   b. estradio-17β
   c. müllerian-inhibiting factor
   d. testosterone

7–81. The gene encoding for androgen receptor has had over 100 mutations identified and is located on which chromosome?

   a. 6
   b. 16
   c. X
   d. Y

7–82. Which of the following is a feature of dysgenetic gonads?

   a. Karyotype is variable, often abnormal.
   b. Müllerian-inhibiting substance is produced.
   c. Normal ovaries or testes may be present.
   d. Uterus is usually absent.

Maternal Adaptations to Pregnancy

8–1. What is the average uterine weight at term?

   a. 200 g
   b. 450 g
   c. 780 g
   d. 1100 g

8–2. Uterine enlargement in pregnancy is primarily due to what process involving myocytes?

   a. hyperplasia (new myocyte production)
   b. hypertrophy and stretching
   c. atrophy with replacement by collagen
   d. hyperplasia and hypertrophy play equal roles

8–3. At what gestational age does the uterus become too large to lie totally within the pelvis?

   a. 10 weeks
   b. 12 weeks
   c. 14 weeks
   d. 16 weeks

8–4. What is the approximate uteroplacental blood flow at term?

   a. 100 mL/min
   b. 250 mL/min
   c. 550 mL/min
   d. 800 mL/min

8–5. Uteroplacental blood flow is sensitive to the regulatory effects of which of the following?

   a. catecholamines
   b. estrogens
   c. nitric oxide
   d. all of the above

8–6. Which of the following is a factor responsible for the softening and cyanosis of the cervix in early pregnancy?

   a. increased vascularity
   b. decreased stromal edema

   c. decreased venous oxygen concentration
   d. atrophy of cervical glands

8–7. Surgical removal of the corpus luteum of pregnancy consistently results in spontaneous abortion if performed prior to what gestational age?

   a. 7 weeks
   b. 9 weeks
   c. 11 weeks
   d. 13 weeks

8–8. What is the major biologic target of relaxin in assisting accommodation to pregnancy?

   a. cardiovascular system
   b. musculoskeletal system
   c. nervous system
   d. reproductive tract

8–9. Which of the following is produced by the corpus luteum throughout pregnancy?

   a. progesterone
   b. 17α-hydroxyprogesterone
   c. relaxin
   d. prolactin

8–10. How does hyperreactio luteinalis differ from a pregnancy luteoma?

   a. It is cystic.
   b. It may cause maternal virilization.
   c. It has a different cellular pattern.
   d. It is associated with very low serum chorionic gonadotropin levels.

8–11. What is pigmentation of the midline of abdominal skin during pregnancy called?

   a. striae gravidarum
   b. linea nigra
   c. chloasma
   d. melasma

8–12. What is the average weight gain during pregnancy?

    a. 5.5 kg
    b. 9.5 kg
    c. 12.5 kg
    d. 15.5 kg

8–13. What is the minimum amount of extra water that the average woman retains during normal pregnancy?

    a. 1.0 L
    b. 3.5 L
    c. 6.5 L
    d. 8.0 L

8–14. Of the total 1000 g net gain of protein in normal pregnancy, how much is utilized by the fetus and placenta?

    a. 100 g
    b. 300 g
    c. 500 g
    d. 750 g

8–15. Which of the following characterizes carbohydrate metabolism in pregnancy relative to the nonpregnant state?

    a. hypoinsulinemia
    b. mild fasting hypoglycemia
    c. postprandial hypoglycemia
    d. fasting hyperglycemia

8–16. Which of the following shows a continuous increase in plasma levels into the late third trimester of pregnancy?

    a. high density lipoprotein (HDL) cholesterol
    b. HDL-2 cholesterol
    c. HDL-3 cholesterol
    d. low density lipoprotein (LDL) cholesterol

8–17. What causes the increase in HDL-cholesterol noted in the first half of pregnancy?

    a. prolactin
    b. estrogen
    c. progesterone
    d. human chorionic gonadotropin

8–18. What is the average plasma bicarbonate level during pregnancy?

    a. 29 mmol/L
    b. 26 mmol/L
    c. 22 mmol/L
    d. 16 mmol/L

8–19. Which of the following best characterizes the acid-base status during pregnancy?

    a. mild respiratory alkalosis
    b. mild respiratory acidosis
    c. mild metabolic alkalosis
    d. mild metabolic acidosis

8–20. What is the average increase in maternal blood volume during pregnancy?

    a. 10%
    b. 25%
    c. 40%
    d. 75%

8–21. What is the average increase in the volume of circulating erythrocytes during pregnancy?

    a. 100 mL
    b. 250 mL
    c. 450 mL
    d. 700 mL

8–22. Which of the following hematologic changes does NOT occur during normal pregnancy?

    a. The mean age of circulating red cells is increased.
    b. The mean red cell volume is increased.
    c. There is moderate erythroid hyperplasia.
    d. There is an increase in plasma erythropoietin.

8–23. Which of the following is an effect of atrial natriuretic peptide?

    a. increased renin secretion
    b. postpartum volume expansion
    c. decreased basal release of aldosterone
    d. increased vascular smooth muscle tone

8–24. What are the average iron stores of normal young women?

    a. 300 mg
    b. 500 mg
    c. 4 g
    d. 6 g

8–25. What are the iron requirements of normal pregnancy?

    a. 300 mg
    b. 500 mg
    c. 1 g
    d. 4 g

8–26. Approximately how much iron is required by the fetus and placenta during pregnancy?

    a. 150 mg
    b. 300 mg
    c. 500 mg
    d. 1 g

8–27. What is the average daily iron requirement during the second half of pregnancy?

   a. 1 to 2 mg/d
   b. 3 to 4 mg/d
   c. 6 to 7 mg/d
   d. 15 to 20 mg/d

8–28. What volume of blood is lost on average with a singleton vaginal delivery?

   a. 250 mL
   b. 500 mL
   c. 750 mL
   d. 1000 mL

8–29. What is the average blood loss with cesarean delivery of a singleton fetus?

   a. 500 mL
   b. 750 mL
   c. 1000 mL
   d. 1500 mL

8–30. Which of the following is NOT increased in pregnancy?

   a. blood leukocyte count
   b. C-reactive protein
   c. leukocyte alkaline phosphate activity
   d. interferon

8–31. What is the average increase in fibrinogen concentration during pregnancy?

   a. 10%
   b. 25%
   c. 50%
   d. 75%

8–32. Which of the following coagulation factors is NOT increased during pregnancy?

   a. factor VII
   b. factor VIII
   c. factor IX
   d. factor XI

8–33. Factor V Leiden mutation causes resistance to which of the following?

   a. activated protein C
   b. free protein S
   c. anti-thrombin III
   d. none of the above

8–34. What is the average increase in the resting pulse during pregnancy?

   a. 0 bpm
   b. 5 bpm
   c. 10 bpm
   d. 20 bpm

8–35. Which of the following is least likely responsible for the increase in the cardiac silhouette noted in radiographs in pregnant women?

   a. displacement of the heart to the left and upward
   b. cardiomegaly of pregnancy
   c. increase in left ventricular mass
   d. pericardial effusion of pregnancy

8–36. Which of the following changes in cardiac sounds is found during pregnancy?

   a. blunting of the first heart sound
   b. wide splitting of the second heart sound
   c. a systolic murmur in 90 percent of women
   d. a loud diastolic murmur in 90 percent of women

8–37. What is the most characteristic electrocardiographic finding in normal pregnancy?

   a. shortening of the QRS complex
   b. shortening of the ST segment
   c. slight depression of the ST segment
   d. slight left axis deviation

8–38. In which of the following positions is cardiac output increased in the pregnant patient?

   a. left lateral recumbent
   b. sitting with knees and hips flexed
   c. right lateral recumbent
   d. supine

8–39. Which of the following hemodynamic values remain unchanged in pregnancy?

   a. systemic vascular resistance
   b. pulmonary vascular resistance
   c. colloid osmotic pressure
   d. pulmonary capillary wedge pressure

8–40. Which of the following is decreased in normotensive pregnant women?

   a. renin activity and renin concentration
   b. angiotensinogen
   c. sensitivity to pressor effects of angiotensin II
   d. aldosterone

8–41. Which of the following is least likely to be involved in the control of vascular reactivity during pregnancy?

   a. prostaglandins
   b. estrogens
   c. alteration in cyclic adenosine monophosphate
   d. changes in intracellular calcium concentrations

8–42. Which of the following characterizes arterial blood pressure in normal pregnancy?

    a. nadir in midpregnancy
    b. nadir in the first trimester, rising thereafter
    c. peaks in the first trimester, falling thereafter
    d. peaks in the second trimester

8–43. What is the average elevation of the diaphragm during normal pregnancy?

    a. 0 to 1 cm
    b. 2 cm
    c. 4 cm
    d. 6 cm

8–44. Which of the following is decreased in normal pregnancy?

    a. arteriovenous oxygen difference
    b. cardiac output
    c. diaphragmatic excursion
    d. hemoglobin in circulation

8–45. Which of the following is decreased in normal pregnancy?

    a. tidal volume
    b. minute ventilatory volume
    c. minute oxygen uptake
    d. functional residual capacity

8–46. Which of the following is decreased during normal pregnancy?

    a. glomerular filtration rate
    b. renal plasma flow
    c. creatinine clearance
    d. plasma concentration of urea

8–47. Which of the following is least likely to be excreted in large amounts in the urine of a normal pregnant woman?

    a. amino acids
    b. glucose
    c. protein
    d. water-soluble vitamins

8–48. Which of the following organs physically enlarges during pregnancy?

    a. appendix
    b. kidneys

    c. liver
    d. lungs

8–49. With regard to liver function in pregnancy, which of the following is normally decreased?

    a. total serum alkaline phosphatase activity
    b. bilirubin levels
    c. plasma albumin concentration
    d. plasma globulins

8–50. Pruritis gravidarum is caused by elevated tissue levels of which of the following?

    a. bile salts
    b. bile acids
    c. bilirubin, direct
    d. bilirubin, indirect

8–51. Which of the following is most likely to cross the placenta?

    a. thyroxine
    b. triiodothyronine
    c. reverse triiodothyronine
    d. thyroid-releasing hormone

8–52. Which of the following is decreased during pregnancy?

    a. parathyroid hormone
    b. serum calcium
    c. calcitonin
    d. size of the thyroid gland

8–53. Which of the following is decreased during normal pregnancy?

    a. serum concentration of circulating cortisol
    b. rate of cortisol secretion by the maternal adrenal
    c. aldosterone secretion
    d. maternal levels of testosterone

8–54. What is the level of testosterone in umbilical venous plasma likely to be in a pregnant woman with an androgen-secreting tumor?

    a. very high
    b. too low to be detected
    c. the same as in maternal serum
    d. none of the above

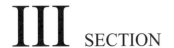

SECTION

*Pregnancy Planning and
Antepartum Management*

Preconceptional Counseling

9–1. Which of the following is an important goal of preconceptional counseling?

   a. prevent unintended pregnancy
   b. initiate preventive care measures
   c. identify genetic and obstetrical risk factors
   d. all of the above

9–2. Approximately what percentage of pregnancies in the United States are unplanned and, therefore, at greater risk of preventable complications?

   a. 10
   b. 20
   c. 30
   d. 50

9–3. Preconceptional counseling of diabetics has been shown to have what effect on subsequent pregnancy?

   a. decreased fetal malformations
   b. lower maternal hemoglobin A_{1c} levels
   c. less fetal growth restriction and macrosomia
   d. all of the above

9–4. What is the increased risk of fetal anomalies if the mother is epileptic?

   a. 2 to 3×
   b. 5×
   c. 7 to 8×
   d. none if not on anticonvulsants

9–5. Which preconceptional intervention is recommended for epileptic women using antiseizure medications?

   a. Control seizures with smaller doses of multiple medications.
   b. Switch to the least teratogenic monotherapy and dose.
   c. Discontinue antiseizure medications in all cases and treat periodically.
   d. Prescribe thiamine supplementation prior to conception.

9–6. What is the leading cause of infant death?

   a. birth defects
   b. sudden infant death syndrome
   c. prematurity and its complications
   d. infections

9–7. What is the incidence of neural tube defects?

   a. 1 to 2 per 10,000 livebirths
   b. 8 per 10,000 livebirths
   c. 1 to 2 per 1000 livebirths
   d. 8 per 1000 livebirths

9–8. Women with a prior child with a neural tube defect can reduce the rate of recurrence in subsequent pregnancy by taking preconceptional folic acid supplementation. What is the magnitude of this reduction?

   a. 10%
   b. 30%
   c. 50%
   d. 70%

9–9. Which of the following is the best approach to preconceptional counseling of women with phenylketonuria (PKU)?

   a. Only a fetus hetero- or homozygous for PKU is at risk for birth defects.
   b. The fetus is at no increased risk.
   c. Strict preconceptional dietary control decreases fetal risk.
   d. Women with PKU should not reproduce under any circumstances.

9–10. The incidence of which genetic disorder has plummeted as a result of preconceptional screening and counseling?

   a. phenylketonuria
   b. sickle cell anemia
   c. Tay-Sachs disease
   d. polycystic kidney disease

9–11. What percentage of the world's population carries a gene for a hemoglobinopathy?

   a. 0.004%
   b. 0.05%
   c. 0.4%
   d. 4.5%

9–12. Which group has been successfully targeted for preconceptional counseling regarding the risk of β-thalassemia?

   a. African descent
   b. Asian descent
   c. Mediterranean descent
   d. Jewish descent

9–13. Teenagers are at higher risk for which of the following?

   a. preterm labor
   b. gestational diabetes
   c. placental abruption
   d. urinary tract infection

9–14. What is the relation between advanced paternal age and the risk of birth defects?

   a. none
   b. increased
   c. slightly decreased
   d. unclear

9–15. Currently, what is the most important cause of dyzygotic twinning?

   a. advanced maternal age
   b. high parity
   c. racial predisposition
   d. assisted reproductive technology

9–16. Which of the following is NOT increased by smoking during pregnancy?

   a. attention deficit hyperactivity disorder
   b. birth defects
   c. fetal growth restriction
   d. preterm labor

9–17. Maternal obesity is related to an increase in which of the following obstetrical complications?

   a. hypertension
   b. gestational diabetes
   c. thrombophlebitis
   d. all of the above

9–18. What is the increased caloric demand of pregnancy?

   a. 100 kcal/d
   b. 300 kcal/d
   c. 600 kcal/d
   d. 1200 kcal/d

9–19. Risk from domestic abuse shows what general pattern during pregnancy as compared with before pregnancy?

   a. decreases
   b. approximately the same
   c. increases
   d. difficult to draw conclusions from available studies

9–20. Which of the following types of malformations are increased in the infants of overt diabetic mothers?

   a. cardiac
   b. neural tube
   c. renal
   d. all of the above

9–21. What is the rate of major fetal anomalies with a preconceptional maternal glycosylated hemoglobin greater than 10.6 percent?

   a. 5%
   b. 10%
   c. 25%
   d. 50%

9–22. What is the usual dose of folic acid recommended to reduce the risk of neural tube defects in the normal female population?

   a. 0.4 mg/d
   b. 4 mg/d
   c. 40 mg/d
   d. 400 mg/d

9–23. What dose of folic acid is recommended for women with a positive personal or positive family history of neural tube defects?

    a. 0.4 mg/d
    b. 4 mg/d
    c. 40 mg/d
    d. 400 mg/d

9–24. In the presence of maternal renal disease, the best predictor of perinatal outcome is which of the following?

    a. maternal serum creatinine
    b. length of time since diagnosed
    c. type of renal disease
    d. blood pressure

9–25. Which group of drugs causes fetal renal tubular dysgenesis?

    a. ACE inhibitors
    b. β-blockers
    c. calcium channel blockers
    d. thiazide diuretics

9–26. An increase in seizure incidence is seen in what proportion of epileptic women during pregnancy?

    a. 1 in 10
    b. 1 in 5
    c. 1 in 3
    d. 1 in 2

9–27. What percentage of nonpregnant epileptic women on monotherapy without seizures will remain seizure-free after discontinuing their medication?

    a. 10
    b. 20
    c. 33
    d. 66

9–28. Which of the following cardiac abnormalities is associated with maternal risk so high as to warrant recommendation against pregnancy?

    a. aortic coarctation (complicated)
    b. Marfan syndrome with aortic involvement
    c. pulmonary hypertension
    d. all of the above

9–29. What is the maternal mortality rate for women with pulmonary hypertension and Eisenmenger syndrome?

    a. 1 to 2%
    b. 5 to 10%
    c. 20 to 30%
    d. 40 to 50%

9–30. Fetal outcome in the presence of maternal cyanotic heart disease correlates LEAST strongly with which of the following?

    a. arterial oxygen saturation
    b. hemoglobin level
    c. resting pulse and blood pressure
    d. type of cardiac lesion

9–31. What is the approximate risk of recurrent thromboembolism in pregnancy?

    a. up to 10%
    b. 20%
    c. 30%
    d. 40%

9–32. Which connective tissue disease is most likely to remit during pregnancy?

    a. lupus
    b. rheumatoid arthritis
    c. ankylosing spondylitis
    d. scleroderma

9–33. What is the recurrence rate of permanent congenital heart block if a woman with lupus has already had an affected child?

    a. 5%
    b. 15%
    c. 50%
    d. 75%

9–34. Which of the following factors may increase the risk of exacerbation of psychiatric illness during pregnancy?

    a. misguided discontinuance of medications
    b. coexistent substance abuse
    c. change in eating and sleeping patterns
    d. all of the above

9–35. A history of which of the following confers the highest risk of postpartum psychosis?

    a. bipolar disorder
    b. episode of postpartum psychosis after prior pregnancy
    c. major depressive disorder
    d. premenstrual dysphoric disorder

9–36. How does pregnancy affect the risk of relapses in schizophrenia?

    a. decreased
    b. unchanged
    c. slightly increased
    d. markedly increased

9–37. In general, what group of medications is the most teratogenic?

    a. anticonvulsants
    b. nonsteroidal antiinflammatory drugs
    c. antipsychotic drugs
    d. narcotic analgesics

9–38. How should a woman be counseled if she inadvertently becomes pregnant within 3 months of receiving a live virus vaccine?

    a. no fetal risk
    b. theoretical but no definite risks

    c. serious fetal risks but are uncommon
    d. significant risk and pregnancy termination is recommended

9–39. How should a woman be counseled when exposed to diagnostic x-rays during pregnancy?

    a. slightly increased risk of fetal malformations
    b. definite increased risk of childhood leukemias
    c. slightly increased risk of fetal growth restriction and stillbirth
    d. no adverse effects are expected

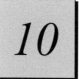

10

Prenatal Care

10–1. In 1998, what was the median number of prenatal visits per pregnancy?

    a. 6
    b. 8
    c. 10
    d. 12

10–2. In 1998, approximately what percentage of pregnant women in the United States received no prenatal care?

    a. 1.2
    b. 4.8
    c. 8.2
    d. 12.0

10–3. What is a primipara?

    a. a woman who was pregnant once, regardless of outcome
    b. a woman delivered once of a viable fetus of at least 24 weeks gestation
    c. a primate model for human pregnancy
    d. a woman who has had one pregnancy lasting at least 12 weeks

10–4. A woman's parity is determined by the number of which of the following?

    a. pregnancies she has had
    b. live fetuses delivered
    c. fetuses reaching viability
    d. pregnancies reaching viability including stillbirths

10–5. A woman is classified as a nulligravida if she has

    a. never delivered a live-born baby
    b. had one miscarriage
    c. never been pregnant
    d. had only one pregnancy

10–6. An obstetrical notation showing a woman to be a gravida 4 para 3-1-0-2 indicates a history of which of the following?

    a. 2 abortions
    b. 3 living children
    c. 3 term deliveries
    d. 0 preterm deliveries

10–7. What is the mean duration of pregnancy from the first day of the last menstrual period (LMP)?

    a. 250 days
    b. 260 days
    c. 270 days
    d. 280 days

10–8. Naegele's rule estimates gestational age based on which of the following formulas?

    a. Add 7 days to LMP and count back 3 months.
    b. Subtract 7 days from LMP and count back 3 months.
    c. Add 21 days to LMP and count back 3 months.
    d. Subtract 21 days from LMP and count back 3 months.

10–9. By convention, pregnancy trimesters divide which of the following gestational time periods (weeks) into 3 equal parts?

    a. 36
    b. 39
    c. 40
    d. 42

10–10. Duration of pregnancy is most appropriately and precisely measured by which of the following units?

    a. completed weeks since first day of LMP
    b. number of weeks, rounded to the nearest whole week, since the first day of LMP
    c. completed weeks since estimated date of conception
    d. number of weeks, rounded to the nearest whole week, since estimated date of conception

10–11. Which of the following is LEAST important in determining gestational age at the first prenatal visit?

    a. presence of an intrauterine contraceptive device
    b. history of recent oral contraceptive use
    c. menstrual history
    d. uterine size on physical exam

10–12. As of 1998, what percentage of adult women are smokers (Ventura and colleagues, 2000)?

    a. 9
    b. 13
    c. 17
    d. 21

10–13. According to the Centers for Disease Control and Prevention (1995), what percentage of women use alcohol in pregnancy?

    a. 3
    b. 5
    c. 9
    d. 15

10–14. Which of the following should NOT be routinely included at the first prenatal visit?

    a. complete history and physical
    b. human immunodeficiency virus testing
    c. hemoglobin A_{1c} determination
    d. urinalysis for glucose, protein, and culture

10–15. The presence of foamy, yellow discharge in the vagina is most suggestive of which of the following?

    a. normal vaginal secretions
    b. *Candida* vaginitis
    c. *Trichomonas vaginalis*
    d. leukorrhea of pregnancy

10–16. There is good correlation of fundal height in centimeters and gestational age during which weeks of gestation?

    a. 14 to 30
    b. 16 to 34
    c. 18 to 32
    d. 20 to 38

10–17. At what gestational age (weeks) are audible fetal heart sounds present in 100 percent of live pregnancies?

    a. 16
    b. 18
    c. 20
    d. 22

10–18. Which of the following is NOT a midpregnancy event that enhances the reliability of the estimated gestational age?

    a. audible fetal heart tones with a DeLee stethoscope by 20 weeks
    b. fundal height at umbilicus at 20 weeks
    c. serum human chorionic gonadotropin (hCG) level greater than 50,000 m/U
    d. fetal movement by 20 to 21 weeks' gestation

10–19. At what gestational age (weeks) should routine screening tests for gestational diabetes be performed?

    a. 10 to 16
    b. 20 to 24
    c. 24 to 28
    d. 32 to 36

10–20. In high risk women of low socioeconomic status, chlamydia infection at 24 weeks increases the likelihood of preterm birth by how much?

    a. none
    b. twofold
    c. threefold
    d. fourfold

10–21. For which of the following is universal prenatal screening currently recommended?

    a. anemia
    b. bacterial vaginosis
    c. fetal fibronectin
    d. herpes

10–22. Which of the following is the consensus regarding prenatal screening for group B *Streptococcus* colonization of the genitourinary tract?

    a. All pregnant women should be screened at the initial visit.
    b. Cultures should be done every trimester in high risk women.
    c. Screening is of no value in any population.
    d. There is currently no consensus of opinion.

10–23. A couple of Indian or Pakistani descent is at highest risk for which of the following genetic diseases?

    a. α-thalassemia
    b. β-thalassemia
    c. cystic fibrosis
    d. Tay-Sachs disease

10–24. A total maternal weight gain of less than 16 lb is associated with which of the following?

    a. fetal malformations
    b. impaired mental development of the infant or child
    c. low birthweight infants
    d. pregnancy-induced hypertension

10–25. What is the average total weight gain in healthy primigravidas (Hytten, 1991)?

    a. 20.0 lb
    b. 27.5 lb
    c. 35.0 lb
    d. 42.5 lb

10–26. What is the average weight gain from 20 weeks' gestation to term?

    a. $\frac{1}{2}$ lb/wk
    b. 1 lb/wk
    c. $1\frac{1}{2}$ lb/wk
    d. 2 lb/wk

10–27. Excessive maternal weight gain is associated with which of the following?

    a. increase in cesarean delivery rate
    b. increase in preterm deliveries
    c. increase in incidence of placental abruption
    d. none of the above

10–28. Which nutrient during pregnancy is NOT adequately provided in diet alone?

    a. calcium
    b. magnesium
    c. iron
    d. folate

10–29. For pregnancy, the National Research Council (1989) recommends a daily caloric increase of how much?

    a. 100 kcal
    b. 300 kcal
    c. 500 kcal
    d. 1000 kcal

10–30. What are the average daily iron requirements during the latter half of pregnancy?

    a. 1 mg/d
    b. 3 mg/d
    c. 5 mg/d
    d. 7 mg/d

10–31. To minimize the gastrointestinal side effects of iron, when is it recommended that patients take iron?

    a. at bedtime
    b. with breakfast
    c. during the first trimester
    d. only if the hemoglobin is less than 10 mg/dL

10–32. What characterizes intestinal calcium absorption during pregnancy?

    a. It decreases.
    b. It remains the same.
    c. It increases.
    d. It increases with vitamin E.

10–33. During pregnancy, how much calcium is retained?

    a. 30 g
    b. 60 g
    c. 90 g
    d. 120 g

10–34. Which of the following is NOT associated with zinc deficiency?

    a. impaired wound healing
    b. poor appetite
    c. dwarfism
    d. diarrhea

10–35. What are the current recommendations for daily zinc intake?

    a. <1 mg
    b. 5 mg
    c. 15 mg
    d. 30 mg

10–36. Subclinical maternal hypothyroidism has been linked to an increase in which of the following?

    a. stillbirths
    b. preterm deliveries
    c. mental retardation in children
    d. molar pregnancies

10–37. In general, iodine intake has shown what trend in the United States in the past 15 years?

    a. stable
    b. increasing
    c. decreasing
    d. unknown

10–38. Which of the following minerals is often deficient in pregnancy?

    a. chromium
    b. copper
    c. manganese
    d. none of the above

10–39. For what enzyme or compound is selenium an essential compound?

    a. glutathione peroxidase
    b. glycosyltransferases
    c. cytochrome oxidase
    d. insulin

10–40. In the People's Republic of China, selenium deficiency is associated with which of the following in children?

    a. cardiomyopathy
    b. renal failure
    c. seizures
    d. short stature

10–41. What cofactor for insulin facilitates the hormone's attachment to its peripheral receptors?

    a. selenium
    b. sodium
    c. manganese
    d. chromium

10–42. What percentage of neural tube defects are related to folic acid metabolism and, therefore, preventable by folic acid supplementation?

    a. 5
    b. 15
    c. 25
    d. 50

10–43. What amount of daily folic acid intake is currently recommended during the preconceptual period and early pregnancy?

    a. 40 μg
    b. 100 μg
    c. 400 μg
    d. 1000 μg

10–44. Excessive intake of vitamin A in pregnancy is suspected of causing which of the following in the fetus?

    a. blindness
    b. congenital heart block
    c. malformations
    d. seizures

10–45. Strict vegetarianism may cause maternal and fetal deficiencies of which of these nutrients?

    a. vitamin K
    b. cobalamin (B_{12})
    c. selenium
    d. phosphorus

10–46. Excessive ingestion of which vitamin can lead to vitamin B_{12} deficiency?

    a. A
    b. B_6
    c. C
    d. D

10–47. What is the recommended daily dietary allowance for vitamin C during pregnancy?

    a. 10 mg
    b. 30 mg
    c. 50 mg
    d. 70 mg

10–48. What are the results of continuation of running and aerobic exercise programs during pregnancy?

    a. reduced birthweight
    b. longer labors
    c. more midtrimester losses
    d. more fetal distress during labor

10–49. What are the hazards for pregnant women who work at jobs that require prolonged standing?

    a. delivering preterm
    b. fetal growth retardation
    c. preeclampsia
    d. preterm rupture of fetal membranes

10–50. What are the hazards of travel to the healthy pregnancy?

    a. decreased birthweight
    b. increased chorioamnionitis
    c. increased hypertensive complications
    d. no identifiable risks

10–51. Which of the following is true regarding safe automobile use during pregnancy?

    a. Air bags increase the risk of fetal injury.
    b. Three-point belt restraints should be used.
    c. Lap belts should not be used.
    d. Shoulder belts should not be used.

10–52. What is the recommendation for the administration of hepatitis A and B vaccines to pregnant women?

    a. contraindicated
    b. same as for nonpregnant women
    c. for postexposure only
    d. only if risk factors are present

10–53. What is the recommendation for the administration of rabies hyperimmune globulin to pregnant women?

    a. contraindicated
    b. the same as for nonpregnant women
    c. for postexposure prophylaxis only
    d. only if risk factors present

10–54. What is the recommendation for the administration of tetanus toxoid to pregnant women?

    a. contraindicated
    b. same as for nonpregnant women
    c. only if traveling to endemic area
    d. only if risk factors are present

10–55. What is the recommendation for the administration of measles vaccine to pregnant women?

    a. contraindicated
    b. same as for nonpregnant women
    c. for postexposure only
    d. only if risk factors are present

10–56. What is the recommendation for the administration of pneumococcus vaccine to pregnant women?

    a. contraindicated
    b. same as for nonpregnant women

    c. for postexposure only
    d. only if risk factors are present

10–57. What is the recommendation for the administration of varicella-zoster vaccine to pregnant women?

    a. contraindicated
    b. same as for nonpregnant women
    c. for postexposure only
    d. only if risk factors are present

10–58. Smoking during pregnancy increases the risk of which of the following adverse pregnancy outcomes?

    a. fetal growth restriction
    b. preterm delivery
    c. placental abruption
    d. all of the above

10–59. What is the maximum daily amount of alcohol considered safe for ingestion during pregnancy after the first trimester?

    a. 2 oz
    b. 1.5 oz
    c. 1 oz
    d. no amount considered safe

10–60. Which of the following statements regarding caffeine consumption during pregnancy is most strongly supported by research?

    a. It is iatrogenic in laboratory animals.
    b. It is positively correlated with pregnancy-induced hypertension.
    c. It causes transient fetal tachycardia.
    d. It may increase the risk of spontaneous abortion at extremely high levels.

10–61. Ninety percent of women with nausea and vomiting of pregnancy have resolution of this problem by what gestational age (weeks)?

    a. 10
    b. 14
    c. 18
    d. 22

10–62. While high levels of hCG have been implicated in the past as the etiology of nausea during pregnancy, which hormone is currently suspected to be the culprit?

    a. estrogen
    b. human placental lactogen
    c. progesterone
    d. prolactin

10–63. Which of the following cravings is NOT seen in association with severe iron deficiency anemia?

    a. ice
    b. dry lump starch
    c. clay
    d. pickles

10–64. What is the current recommendation for treatment of bacterial vaginosis in pregnancy?

    a. Defer treatment with metronidazole until postpartum.
    b. Screen for and treat all cases to prevent preterm labor.
    c. Treat symptomatic women.
    d. Treat the partner only.

11

Parturition

11–1. What is the characteristic of myometrial contractions that do not cause labor?

    a. not intense
    b. brief in duration
    c. unpredictable
    d. all of the above

11–2. Which of the following is essential for myometrial contractions?

    a. tubulin-actin
    b. actin-myosin
    c. myosin-tubulin
    d. all of the above

11–3. Which of the following is essential for the generation of smooth muscle contractions?

    a. prostaglandins
    b. intracellular free calcium
    c. extracellular free calcium
    d. oxytocin

11–4. Which of the following activates the phosphorylation reaction responsible for myometrial contractions?

    a. free intracellular calcium
    b. adenosine triphosphatase
    c. adenosine triphosphate hydrolysis
    d. myosin light chain kinase

11–5. The first stage of labor is best characterized by which of the following?

    a. cervical effacement and dilatation
    b. delivery of the fetus
    c. uterine preparedness for labor
    d. separation and expulsion

11–6. Which of the following characterizes active labor?

	contraction duration (sec)	amniotic fluid pressure (mm)
a.	30	10
b.	30	20
c.	60	40
d.	90	80

11–7. What is the most attractive hypothesis for the cause of labor pain?

    a. myometrial hypoxia
    b. cervical stretching
    c. peritoneum stretching
    d. compression of nerve ganglia in the cervix

11–8. What is the average amnionic fluid pressure generated by uterine contractions?

    a. 1 mm Hg
    b. 10 mm Hg
    c. 40 mm Hg
    d. 100 mm Hg

11–9. What causes the pathological Bandl ring?

    a. thinning of lower uterine segment
    b. thinning of upper uterus
    c. thickness of lower uterine segment
    d. a band of fibromuscular tissue at the level of the internal os

11–10. What is the most important force in the expulsion of the fetus?

    a. cervical softening
    b. uterine contractions
    c. maternal intra-abdominal pressure
    d. oxytocin concentration

11–11. Which of the following is NOT a vital force concerned in labor?

   a. intra-abdominal pressure
   b. cervical position
   c. resistance
   d. uterine contractions

11–12. According to Friedman (1978), what is the most important measure of labor progression?

   a. contraction frequency
   b. contraction intensity
   c. cervical effacement
   d. cervical dilatation

11–13. During the preparatory division of labor, which of the following inhibits uterine contractions?

   a. sedation
   b. antibiotics
   c. bedrest
   d. warm baths

11–14. What term refers to a fetus born surrounded by amniotic membranes?

   a. intact
   b. caul
   c. encapsulated
   d. en membranacio

11–15. Which of the following is a part of the urogenital diaphragm?

   a. deep transverse perineal muscle
   b. levator ani muscle
   c. coccygeus muscle
   d. ischiorectal fossa

11–16. What is the most important muscle of the pelvic floor?

   a. bulbocavernosus
   b. ischiocavernosus
   c. levator ani
   d. superficial transverse perineal muscle

11–17. What mechanism refers to peripheral separation of the placenta so that blood collects between the membranes and uterine wall and escapes from the vagina?

   a. Schultze
   b. Duncan
   c. Cunningham
   d. Pritchard

11–18. What is the major site of estrogen formation during pregnancy?

   a. peripheral conversion
   b. ovary
   c. corpus luteum
   d. placenta

11–19. In most mammals the implementation of phase 1 of parturition is due to which of the following?

   a. cortisol withdrawal
   b. progesterone withdrawal
   c. increase in oxytocin receptors
   d. inflammatory responses

11–20. What is the fetal signal for commencement of parturition?

   a. withdrawal of progesterone
   b. deficient placenta estrogen
   c. increased fetal cortisol production
   d. no fetal signal

11–21. Which of the following characterizes phase 0 of parturition?

   a. myometrial tranquility
   b. uterine awakening
   c. cervical effacement
   d. cervical dilatation

11–22. What is an agent that helps bring about the "awakening" of the uterus in terms of its ability to contract?

   a. contracting agent
   b. uterotropin
   c. uterotonin
   d. growth factor

11–23. Which of the following is NOT considered a structural component of the cervix?

   a. smooth muscle
   b. collagen
   c. ground substance
   d. oncofibronectin

11–24. At term, which of the following cervical components is increased?

   a. hyaluronic acid
   b. dermatan sulfate
   c. collagen
   d. endocervical glands

11–25. Which of the following is NOT associated with phase 3 of parturition?

   a. uterine contractions
   b. milk ejection
   c. restoration of fertility
   d. uterine inversion

11–26. What does the uterus weigh at term?

    a. 60 g
    b. 500 to 600 g
    c. 1000 g
    d. 1500 g

11–27. What is gap junction protein?

    a. actin
    b. myosin
    c. connexin
    d. laminin

11–28. The human oxytocin receptor gene is located on which chromosome?

    a. 3
    b. 11
    c. 16
    d. X

11–29. Which of the following can block progesterone action?

    a. steroids
    b. RU-486
    c. aspirin
    d. β-blockers (i.e., inderal)

11–30. During what weeks of gestation are plasma relaxin levels the highest?

    a. week 4 to 6
    b. week 8 to 12
    c. week 16 to 20
    d. week 24 to 28

11–31. What is the possible action of parathyroid hormone-related protein (PTH-γP)?

    a. vasorelaxant
    b. vasoconstrictor
    c. increases oxytocin receptors
    d. stimulates cervical ripening

11–32. Nitric oxide reacts with what element to produce cyclic guanosine monophosphate?

    a. iron
    b. lithium
    c. magnesium
    d. calcium

11–33. Which of the following enzymes catalyzes the degradation of endothelin-1?

    a. endothelinase
    b. oxytocinase
    c. placental sulfatase
    d. enkephalinase

11–34. Which of the following is NOT a uterotonin?

    a. endothelin-1
    b. prostaglandins
    c. oxytocin
    d. calcium

11–35. Where is oxytocin primarily synthesized?

    a. adrenal gland
    b. placenta
    c. posterior pituitary
    d. ovary

11–36. What is the carrier protein for oxytocin transport to the posterior pituitary?

    a. neurophysin
    b. relaxin
    c. binding globulin
    d. actin

11–37. Which of the following is NOT evidence for a role of prostaglandins in human parturition?

    a. It will cause abortion at any stage of gestation.
    b. It will cause labor at any stage of gestation.
    c. Levels in the forebag are increased during labor.
    d. It can cause contractions of smooth muscle cells in vitro.

11–38. What major prostaglandin is produced by the amnion?

    a. PGE_2
    b. PGF_2
    c. PGI
    d. PGG

11–39. What prostaglandin is preferentially produced by the decidua?

    a. PGE_1
    b. $PGF_{2\alpha}$
    c. PGI
    d. PGG

11–40. What prostaglandin is produced by the chorion laeve in vitro?

    a. PGE_2
    b. $PGF_{2\alpha}$
    c. PGG
    d. PGI

11–41. What is the initial and rate-limiting enzyme in prostaglandin inactivation?

    a. cyclooxygenase
    b. prostaglandin dehydrogenase
    c. enkephalinase
    d. oxytocinase

11–42. Which of the following is the action of platelet-activating factor (PAF) on myometrial cell?

    a. no effects on the myometrial cell
    b. decreases myosin light chain kinase
    c. decreases Ca^{2+}
    d. increases Ca^{2+}

11–43. What is the action of endothelin-1 on myometrial cells?

    a. decrease K+ intracellular
    b. decrease Ca^{2+} intracellular
    c. increase K+ intracellular
    d. increase Ca^{2+} intracellular

11–44. Which of the following tissues is avascularized?

    a. amnion
    b. syncytium
    c. decidua
    d. placenta

11–45. Which of the following bioactive agents is NOT a normal constituent of amnionic fluid?

    a. IL-1β
    b. IL-6
    c. macrophage colony stimulating factor
    d. prostaglandins

11–46. How often is interleukin-1β found in amnionic fluid of preterm pregnancies?

    a. 0%
    b. 25%
    c. 33%
    d. 50%

11–47. What is the cell source of interleukin-1β in amnionic fluid?

    a. amnion
    b. chorion laeve
    c. cytotrophoblast
    d. mononuclear phagocytes

11–48. Which of the following is a normal constituent of amnionic fluid?

    a. IL-1
    b. IL-2
    c. IL-4
    d. IL-8

11–49. What are the likely sources of the bioactive agent set in the amnionic fluid?

    a. chorion laeve; mononuclear cells
    b. chorion laeve; amnion
    c. decidual cells; mononuclear cells
    d. decidual cells; amnion

12

Mechanisms of Normal Labor

12–1. What is the relation of the long axis of the fetus to that of the mother called?

    a. presentation of the fetus
    b. lie of the fetus
    c. fetal attitude
    d. fetal posture

12–2. What is the lie if the fetal and maternal axes cross at a 45 degree angle?

    a. longitudinal
    b. breech
    c. oblique
    d. transverse

12–3. What percentage of term labors present with a longitudinal lie?

a. 20
b. 50
c. 70
d. 99

12–4. Which of the following factors is NOT associated with transverse lie?

a. multiparity
b. abruptio placentae
c. placenta previa
d. uterine anomalies

12–5. What is the presentation when the fetal head is flexed and the occipital fontanel is presenting?

a. vertex
b. face
c. brow
d. sinciput

12–6. What is the presentation when the fetal neck is extended and the back and occiput are in contact?

a. vertex
b. face
c. brow
d. sinciput

12–7. What is the presentation when the fetal head is partially flexed and a large anterior fontanel is presenting?

a. vertex
b. face
c. brow
d. sinciput

12–8. What type of breech presents with the thighs flexed on the abdomen and legs upon the thighs?

a. complete
b. incomplete
c. frank
d. double footling

12–9. In which of the following presentations does the fetal attitude (vertebral column) become concave (extended)?

a. face
b. shoulder
c. cephalic
d. breech

12–10. In shoulder presentations, what portion of the fetus is used to orient it with the maternal pelvis?

a. humerus
b. vertex

c. acromion
d. clavicle

12–11. Approximately what percentage of fetuses are in the occiput presentation at term?

a. 50
b. 65
c. 80
d. 95

12–12. What is the incidence of breech presentation at 29 to 32 weeks' gestation?

a. 5%
b. 14%
c. 31%
d. 48%

12–13. What components make up the podalic pole?

a. breech only
b. extremities only
c. breech and extremities
d. none of the above

12–14. What Leopold maneuver involves fundal palpation to define the fetal pole present in the fundus?

a. 1st
b. 2nd
c. 3rd
d. 4th

12–15. What Leopold maneuver involves grasping the lower portion of abdomen just above the symphysis?

a. 1st
b. 2nd
c. 3rd
d. 4th

12–16. What Leopold maneuver involves placing the palms of the hands on each side of the abdomen to determine the location of the back and small parts?

a. 1st
b. 2nd
c. 3rd
d. 4th

12–17. Breech presentations are best identified by palpation of which of the following?

a. fetal sacrum
b. maternal ischial tuberosities
c. umbilical cord
d. a and b only

12–18. With which of the following presentations will the fetal heart sounds be best heard a short distance from the midline?

   a. occipitoanterior
   b. occipitoposterior
   c. transverse
   d. breech

12–19. In transverse lie presentations, where are the fetal heart sounds best heard?

   a. midway between the maternal umbilicus and anterior spine of the maternal ilium
   b. slightly above or below the umbilicus
   c. a short distance from the midline
   d. laterally on abdomen

12–20. What is the most common presentation of the fetus as it enters the pelvis?

   a. right occiptoanterior (ROA)
   b. right occiptotransverse (ROT)
   c. left occiptoanterior (LOA)
   d. left occiptotransverse (LOT)

12–21. Posterior presentations are associated more commonly with which of the following?

   a. narrow forepelvis
   b. normal forepelvis
   c. wide forepelvis
   d. no association with forepelvis type

12–22. What are the cardinal movements of labor (in order)?

   a. descent, engagement, flexion, internal rotation, extension, external rotation, expulsion
   b. descent, flexion, engagement, internal rotation, extension, external rotation, expulsion
   c. engagement, descent, flexion, internal rotation, extension, external rotation, expulsion
   d. engagement, flexion, descent, internal rotation, extension, external rotation, expulsion

12–23. What is the mechanism where the biparietal diameter passes through the pelvic inlet?

   a. flexion
   b. engagement
   c. descent
   d. internal rotation

12–24. Which of the following is characteristic of asynclitism?

   a. Sagittal suture is not parallel to the transverse axis of the inlet.
   b. Sagittal suture lies midway between the symphysis and sacral promontory.

   c. Sagittal suture, although parallel to the transverse axis of the inlet, does not lie exactly midway between the symphysis and sacral promontory.
   d. Sagittal suture rotates 45 degrees from the sacral spines.

12–25. What part of the fetal anatomy is palpated easily when the presentation is Litzman obliquity (extreme posterior asynclitism)?

   a. nose
   b. mouth
   c. ear
   d. shoulder

12–26. Which of the following is NOT one of the four forces of descent?

   a. pressure of amnionic fluid
   b. direct fundal pressure on the breech
   c. myometrial contractions
   d. contraction of abdominal muscles

12–27. The chin is brought into intimate contact with the fetal thorax during which cardinal movement of labor?

   a. flexion
   b. extension
   c. engagement
   d. descent

12–28. The anterior shoulder appears under the symphysis during which cardinal movement of labor?

   a. extension
   b. expulsion
   c. external rotation
   d. descent

12–29. During which cardinal movement of labor is the head returned to the oblique position?

   a. internal rotation
   b. extension
   c. external rotation
   d. expulsion

12–30. The base of the occiput is brought into contact with the inferior margin of the symphysis during which cardinal movement of labor?

   a. extension
   b. expulsion
   c. descent
   d. flexion

12–31. During labor in the occiput posterior position, the occiput has to rotate to the symphysis pubis how many degrees?

    a. 45 degrees
    b. 90 degrees
    c. 135 degrees
    d. 180 degrees

12–32. What is the most common cause of persistent occiput posterior presentation?

    a. malrotation
    b. android pelvis
    c. fetopelvic disproportion
    d. prematurity

12–33. What is edematous swelling of the fetal scalp during labor?

    a. molding
    b. caput succedaneum
    c. subdural hematoma
    d. erythema nodosum

12–34. What is a change in the fetal head from external forces called?

    a. squashing
    b. forming
    c. shaping
    d. molding

13

Conduct of Normal Labor and Delivery

13–1. Which of the following is characteristic of true labor?

    a. irregular contractions
    b. discomfort restricted to lower abdomen
    c. cervical dilatation
    d. discomfort relieved by sedation

13–2. When should the fetal heart rate be auscultated during observation for labor?

    a. before the contraction
    b. during the contraction
    c. at the end and immediately after a contraction
    d. anytime

13–3. In which situation should standard vaginal examination be deferred or modified when admitting a woman to the labor unit?

    a. bleeding in excess of a bloody show
    b. maternal fever
    c. patient nervousness
    d. suspected ruptured membranes

13–4. What is the station where the presenting part is at the level of the ischial spines?

    a. −2
    b. −1
    c. 0
    d. +1

13–5. What is the station where the fetal head is visible at the introitus (based on centimeters)?

    a. +2
    b. +3
    c. +4
    d. +5

13–6. What is the station of the leading part of the fetal head when engagement (biparietal diameter is past the pelvic inlet) has occurred?

    a. −2
    b. +1
    c. −1
    d. 0

13–7. What is the most reliable indicator of rupture of the fetal membranes?

    a. fluid per cervical os
    b. positive nitrazine test
    c. positive ferning
    d. positive oncofetal fibronectin

13–8. What is the usual pH of amniotic fluid?

    a. 4.5 to 5.5
    b. 5.5 to 6.5
    c. 7.0 to 7.5
    d. 8.0 to 8.5

13–9. The nitrazine test for rupture of membranes may be false-positive if which of the following is present?

    a. candida
    b. vaginal bleeding
    c. cervical mucus
    d. scant amniotic fluid

13–10. What is the average duration (hours) of the first stage of labor in nulliparous women?

    a. 5
    b. 7
    c. 12
    d. 20

13–11. What is the average duration (hours) of the first stage of labor in parous women?

    a. 4
    b. 6
    c. 8
    d. 12

13–12. How often during the first stage of labor should the fetal heart rate be auscultated in a low risk pregnancy?

    a. every 15 min, before a contraction
    b. every 15 min, after a contraction
    c. every 30 min, before a contraction
    d. every 30 min, after a contraction

13–13. How often during the first stage of labor should the fetal heart rate be monitored in a high-risk pregnancy?

    a. every 15 min, before a contraction
    b. every 15 min, after a contraction
    c. every 30 min, before a contraction
    d. every 30 min, after a contraction

13–14. How often should the fetal heart rate be auscultated during the second stage of labor in low versus high-risk patients?

    a. 5 min/5 min
    b. 10 min/5 min
    c. 15 min/5 min
    d. 30 min/5 min

13–15. For the purpose of administering antimicrobial prophylaxis for group B streptococcus, prolonged membrane rupture is defined as duration greater than how many hours?

    a. 10
    b. 12
    c. 18
    d. 24

13–16. In a 1998 study of over 1000 women, walking during labor had what effect?

    a. prolonged first phase of labor
    b. shortened period of latency and second stage of labor
    c. increased incidence of dysfunctional labor, two intrapartum deaths
    d. no effect on active labor; not harmful

13–17. What is the median duration of the second stage of labor in multiparas?

    a. 5 min
    b. 10 min
    c. 20 min
    d. 30 min

13–18. What is the median duration of the second stage of labor in primiparas?

    a. 5 min
    b. 20 min
    c. 50 min
    d. 100 min

13–19. Which of the following may be associated with a shortened second stage of labor?

    a. standing position
    b. squatting position
    c. supine position
    d. left lateral position

13–20. What is the term for encirclement of the largest diameter of the fetal head by the vulvar ring?

    a. Bandl's ring
    b. crowning
    c. complete dilatation or beginning of second stage
    d. beginning of third stage of labor

13–21. Which of the following is true regarding the routine use of episiotomy?

    a. It decreases the risk of anal sphincter laceration.

    b. It increases the risk of anal sphincter laceration.

    c. It does not affect the risk of urethral lacerations.

    d. It increases the risk of urethral lacerations.

13–22. What is the maneuver used to facilitate delivery of the fetal head over the perineum in a controlled manner?

    a. MacRoberts

    b. Ragu

    c. Ritgen

    d. Woods

13–23. What percentage of deliveries are complicated by a nuchal cord?

    a. 1

    b. 5

    c. 10

    d. 25

13–24. If the umbilical cord is left unclamped, what volume of blood can be transfused into the newborn, on average?

    a. 10 mL

    b. 30 mL

    c. 50 mL

    d. 80 mL

13–25. During the third stage of labor, which of the following is NOT a sign of placental separation?

    a. a gush of blood

    b. uterus rises in the abdomen

    c. umbilical cord protrudes farther out of the vagina

    d. painful uterine tetany

13–26. Which of the following is a complication of the third stage of labor associated with forced placental separation?

    a. endometritis

    b. uterine atony

    c. Asherman syndrome

    d. uterine inversion

13–27. In the absence of excessive bleeding, after how much time should manual removal of the placenta be performed if spontaneous separation does not occur?

    a. 5 min

    b. 15 min

    c. 25 min

    d. unclear

13–28. How long does the so-called "fourth stage" of labor, when risk of postpartum hemorrhage is greatest, last?

    a. 15 min

    b. 1 hr

    c. 2 hr

    d. 4 hr

13–29. What is the primary mechanism of placental site hemostasis?

    a. vasoconstriction by contracted myometrium

    b. prostaglandin secretion

    c. maternal hypotension

    d. decreased cardiac output

13–30. What is the half-life of oxytocin?

    a. <1 min

    b. 3 min

    c. 10 to 15 min

    d. 20 to 30 min

13–31. Which deleterious effect is associated with oxytocin when given intravenously as a 10-U bolus?

    a. bradycardia

    b. hypotension

    c. oliguria

    d. cardiac arrhythmia

13–32. At what dosage of oxytocin should you expect to see a decrease in urine output?

    a. 10 mU/min

    b. 20 mU/min

    c. 30 mU/min

    d. 40 mU/min

13–33. Which of the following is associated with ergonovine and methylergonovine?

    a. seizures

    b. hypertension

    c. oliguria

    d. thrombocytopenia

13–34. What is a laceration involving the skin, mucous membrane, perineal body, anal sphincter, and rectal mucosa called?

    a. first degree

    b. second degree

    c. third degree

    d. fourth degree

13–35. What is a laceration involving the fourchette or perineal skin, but not the muscle, called?

    a. first degree
    b. second degree
    c. third degree
    d. fourth degree

13–36. What is a laceration involving the skin, mucous membrane, perineal body, and anal sphincter called?

    a. first degree
    b. second degree

    c. third degree
    d. fourth degree

13–37. What is the major advantage of a mediolateral episiotomy?

    a. easy surgical repair
    b. less postoperative pain
    c. less blood loss
    d. fewer extensions

Intrapartum Assessment

14–1. What percentage of livebirths in the United States undergo electronic fetal monitoring?

    a. 40 to 50
    b. 60 to 70
    c. 80 to 90
    d. ~100

14–2. What portion of the fetal electrocardiogram is most reliably detected?

    a. p wave
    b. QRS complex
    c. R wave peak
    d. T wave

14–3. During electronic fetal monitoring how is a premature atrial contraction recorded?

    a. pause
    b. acceleration
    c. deceleration
    d. not detected

14–4. What term indicates that fetal heart rate has regularity whereas noise is random?

    a. autoregulation
    b. automation

    c. autocorrelation
    d. randomization

14–5. What are the usual settings for vertical and horizontal scaling during electronic monitoring?

    a. 30 bpm; 1 cm/min
    b. 30 bpm; 3 cm/min
    c. 60 bpm; 1 cm/min
    d. 60 bpm; 3 cm/min

14–6. Which of the following is responsible for the baseline fetal heart rate decreasing from 16 weeks to term?

    a. maturation of sympathetic response
    b. maturation of parasympathetic response
    c. increasing size of fetus
    d. hormonal alterations

14–7. What is baseline bradycardia?

    a. <90 bpm
    b. <100 bpm
    c. <110 bpm
    d. <120 bpm

14–8. What is baseline tachycardia?

    a. >160 bpm

    b. >170 bpm

    c. >180 bpm

    d. >190 bpm

14–9. What is the normal average baseline fetal heart rate at term?

    a. 100 to 140 bpm

    b. 110 to 150 bpm

    c. 120 to 160 bpm

    d. 120 to 140 bpm

14–10. Which of the following defines severe bradycardia?

    a. <60 bpm for 1 min

    b. <80 bpm for 1 min

    c. <60 bpm for 3 min

    d. <80 bpm for 3 min

14–11. Which of the following is NOT associated with fetal bradycardia?

    a. head compression

    b. congenital heart block

    c. fetal compromise

    d. aminophylline

14–12. What is severe tachycardia?

    a. >160 bpm

    b. >180 bpm

    c. >200 bpm

    d. >220 bpm

14–13. What is the most common cause of fetal tachycardia?

    a. drug-induced

    b. maternal fever

    c. thyroid storm

    d. cardiac arrhythmias

14–14. What is the single most reliable sign of fetal compromise?

    a. fetal bradycardia

    b. fetal tachycardia

    c. reduced baseline variability

    d. repetitive severe variable decelerations

14–15. Which of the following is NOT a common cause of diminished beat-to-beat variability?

    a. magnesium sulfate

    b. tranquilizers

    c. antibiotics

    d. analgesic drugs

14–16. Which of the following is characteristic of sinusoidal fetal heart rate patterns?

    a. stable baseline with oscillation of 6 cycles/min

    b. stable baseline; amplitude of 5 to 15 bpm; and 2 to 5 cycles/min long-term variability

    c. unstable baseline with oscillation of 6 cycles/min

    d. unstable baseline; amplitude of 5 to 15 bpm and 2 to 5 cycles/min long-term variability

14–17. What is the frequency of sine waves when caused by maternal meperidine?

    a. 1 cycle/min

    b. 3 cycles/min

    c. 6 cycles/min

    d. 12 cycles/min

14–18. An acceleration is defined as an increase in fetal heart rate of what magnitude above baseline?

    a. 10 bpm for 10 sec

    b. 15 bpm for 10 sec

    c. 10 bpm for 15 sec

    d. 15 bpm for 15 sec

14–19. What is a drop in the fetal heart rate that coincides with a uterine contraction called?

    a. early deceleration

    b. late deceleration

    c. variable deceleration

    d. acceleration

14–20. What is a gradual, smooth descent of the fetal heart rate after the peak of the contraction called?

    a. early deceleration

    b. late deceleration

    c. variable deceleration

    d. acceleration

14–21. What is the most common deceleration pattern encountered during labor?

    a. late

    b. early

    c. variable

    d. mixed

14–22. What is the cause of variable decelerations?

    a. head compression

    b. acidemia

    c. cord compression

    d. hypoxia

14–23. What are significant variable decelerations?

    a. fetal heart rate <90 bpm for >30 sec
    b. fetal heart rate <70 bpm for >30 sec
    c. fetal heart rate <90 bpm for >60 sec
    d. fetal heart rate <70 bpm for >60 sec

14–24. What percentage of women given epidural analgesia have a prolonged deceleration?

    a. 4
    b. 8
    c. 16
    d. 32

14–25. Which fetal heart rate pattern is NOT associated with an increase in fetal compromise?

    a. abnormal baseline rate less than 120
    b. absent beat-to-beat variability
    c. abnormal baseline rate more than 160
    d. repetitive mild variable decelerations

14–26. For which of the following is amnioinfusion NOT employed?

    a. meconium
    b. amniotic fluid index <3
    c. chorioamnionitis
    d. variable decelerations during labor

14–27. Which of the following pregnancy complications is NOT associated with intrapartum amnioinfusion?

    a. seizures
    b. uterine hypertonus
    c. chorioamnionitis
    d. cord prolapse

14–28. Which of the following is NOT linked to an abnormal fetal heart rate pattern?

    a. low 5 min Apgar
    b. fetal death
    c. neonatal death
    d. abnormal neurological outcomes

14–29. Approximately what percentage of laboring women's fetuses have intermittent oxygen saturation <30 percent?

    a. 10
    b. 30
    c. 50
    d. 70

14–30. What is the definition of asphyxia?

    a. fetal distress
    b. hypoxia leading to acidemia
    c. acidemia alone
    d. severe variable decelerations

14–31. Which of the following is NOT microscopic findings associated with perinatal brain damage?

    a. neuronal necrosis with lysis
    b. neuronal necrosis with eosinophilia
    c. neuronal necrosis with macrophage response
    d. neuronal necrosis with astrocytic response

14–32. What are the effects of using electronic fetal monitoring?

    a. improved perinatal outcome
    b. increased incidence of forceps delivery
    c. increased incidence of primary cesarean sections
    d. improved care of the mother during labor

14–33. What are the current recommendations for auscultation of fetal heart rate in high-risk pregnancies?

    a. first stage labor every 30 min; second stage every 15 min
    b. first stage labor every 30 min; second stage every 5 min
    c. first stage labor every 15 min; second stage every 15 min
    d. first stage labor every 15 min; second stage every 5 min

14–34. How is a Montevideo unit defined?

    a. an increased pressure above baseline multiplied by the contraction frequency in 10 min
    b. the number of contractions in 1 hr times the peak contraction pressure
    c. the minimum contraction frequency in 10 min times the average contraction pressure
    d. the number of contractions in 10 min times the amount of pitocin infused per hour

14–35. At what intensity are uterine contractions clinically palpable?

    a. 5 mm Hg
    b. 10 mm Hg
    c. 20 mm Hg
    d. 30 mm Hg

14–36. At what intensity are uterine contractions associated with pain?

    a. 5 mm Hg
    b. 10 mm Hg
    c. 15 mm Hg
    d. 20 mm Hg

14–37. Where is the uterine contraction "pacemaker"?

    a. cervix, laterally
    b. low uterine segment, centrally
    c. fundus, anteriorly
    d. fallopian tubes, uterine end

14–38. In humans, at what speed does the contraction spread from the pacemaker area throughout the uterus?

    a. 0.5 cm/sec
    b. 1.0 cm/sec
    c. 2.0 cm/sec
    d. 4.0 cm/sec

14–39. Before one decides to perform a cesarean section for dystocia there should be how much uterine activity?

    a. 75 to 100 Montevideo units
    b. 150 to 175 Montevideo units
    c. 200 to 225 Montevideo units
    d. 300 to 325 Montevideo units

15

Analgesia and Anesthesia

15–1. What percentage of direct maternal deaths are secondary to anesthesia complications?

    a. <1
    b. 3 to 4
    c. 6 to 8
    d. 12 to 16

15–2. Which maternal finding is NOT an anesthesia risk factor?

    a. anatomical anomaly of the face
    b. asthma
    c. morbid obesity
    d. mild hypertension

15–3. Which of the following characterizes women who receive continuous emotional support during labor?

    a. deliver by cesarean section more often
    b. request epidural analgesia more often

    c. need oxytocin during labor more often
    d. experience less pain

15–4. When does the peak analgesic effect of meperidine given intramuscularly occur?

    a. <5 min
    b. 20 min
    c. 45 min
    d. 60 min

15–5. When does the peak analgesic effect of meperidine given intravenously occur?

    a. <5 min
    b. 20 min
    c. 45 min
    d. 60 min

15–6. What is the half-life of meperidine in the newborn?

    a. <1 hr
    b. 2 to 3 hr
    c. 6 to 8 hr
    d. 12 to 14 hr

15–7. Butorphanol administration has been associated with which fetal heart rate abnormality?

    a. repetitive late decelerations
    b. fetal tachycardia
    c. sinusoidal rhythm
    d. saltatory patter

15–8. What dose of butorphanol is comparable to 50 mg of meperidine?

    a. 0.5 mg intravenously (IV)
    b. 1 to 2 mg IV
    c. 4 to 5 mg IV
    d. 10 mg IV

15–9. What is the mechanism of action of naloxone hydrochloride?

    a. stimulates acetylcholinesterase
    b. displaces narcotic from specific receptors
    c. inhibits muscarinic receptors
    d. blocks β receptors

15–10. Which physiological event causes the concentration of inhalation anesthetic to increase more rapidly in a pregnant woman's lungs?

    a. increased tidal volume
    b. decreased functional residual capacity
    c. increased residual volume
    d. decreased total lung capacity

15–11. Which of the following is a rare side effect of halothane anesthesia?

    a. anemia
    b. thrombocytopenia
    c. hypertension
    d. hepatitis

15–12. During balanced general anesthesia, which agent can decrease maternal awareness?

    a. 1% halogenated agent
    b. lidocaine
    c. valium
    d. morphine

15–13. Which of the following is NOT associated with general anesthesia?

    a. decreased blood loss at cesarean section
    b. neonatal depression

    c. a significantly increased risk of early pregnancy loss in operating room personnel
    d. prolonged hospitalization

15–14. What is the advantage of ketamine when compared to thiopental?

    a. not associated with hypotension
    b. causes delirium
    c. causes hallucinations
    d. induces general anesthesia at very low doses (<0.5 mg/kg)

15–15. What is one of the most common causes of anesthetic death in obstetrics?

    a. esophageal intubation
    b. hemorrhage
    c. pneumonitis
    d. stroke

15–16. What is pressure on the cricoid cartilage (to occlude esophagus) called?

    a. Heimlich maneuver
    b. Circus maneuver
    c. Sellick maneuver
    d. Hawaiian maneuver

15–17. What amount of time is required after intravenously administered cimetidine to decrease gastric acidity?

    a. 15 min
    b. 60 min
    c. 2 hr
    d. 4 hr

15–18. Chemical pneumonitis develops if the gastric pH that is aspirated is less than which of the following?

    a. 2.5
    b. 3.0
    c. 4.0
    d. 5.0

15–19. What are the signs of aspiration of acidic liquid?

    a. bradycardia, decreased respiratory rate, hypotension
    b. bradycardia, tachypnea, hypertension
    c. tachycardia, decreased respiratory rate, hypotension
    d. tachycardia, tachypnea, hypotension

15–20. All EXCEPT which of the following is included in the treatment of aspiration?

 a. mouth suction
 b. bronchoscopy for removal of large particulate matter
 c. corticosteroids
 d. mechanical ventilation for respiratory distress

15–21. Which nerve roots are predominantly responsible for early first-stage labor pain?

 a. T10, T11
 b. T11, T12
 c. T10, T11, T12, L1
 d. S2, S3, S4

15–22. Which nerve roots are responsible for the pain of vaginal delivery?

 a. T10, T11
 b. T11, T12
 c. T10, T11, T12, L1
 d. S2, S3, S4

15–23. Which of the following is NOT a sign of central nervous system (CNS) toxicity from local anesthetics?

 a. slurred speech
 b. tinnitus
 c. paresthesia (mouth)
 d. hypertension

15–24. Which central acting agent is used to control convulsions caused by anesthetic-induced CNS toxicity?

 a. succinylcholine
 b. thiopental
 c. magnesium sulfate
 d. phenytoin

15–25. Which of the following is generally true concerning cardiovascular manifestations of local anesthetic toxicity?

 a. They develop before CNS toxicity.
 b. They develop with CNS toxicity.
 c. They develop later than CNS toxicity.
 d. There are no cardiovascular manifestations from local anesthetic toxicity.

15–26. What is the most common complication of paracervical block?

 a. maternal hypotension
 b. central nervous system toxicity
 c. fetal bradycardia
 d. bleeding

15–27. What is the etiology of spinal headaches?

 a. puncture of meninges followed by leaking fluid
 b. hypotension after spinal block
 c. vasodilation of cerebral vessels
 d. drug-induced hormonal changes

15–28. Which of the following is an absolute contraindication to spinal analgesia?

 a. preeclampsia
 b. infected skin at site of needle entry
 c. convulsions secondary to seizure disorder
 d. diabetes

15–29. Which of the following nerve blocks would provide complete analgesia for labor pain and vaginal delivery?

 a. T8-S2
 b. T10-S5
 c. T12-S2
 d. T8-L4

15–30. What is the most common side effect of epidural anesthesia?

 a. maternal hypertension
 b. maternal hypotension
 c. CNS stimulation
 d. ineffective block

15–31. What is the cause of intrapartum fever in women with epidurals?

 a. pain
 b. analgesics
 c. placental inflammation
 d. meningitis

15–32. What is the major advantage of using combination opiate and local anesthetic for epidural blockade?

 a. denser motor block
 b. less toxicity
 c. rapid onset of pain relief
 d. increase in shivering

15–33. What is the most common side effect in combined opiate-epidural anesthesia?

 a. urinary retention
 b. nausea and vomiting
 c. pruritis
 d. headaches

16

The Newborn Infant

16–1. Which of the following characterizes fetal breathing?

    a. deep, regular breathing
    b. shallow, episodic breathing
    c. deep inhalations
    d. long expirations

16–2. Which of the following contributes to transient tachypnea of the newborn?

    a. delay in removal of fluid from alveoli
    b. hypoxia
    c. hypercapnea
    d. hypothermia

16–3. What physiological process is associated with closure of the ductus arteriosus?

    a. increased systemic blood pressure
    b. decreased systemic blood pressure
    c. increased pulmonary arterial pressure
    d. decreased pulmonary arterial pressure

16–4. What causes respiratory distress syndrome?

    a. increased lung fluid
    b. decreased lung fluid
    c. lack of surfactant
    d. increased surfactant

16–5. Which of the following stimulates newborn respiration?

    a. O_2 accumulation and CO_2 accumulation
    b. O_2 accumulation and CO_2 deprivation
    c. O_2 deprivation and CO_2 deprivation
    d. O_2 deprivation and CO_2 accumulation

16–6. A low 1-min Apgar score helps identify which of the following?

    a. infant who needs special attention
    b. infant with birth asphyxia
    c. infant destined to develop neurological problems
    d. normal infant

16–7. What is the Apgar score of a male infant at 5 min of life whose respiratory effort is irregular, pulse is 90, who is floppy and blue and with only minimal grimaces?

    a. 1
    b. 3
    c. 5
    d. 7

16–8. Which of the following is NOT part of the Apgar score?

    a. heart rate
    b. respiratory effort
    c. color
    d. amniotic fluid consistency

16–9. What does the change in 1-min to 5-min Apgar scores represent?

    a. likelihood of cerebral palsy
    b. index of effectiveness of resuscitation
    c. early neonatal maturity
    d. incidence of birth asphyxia

16–10. What is the risk of cerebral palsy in an infant with a 5-min Apgar score less than or equal to 3?

    a. no increased risk
    b. 1%
    c. 3%
    d. 10%

16–11. What percentage of children with cerebral palsy had normal Apgar scores?

    a. 10
    b. 25
    c. 50
    d. 75

16–12. Which of the following is NOT a criterion for intrapartum hypoxia associated with cerebral palsy?

    a. Apgar <3 at 10 min
    b. seizures
    c. hypotonia
    d. respiratory acidemia

16–13. Which of the following neurological deficits is most clearly related to perinatal asphyxia?

    a. mental retardation
    b. epilepsy
    c. hypotonia
    d. cerebral palsy

16–14. How is neonatal acidemia defined?

    a. pH 6.94 to 7.00
    b. pH 7.04 to 7.10
    c. pH 7.14 to 7.20
    d. pH 7.24 to 7.30

16–15. What pH is considered clinically significant for fetal acidemia?

    a. pH <7.20
    b. pH <7.15
    c. pH <7.10
    d. pH <7.0

16–16. Which umbilical artery blood gas represents the mean expected in a normal term infant?

    a. pH 7.35, pCO_2 49 mm Hg, HCO_3 10 mEq/L
    b. pH 7.35, pCO_2 49 mm Hg, HCO_3 23 mEq/L
    c. pH 7.28, pCO_2 49 mm Hg, HCO_3 10 mEq/L
    d. pH 7.28, pCO_2 49 mm Hg, HCO_3 23 mEq/L

16–17. Which of the following represents the mean umbilical vein blood gas analysis in a normal term infant?

    a. pH 7.35, pCO_2 49 mm Hg, HCO_3 10 mEq/L
    b. pH 7.35, pCO_2 40 mm Hg, HCO_3 21 mEq/L
    c. pH 7.28, pCO_2 49 mm Hg, HCO_3 10 mEq/L
    d. pH 7.28, pCO_2 40 mm Hg, HCO_3 21 mEq/L

16–18. A blood gas analysis result of Ua pH 7.1; pCO_2 65 mm Hg; HCO_3 24 mEq/L corresponds to which acidosis type?

    a. metabolic
    b. mixed
    c. respiratory
    d. normal

16–19. A blood gas analysis result of Ua pH 7.1; pCO_2 65 mm Hg; HCO_3 14 mEq/L corresponds to which acidosis type?

    a. metabolic
    b. mixed
    c. respiratory
    d. normal

16–20. A blood gas analysis result of Ua pH 7.1; pCO_2 49 mm Hg; HCO_3 10 mEq/L corresponds to which acidosis type?

    a. metabolic
    b. mixed
    c. respiratory
    d. normal

16–21. By how much will the pH be lowered if the pCO_2 is increased by 30 U?

    a. 0.08
    b. 0.16
    c. 0.24
    d. 0.32

16–22. Which of the following is NOT part of neonatal resuscitation?

    a. prevent heat loss
    b. open airway
    c. positive pressure ventilation if needed
    d. oxygen for peripheral cyanosis

16–23. What is the pressure needed to effectively deliver O_2 via a face mask to a newborn?

    a. 1 to 5 cm H_2O
    b. 10 to 20 cm H_2O
    c. 25 to 35 cm H_2O
    d. 50 to 60 cm H_2O

16–24. In a male neonate, all EXCEPT which of the following are important in assessing gestational age?

    a. testes
    b. breasts
    c. ear lobes
    d. fingernails

16–25. All EXCEPT which of the following are currently acceptable recommendations from the Centers for Disease Control and Prevention for prevention of neonatal *Neisseria gonorrhoeae?*

    a. aqueous silver nitrate (1%)
    b. erythromycin ointment (0.5%)
    c. azithromycin ointment (0.25%)
    d. tetracycline ophthalmic ointment (1%)

16–26. Which of the following is effective prophylaxis against chlamydial conjunctivitis in the newborn?

    a. 1% silver nitrate
    b. 2.5% povidone-iodine solution
    c. 0.5% erythromycin ointment
    d. none of the above

16–27. Which of the following will NOT be prevented by circumcision?

   a. phimosis
   b. epiphimosis
   c. paraphimosis
   d. balanoposthitis

16–28. What is the ideal recommended analgesia for neonatal circumcision?

   a. dorsal penile nerve block
   b. local analgesic infiltration
   c. ring block
   d. general anesthesia

17

The Puerperium

17–1. What is the anterior uterine wall thickness immediately after expulsion of the placenta?

   a. <1 cm
   b. 2 to 3 cm
   c. 4 to 5 cm
   d. 8 cm

17–2. How many weeks does it take the uterus to return to its nonpregnant size postpartum?

   a. 2
   b. 4
   c. 6
   d. 12

17–3. When does the lochia become lochia serosa?

   a. 1 to 2 days
   b. 3 to 4 days
   c. 7 to 8 days
   d. >10 days

17–4. What is the order of the stages of lochia (beginning with early postpartum)?

   a. lochia rubra, lochia alba, lochia serosa
   b. lochia rubra, lochia serosa, lochia alba
   c. lochia serosa, lochia alba, lochia rubra
   d. lochia alba, lochia serosa, lochia rubra

17–5. By what week postpartum is the endometrium restored?

   a. 1
   b. 2

   c. 3
   d. 4

17–6. How long (weeks) does it take for complete extrusion of the placental bed?

   a. 2
   b. 4
   c. 6
   d. 12

17–7. Placental site exfoliation is brought about by what process?

   a. hypertrophic repair
   b. decrease in myometrial cell size
   c. proliferation of new endometrial glands
   d. necrotic sloughing

17–8. Which of the following are characteristics of the puerperal bladder?

   a. underdistension; complete emptying
   b. underdistension; incomplete emptying
   c. overdistension; complete emptying
   d. overdistension; incomplete emptying

17–9. Which is NOT associated with postpartum stress urinary incontinence?

   a. prolonged second stage
   b. size of infant's head
   c. episiotomy
   d. cesarean delivery

17–10. At what time in the puerperium do the renal pelves and ureters return to prepregnant size?

    a. 1 day
    b. 5 days
    c. 10 days
    d. 2 to 8 weeks

17–11. Most women return to their prepregnancy weight by what month postpartum?

    a. second
    b. third
    c. fourth
    d. sixth

17–12. What breast cell type synthesizes milk?

    a. secretory epithelium
    b. mucous epithelium
    c. myoepithelium
    d. glandular cell

17–13. During thelarche, which hormone stimulates development of the alveoli?

    a. estrogen
    b. cortisol
    c. progesterone
    d. growth hormone

17–14. Compared to breast milk, colostrum contains more of which of the following?

    a. fat
    b. minerals
    c. sugar
    d. immunoglobulin M

17–15. How much human milk is made per day by a nursing mother?

    a. 200 mL
    b. 400 mL
    c. 600 mL
    d. 800 mL

17–16. Which of the following factors has NOT been identified in breast milk?

    a. interleukin-6
    b. prolactin
    c. epidermal growth factor
    d. somatostatin

17–17. Which vitamin is NOT found in breast milk?

    a. B
    b. C
    c. D
    d. K

17–18. Which hormone is responsible for causing contractions in myoepithelial cells?

    a. oxytocin
    b. prolactin
    c. progesterone
    d. placental lactogen

17–19. Which of the following is a direct benefit of breastfeeding to the newborn?

    a. increase in protein
    b. increase in vitamin D
    c. decrease in enteric infection
    d. decrease in fat content

17–20. What are the effects of oral contraceptives on lactation?

    a. block milk secretion
    b. decrease the volume of milk produced
    c. inhibit milk release
    d. block secretion of oxytocin

17–21. Which of the following maternal infections is NOT a relative contraindication to breastfeeding?

    a. cytomegalovirus
    b. chronic hepatitis B
    c. human immunodeficiency virus infection
    d. herpes simplex infection of the cervix

17–22. What is the frequency of human immunodeficiency virus transmission via breast milk?

    a. 4%
    b. 8%
    c. 16%
    d. 32%

17–23. Which of the following psychiatric medications is contraindicated during breastfeeding?

    a. lithium
    b. sertraline
    c. nefazodone
    d. bupropion

17–24 Which of the following drugs is concentrated in human milk?

    a. bromocriptine
    b. cocaine
    c. doxorubicin
    d. lithium

17–25. Fever owing to breast engorgement is self-limited and generally, at the most, lasts how long?

    a. 4 to 16 hr
    b. 24 hr
    c. 48 hr
    d. 72 hr

17–26. Approximately what percentage of postpartum women will manifest transient fever from breast engorgement?

    a. <1
    b. 15
    c. 25
    d. 35

17–27. Approximately what percentage of women with mastitis will develop a breast abscess?

    a. <1
    b. 5
    c. 10
    d. 20

17–28. What is the most common etiologic agent for mastitis?

    a. *Staphylococcus aureus*
    b. *Staphylococcus epidermitis*
    c. enterococci
    d. group A streptococci

17–29. What is the treatment of choice for a postpartum breast abscess?

    a. vancomycin
    b. doxycycline
    c. drainage
    d. erythromycin

17–30. Which of the following is recommended to minimize episiotomy discomfort immediately postpartum?

    a. codeine 30 mg every 8 hr
    b. morphine 10 mg every 2 hr
    c. aspirin 600 mg every 8 hr
    d. ice packs to perineum

17–31. Which of the following is prominent in the genesis of "postpartum blues"?

    a. emotional letdown following the excitement of pregnancy
    b. the discomforts of the early puerperium
    c. lack of rest obtained during the hospital stay
    d. all of the above

17–32. Which of the following immunizations should NOT be given postpartum?

    a. diphtheria-tetanus
    b. anti-D immune globulin
    c. hepatitis B
    d. no restrictions for any that are indicated

17–33. At what point postpartum (weeks) does menstruation normally return in a nonbreastfeeding woman?

    a. 1 to 2
    b. 3 to 4
    c. 6 to 8
    d. 12 or later

18

Dystocia: Abnormal Labor and Fetopelvic Disproportion

18–1. What percentage of women with a prior history of cephalopelvic disproportion subsequently delivery vaginally?

   a. 10
   b. 30
   c. 50
   d. 70

18–2. What is the most common reason for primary cesarean section?

   a. malpresentation
   b. placental abruption
   c. prematurity
   d. dystocia

18–3. According to the American College of Obstetricians and Gynecologists, what is the minimum cervical dilation required before the diagnosis of dystocia can be made?

   a. 2 cm
   b. 3 cm
   c. 4 cm
   d. 5 cm

18–4. In order, what are the cardinal fetal movements of labor?

   a. descent, flexion, internal rotation, extension
   b. flexion, descent, internal rotation, extension
   c. descent, flexion, extension, internal rotation
   d. flexion, descent, extension, internal rotation

18–5. What is active labor?

   a. painless, regular uterine contractions
   b. progressive cervical dilatation and effacement

   c. painful contractions every 2 to 3 min
   d. 3 contractions per 10 min

18–6. Which of the following is characteristic of the preparatory division of labor?

   a. change in cervical connective tissue
   b. irregular contractions
   c. marked cervical dilatation
   d. rupture of membranes

18–7. According to Friedman, what are the phases of cervical dilatation?

   a. preparatory, active
   b. preparatory, latent
   c. latent, active
   d. active, pelvic

18–8. In a primigravida, what is the minimum normal rate of dilation of the cervix in the active phase of labor?

   a. 0.5 cm/hr
   b. 1.2 cm/hr
   c. 1.5 cm/hr
   d. 2.0 cm/hr

18–9. According to Friedman, what is prolongation of the latent phase of labor in a primigravida?

   a. >14 hr
   b. >20 hr
   c. >24 hr
   d. >48 hr

18–10. In the parous woman, how is the prolonged latent phase defined?

    a. >6 hr
    b. >14 hr
    c. >20 hr
    d. >24 hr

18–11. Which factor likely contributes to the prolongation of the latent phase?

    a. excessive sedation
    b. conduction analgesia
    c. uneffaced and undilated cervix
    d. all of the above

18–12. According to Rosen (1990), the active phase of labor begins at what dilatation?

    a. 3 cm
    b. 4 cm
    c. 5 cm
    d. 3 cm, if completely effaced

18–13. What is the mean duration of active phase labor in nulliparous women?

    a. <3 hr
    b. 4 to 5 hr
    c. 6 to 8 hr
    d. ~12 hr

18–14. In a multiparous woman, secondary arrest of dilatation is defined as no cervical dilatation for how long?

    a. >1 hr
    b. >2 hr
    c. >3 hr
    d. >14 hr

18–15. What is the median duration of second-stage labor in nulliparas and multiparas, respectively?

    a. 2 hr, 1 hr
    b. 2 hr, 30 min
    c. 50 min, 50 min
    d. 50 min, 20 min

18–16. Ninety-five percent of women admitted to a hospital in active labor will deliver spontaneously within how many hours?

    a. 4
    b. 6
    c. 10
    d. 14

18–17. Where in the myometrium do uterine contractions of normal labor begin?

    a. laterally in the cornual region
    b. lower uterine segment

    c. cervix
    d. fundus

18–18. What amplitude of a uterine contraction is generally necessary to effect cervical dilatation?

    a. 5 mm Hg
    b. 15 mm Hg
    c. 25 mm Hg
    d. 50 mm Hg

18–19. What is the preferred treatment for a nulliparous patient with prolonged deceleration phase and no signs of cephalopelvic disproportion?

    a. sedation
    b. oxytocin augmentation
    c. cesarean delivery
    d. increased hydration

18–20. What is the anteroposterior diameter in the presence of pelvic inlet contracture?

    a. <8 cm
    b. <9 cm
    c. <10 cm
    d. <12 cm

18–21. In a woman with a contracted pelvic inlet, what is the diagonal conjugate generally less than?

    a. 9.5 cm
    b. 10.5 cm
    c. 11.5 cm
    d. 12.5 cm

18–22. What is the average biparietal diameter of term infants?

    a. 8.5 cm
    b. 9.0 cm
    c. 9.5 cm
    d. >10.0 cm

18–23. What is the incidence of shoulder presentation in women who have a contracted pelvic inlet compared to those whose pelves are normal?

    a. 2 times more frequent
    b. 3 times more frequent
    c. 4 times more frequent
    d. 6 times more frequent

18–24. What is the average interspinous measurement?

    a. 8.0 cm
    b. 9.0 cm
    c. 10.0 cm
    d. 10.5 cm

18–25. What is the average posterior sagittal diameter?

   a. 4 cm
   b. 5 cm
   c. 6 cm
   d. 8 cm

18–26. The midpelvis is likely to be contracted if the sum of the interischial spinous and the posterior sagittal diameter is less or equal to which of the following?

   a. 9.5 cm
   b. 11.5 cm
   c. 12.5 cm
   d. 13.5 cm

18–27. Which of the following factors is amenable to radiographic measurement (x-ray)?

   a. fetal head size
   b. moldability of the fetal head
   c. size of bony pelvis
   d. amount of amniotic fluid

18–28. What is the mean gonadal exposure to the fetus with conventional x-ray pelvimetry?

   a. ~0.001 Gy
   b. ~0.01 Gy
   c. ~0.1 Gy
   d. ~1.0 Gy

18–29. What is a typical fetal dose with computed tomograms?

   a. ~0.0003 Gy
   b. ~0.003 Gy
   c. ~0.03 Gy
   d. ~0.3 Gy

18–30. Which of the following is the most important predictor of neonatal infection in term women with spontaneous rupture of membranes?

   a. length of labor
   b. colonization with group B streptococcus
   c. use of scalp electrodes
   d. latency period >4 hr

18–31. How are Montevideo units calculated?

   a. number of contractions in 10 min × peak amplitude
   b. number of contractions in 20 min × peak amplitude

   c. number of contractions in 30 min × peak amplitude
   d. add the peak amplitude minus the baseline, for each contraction in a 10-min period

18–32. According to American College of Obstetricians and Gynecologists guidelines, when is failure to progress diagnosed?

   a. The active phase of labor exceeds 8 hr.
   b. Montevideo units exceed 200 for 2 hr without cervical change.
   c. There is no cervical change in 2 hr regardless of contraction strength.
   d. The latent phase of labor exceeds 20 hr.

18–33. Rouse and colleagues (1999) suggest that at least how many hours without cervical change are necessary to diagnosis active-phase arrest?

   a. 2
   b. 4
   c. 6
   d. 8

18–34. In a nulliparous woman, how long is a prolonged deceleration phase?

   a. >1 hr
   b. >2 hr
   c. >3 hr
   d. >20 hr

18–35. Which of the following is the LEAST likely to contribute to fetal head molding?

   a. multiparity
   b. oxytocin labor stimulation
   c. vacuum extractor delivery
   d. prolonged labor

18–36. Which of the following is NOT associated with precipitate labor and delivery?

   a. amnionic fluid embolism
   b. intrapartum hemorrhage
   c. increased perinatal mortality and morbidity
   d. chorioamnionitis

18–37. Which of the following is a common postpartum complication of precipitous labor?

   a. hemorrhage
   b. endometritis
   c. mastitis
   d. milk fever

19

Dystocia: Abnormal Presentation, Position, and Development of the Fetus

19–1. What is the approximate incidence of breech presentation at term?

  a. 0.5%
  b. 3.0%
  c. 7.0%
  d. 12.0%

19–2. What is the presenting part with a face presentation?

  a. sinciput
  b. malar eminence
  c. mentum
  d. occiput

19–3. What is the overall incidence of face presentation?

  a. 0.02%
  b. 0.2%
  c. 2.0%
  d. 5.0%

19–4. Which of the following is associated etiologically with a face presentation?

  a. contracted pelvic inlet
  b. oxytocin induction
  c. small for gestational age infant
  d. tight abdominal musculature

19–5. Approximately what percentage of face presentations are associated with inlet contraction?

  a. 5
  b. 20
  c. 40
  d. 65

19–6. In labor, if the presenting part is the sagittal suture midway between the orbital ridge and the anterior fontanelle, what is the presentation?

  a. face
  b. brow
  c. occiput
  d. left occiput anterior

19–7. In which situation is the brow presentation likely to delivery vaginally?

  a. small fetus, large pelvis
  b. small fetus, small pelvis
  c. large fetus, large pelvis
  d. large fetus, small pelvis

19–8. What bony landmark determines the designation of lie in shoulder presentations?

  a. acromion
  b. brow
  c. breech
  d. occiput

19–9. What is the incidence of transverse lie at term?

  a. 0.003%
  b. 0.03%
  c. 0.3%
  d. 3.0%

19–10. Which of the following is a common cause of transverse lie?

  a. placental abruption
  b. normal uterus
  c. postterm pregnancy
  d. contracted pelvis

19–11. What is the best way to deliver a term transverse lie in labor with ruptured membranes?

  a. low transverse cesarean section
  b. vertical cesarean section
  c. version to vertex and vaginal delivery
  d. version to breech and vaginal delivery

19–12. How often is compound presentation identified?

  a. 1 in 400
  b. 1 in 800
  c. 1 in 1000
  d. 1 in 2000

19–13. Which of the following characterizes the incidence of occiput posterior positions in early term labor compared to at delivery?

  a. no change
  b. decreased
  c. markedly decreased
  d. increased

19–14. In the multiparous woman delivering a fetus with an occiput posterior position, labor is prolonged by approximately how long, compared to an occiput anterior position?

  a. 30 min
  b. 1 hr
  c. 2 hr
  d. 4 hr

19–15. During the last decade, what has happened to the incidence of shoulder dystocia?

  a. markedly decreased
  b. decreased slightly
  c. increased slightly
  d. not changed

19–16. What is the mean head-to-body delivery time in deliveries complicated by shoulder dystocia?

  a. ~40 sec
  b. ~60 sec
  c. ~80 sec
  d. ~100 sec

19–17. Which of the following is a maternal risk factor for shoulder dystocia?

  a. nulliparity
  b. obesity
  c. class F diabetes
  d. chronic hypertension

19–18. In which of the following circumstances should a primary cesarean delivery be performed to prevent shoulder dystocia (American College of Obstetricians and Gynecologists guidelines)?

  a. term labor, estimated fetal weight (EFW) 4000 g by Leopold's maneuver
  b. term labor, EFW 4180 g by ultrasound
  c. diabetic (gestational), term, EFW 4200 g by ultrasound
  d. diabetic (gestational), term, EFW 4600 g by ultrasound

19–19. Which of the following is NOT part of the management of shoulder dystocia?

  a. Woods corkscrew maneuver
  b. fundal pressure
  c. McRoberts maneuver
  d. delivery of posterior shoulder

19–20. Of the following methods used for delivery of shoulder dystocia, which is associated with the highest incidence of orthopedic and neurological damage?

  a. suprapubic pressure
  b. McRoberts maneuver
  c. Hibbard maneuver
  d. Woods corkscrew maneuver

20

Induction and Augmentation of Labor

20–1. How many births are there a year in the United States?

    a. 1 million
    b. 2 million
    c. 4 million
    d. 8 million

20–2. Which of the following are increased in nulliparas undergoing elective induction of labor?

    a. preterm infants
    b. endometritis
    c. chorioamnionitis
    d. cesarean births

20–3. Which of the following is most likely to have a successful induction of labor?

    a. primiparous; cervix 1 cm/80% effaced/0 station
    b. primiparous; cervix 2 cm/20% effaced/−1 station
    c. multiparous; cervix 2 cm/80% effaced/−1 station
    d. multiparous; cervix 1 cm/20% effaced/0 station

20–4. Contraindications to induction of labor include all EXCEPT which of the following?

    a. macrosomia
    b. prior classical cesarean birth
    c. placenta previa
    d. fetal renal anomaly

20–5. Which of the following is NOT a component of the Bishop score?

    a. parity
    b. dilation
    c. effacement
    d. station

20–6. What has prostaglandin E_2 (PGE_2) for cervical ripening been shown to do?

    a. increase the chance of successful labor induction
    b. reduce the amount of oxytocin needed
    c. decrease the incidence of prolonged labor
    d. all of the above

20–7. When using PGE_2 for cervical ripening, what percentage of women enter labor?

    a. 10
    b. 25
    c. 50
    d. 75

20–8. What is the Bishop score cutoff for an unfavorable cervix?

    a. ≤2
    b. ≤4
    c. ≤6
    d. ≤8

20–9. What is the minimum safe time interval after PGE_2 administration and initiation of oxytocin?

    a. not yet established
    b. 30 min
    c. 2 hr
    d. 8 hr

20–10. What is the minimum number of uterine contractions in 10 min to be considered hyperstimulation?

    a. 4 or more
    b. 5 or more
    c. 6 or more
    d. 7 or more

20–11. For what purpose has the Food and Drug Administration approved misoprostol?

    a. cervical ripening
    b. labor induction
    c. gastroesophageal reflux
    d. peptic ulcers

20–12. What is the dose of misoprostol that the American College of Obstetricians and Gynecologists (ACOG) recommends be used for cervical ripening?

    a. 25 μg
    b. 50 μg
    c. 100 μg
    d. 200 μg

20–13. In which of the following ways is balloon catheter cervical ripening superior to intracervical PGE_2 gel?

    a. decreases cesarean births
    b. lowers Bishop score after treatment
    c. decreases randomization-to-delivery time
    d. no difference

20–14. What proportion of women who undergo membrane stripping at term gestation enter labor spontaneously within 72 hr?

    a. one-half
    b. one-third
    c. one-fourth
    d. two-thirds

20–15. In what year was oxytocin first synthesized?

    a. 1920
    b. 1931
    c. 1942
    d. 1953

20–16. What is the mean half-life of oxytocin?

    a. 5 min
    b. 10 min
    c. 20 min
    d. 30 min

20–17. How long does it take oxytocin to reach steady-state levels in the plasma?

    a. 5 min
    b. 10 min
    c. 20 min
    d. 40 min

20–18. At what dose of oxytocin is renal free water clearance decreased?

    a. 10 mU/min
    b. 20 mU/min
    c. 40 mU/min
    d. 60 mU/min

20–19. How are Montevideo units calculated?

    a. number of contractions in 10 min × peak amplitude
    b. number of contractions in 20 min × peak amplitude
    c. number of contractions in 30 min × peak amplitude
    d. add the peak amplitude minus the baseline for each contraction in a 10-min period

20–20. What is the mean spontaneous uterine contraction pattern resulting in vaginal delivery?

    a. 100 to 120 Montevideo units
    b. 140 to 150 Montevideo units
    c. 180 to 190 Montevideo units
    d. 220 to 230 Montevideo units

20–21. According to the ACOG guidelines, when is failure to progress diagnosed?

    a. The latent phase of labor has been completed.
    b. Montevideo units exceed 200 for 2 hr.
    c. There is no cervical change in 2 hr.
    d. The latent phase of labor exceeds 20 hr.

20–22. At what cervical dilatation is spontaneous rupture of the membranes likely to occur?

    a. 4 cm
    b. 6 cm
    c. 8 cm
    d. complete

VI SECTION

Operative Obstetrics

21

Forceps Delivery and Vacuum Extraction

21–1. Which of the following is NOT a basic component of a forceps branch?

    a. blade
    b. handle
    c. lock
    d. stem

21–2. Which of the following forceps have crossing shanks?

    a. Tucker-McLane
    b. Simpson
    c. Kielland
    d. Barton

21–3. Which forceps has a sliding lock?

    a. Tucker-McLane
    b. Simpson
    c. Kielland
    d. Piper

21–4. When forceps are applied to the fetal head in which the scalp is visible at the introitus without manual separation of the labia, what type of delivery occurs?

    a. outlet forceps
    b. low forceps
    c. midforceps
    d. either outlet or low

21–5. What is the classification for any forceps rotation at a station of +2 cm or greater?

    a. outlet forceps
    b. low forceps

    c. midforceps
    d. high forceps

21–6. When the fetal head is engaged and at a +1 cm station, how would a forceps delivery be classified?

    a. outlet forceps
    b. low forceps
    c. midforceps
    d. high forceps

21–7. Forceps applied when fetal head (left occiput anterior position) has reached the pelvic floor and is at the perineum should be classified as what type of delivery?

    a. outlet forceps
    b. low forceps
    c. midforceps
    d. high forceps

21–8. What is the incidence of operative vaginal delivery?

    a. 1 to 2%
    b. 4 to 6%
    c. 10 to 12%
    d. ~20%

21–9. Which of the following is NOT associated with regional analgesia?

    a. increased frequency of instrumental deliveries
    b. prolonged second stage of labor
    c. increased frequency of occiput posterior positions
    d. decreased frequency of rotational forceps deliveries

21–10. Which of the following forceps is best suited for low-forceps delivery of a fetus with a molded head?

    a. Simpson
    b. Tucker-McLane
    c. Kielland
    d. Chamberlain

21–11. Which of the following forceps is best suited for low-forceps delivery of a fetus with a rounded head?

    a. Simpson
    b. Tucker-McLane
    c. Kielland
    d. Chamberlain

21–12. The fetal skull may be damaged if pull of the forceps exceeds which of the following forces?

    a. 5 kg
    b. 15 kg
    c. 30 kg
    d. 60 kg

21–13. Which of the following maternal conditions is NOT an indication for termination of labor by forceps?

    a. heart disease
    b. acute pulmonary edema
    c. intrapartum infection
    d. second stage of labor of $1\frac{1}{2}$ hr in nullipara

21–14. Which of the following is a fetal indication for termination of labor by forceps?

    a. prolapse of umbilical cord
    b. meconium-stained amnionic fluid
    c. placenta previa
    d. reactive fetal heart rate pattern

21–15. When exceeded, which of the following is considered a prolonged second stage of labor for the nulliparous patient?

    a. 1 hr without regional anesthesia
    b. 1 hr with regional anesthesia
    c. 2 hr without regional anesthesia
    d. 2 hr with regional anesthesia

21–16. When exceeded, which of the following is the most correct definition of a prolonged second stage in the parous patient?

    a. 1 hr without regional anesthesia
    b. 1 hr with regional anesthesia
    c. 2 hr without regional anesthesia
    d. 2 hr with regional anesthesia

21–17. Forceps should generally NOT be used electively until the fetal head has reached what station?

    a. 0 to +1 station
    b. +2 to +3 station
    c. the perineal floor
    d. at least at 0 station and OA position

21–18. With regard to the use of prophylactic forceps, which of the following statements is correct?

    a. They will prevent episiotomy extension.
    b. They will reduce the incidence of fetal brain damage from prolonged perineal pressure.
    c. They are associated with improved neonatal outcome in low-birthweight infants.
    d. There is no current evidence that they are beneficial in otherwise normal labor and delivery.

21–19. Which of the following is NOT a prerequisite for forceps application?

    a. Head must be engaged.
    b. Fetus must present either by the vertex or by the face with the chin posterior.
    c. Cervix must be completely dilated.
    d. Membranes must be ruptured.

21–20. Which of the following analgesia or anesthesia techniques is least adequate for low-forceps or midpelvic procedures?

    a. pudendal block
    b. spinal block
    c. epidural block
    d. ketamine

21–21. Regarding traction with forceps, which of the following statements is NOT correct?

    a. Gentle traction should be intermittent.
    b. The fetal head should be allowed to recede in intervals.
    c. Delivery should be deliberate and slow.
    d. Traction should be applied between contractions.

21–22. Which of the following pelvic architecture is most likely to be associated with occiput transverse positions?

    a. gynecoid
    b. platypelloid
    c. anthropoid
    d. gynecoid-anthropoid combination

21–23. When rotating the fetal head from posterior positions to anterior positions, it is NOT necessary to flex the head when using which of the forceps below?

 a. Simpson
 b. Tucker-McLane
 c. Simpson-Luikart
 d. Kielland

21–24. Which of the following is the most common maternal complication associated with Kielland forceps delivery?

 a. postpartum hemorrhage
 b. proctoepisiotomy lacerations
 c. chorioamnionitis
 d. manual removal of the placenta

21–25. Which of the following neonatal morbidities is NOT related to Kielland forceps deliveries?

 a. fractured skull
 b. sepsis
 c. nerve palsies
 d. cephalohematomas

21–26. In which of the following are forceps contraindicated?

 a. mentum anterior
 b. mentum posterior
 c. right occiput transverse
 d. left occiput transverse

21–27. In which of the following types of delivery is maternal blood transfusion most likely to be needed?

 a. cesarean delivery
 b. spontaneous vaginal delivery
 c. forceps-assisted delivery
 d. vacuum extraction

21–28. According to Sultan and associates (1993), which of the following is increased significantly in women who undergo a forceps delivery compared to those who had spontaneous vaginal delivery?

 a. bladder neck defects
 b. chorioamnionitis
 c. anal sphincter defects
 d. none of the above, all are equal

21–29. Which of the following is NOT a theoretical advantage of the vacuum extractor over forceps?

 a. not as much vaginal space required
 b. ability to rotate the fetal head without impinging upon maternal soft tissues
 c. less intracranial pressure during traction
 d. can be applied at higher stations than forceps

21–30. What is a chignon?

 a. an artificial caput
 b. a scalp hematoma
 c. an abrasion caused by the metal vacuum cup
 d. an abrasion caused by a soft, silastic vacuum cup

21–31. Which of the following is a relative contraindication for delivery using vacuum extraction?

 a. face presentation
 b. 35-week gestation
 c. chorioamnionitis
 d. post-term pregnancy

21–32. Which of the following is NOT a direct complication of delivery using the vacuum extraction?

 a. cephalohematoma
 b. intracranial hemorrhage
 c. retinal hemorrhage
 d. newborn acidemia

22

Breech Presentation and Delivery

22–1. What is the approximate incidence of breech presentation at term?

    a. 0.1 to 0.5%
    b. 3.0 to 4.0%
    c. 7.0 to 8.0%
    d. 12.0 to 15.0%

22–2. Which of the following is not a risk factor for breech?

    a. multiple fetuses
    b. hydramnios
    c. uterine anomalies
    d. low parity

22–3. Which of the following is NOT associated with persistent breech presentation?

    a. perinatal morbidity and mortality
    b. macrosomia
    c. prolapsed cord
    d. placenta previa

22–4. Which of the following describes a frank breech presentation?

    a. flexion of the hips and extension of the knees
    b. flexion of the hips and flexion of the knees
    c. extension of the hips and flexion of the knees
    d. extension of the hips and extension of the knees

22–5. Which of the following best describes the incomplete breech presentation?

    a. lower extremities flexed at the hips and extended at knees
    b. lower extremities flexed at the hips and one or both knees flexed
    c. one or both hips not flexed or both feet or knees below breech
    d. both feet are in the right fundal area

22–6. Which of the following best describes a complete breech presentation?

    a. lower extremities flexed at the hips and extended at knees
    b. lower extremities flexed at the hips and one or both knees flexed
    c. one or both hips not flexed or both feet or knees below breech
    d. a foot is in the birth canal

22–7. When examining a woman at term, hearing fetal heart tones loudest above the umbilicus suggests which type of presentation?

    a. cephalic presentation
    b. transverse lie
    c. breech presentation
    d. multiple pregnancy

22–8. Cerebral palsy in a breech presenting fetus is more likely related to which of the following delivery events?

    a. vaginal breech delivery
    b. Piper forceps to aftercoming fetal head
    c. cesarean section
    d. not related to mode of delivery

22–9. What percentage of breech deliveries will be complicated by nuchal arm?

    a. <1
    b. 3
    c. 6
    d. 10

22–10. Which of the following pelvis type(s) are favorable configurations for breech vaginal deliveries?

    a. gyneoid
    b. anthropoid
    c. android
    d. a and b

22–11. Approximately what percentage of breech presentations at term will be associated with an extreme hyperextension of the fetal head?

    a. 0.5
    b. 5
    c. 15
    d. 25

22–12. What is the position of the biotrochanteric diameter during engagement and descent of the breech?

    a. oblique
    b. transverse
    c. anterior posterior diameter
    d. a and then c

22–13. Which of the following characterizes partial breech extraction?

    a. infant expelled entirely to shoulder
    b. infant spontaneously delivers to umbilicus
    c. infant buttocks deliver spontaneously
    d. infant is extracted by the attendant

22–14. During early labor in a breech presentation the fetal heart rate should be evaluated how often?

    a. every 5 min
    b. every 15 min
    c. every 30 min
    d. continuously

22–15. How should traction in a breech extraction be employed?

    a. parallel to the floor
    b. 30-degree angle toward the ceiling
    c. gentle and downward
    d. marked downward pull until the axilla are visible

22–16. What is the maneuver that involves intrauterine manipulation of a frank breech to a footling breech?

    a. Prague
    b. Pinard
    c. Bracht
    d. Lemille

22–17. In which maneuver are the index and middle finger applied over the maxilla in order to free the head?

    a. Pinard
    b. Bracht
    c. Mauriceau-Smellie-Veit
    d. Zavanelli

22–18. With breech delivery, which maneuver is suggested when there is persistence of the fetal spine directed toward the maternal sacrum?

    a. Prague
    b. Bracht
    c. Pinard
    d. McRoberts

22–19. In which of the maneuvers is the fetal body held against the maternal symphysis?

    a. Mauriceau-Smellie-Veit
    b. Bracht
    c. Pinard
    d. Prague

22–20. What maneuver is employed during a frank breech presentation to deliver the foot into the vagina?

    a. Mauriceau-Smellie-Veit
    b. Bracht
    c. Pinard
    d. Prague

22–21. During a breech delivery, rotation may occur such that the back of the infant is directed toward the maternal vertebral column. If traction occurs, what may happen to the fetal head?

    a. may flex
    b. may assume a military position
    c. may wedge beneath the symphysis
    d. may extend

22–22. Of successful versions, approximately what percentage will be vertex at delivery?

    a. 30
    b. 50
    c. 70
    d. 90

22–23. What is the best position for the operator in completing an assisted breech delivery or applying Piper forceps?

    a. standing
    b. sitting
    c. kneeling on one knee
    d. squatting

22–24. "Abdominal rescue" of a partially delivered breech is similar to which maneuver?

    a. Prague
    b. Zavanelli
    c. Pinard
    d. Bracht

22–25. According to the American College of Obstetricians and Gynecologists, what is the average success rate of external cephalic version for breech presentations late in pregnancy?

    a. 20%
    b. 40%
    c. 60%
    d. 80%

22–26. Universal application of external cephalic version can reduce the cesarean section rate by how much?

    a. 2%
    b. 10%
    c. 25%
    d. 50%

22–27. Which of the following is most strongly associated with failure of external cephalic version?

    a. frank breech
    b. anteriorly located fetal spine
    c. ample amnionic fluid
    d. descent of breech into the pelvis

22–28. A 21-year-old, nulliparous D-negative patient at 36 weeks undergoes an external version for breech presentation. Which of the following should be given?

    a. anti-D immunoglobulin
    b. magnesium sulfate

    c. oxytocin
    d. nifedipine

22–29. External version is accomplished at 38 weeks. Which of the following is not a risk?

    a. placental abruption
    b. uterine rupture
    c. induction of labor
    d. feto-maternal hemorrhage

22–30. Which of the following is NOT associated with a successful external cephalic version?

    a. postterm gestation
    b. large amniotic fluid volume
    c. unengaged fetus
    d. high parity

22–31. What is the cost effectiveness of external cephalic version?

    a. marked decrease based on decreased cesarean section
    b. marked increase due to cost of version
    c. marked decrease in multiparas only
    d. not established

23

Cesarean Delivery and Postpartum Hysterectomy

23–1. What percentage of women have had a prior cesarean delivery?

    a. 5
    b. 10
    c. 20
    d. 30

23–2. What accounted most for the decrease in the United States cesarean birth rate from 1989 to 1996?

    a. increase in vaginal breech deliveries
    b. active management of labor
    c. vaginal birth after cesarean delivery
    d. increase in midforceps deliveries

23–3. What is the most common indication for a primary cesarean delivery in the United States?

a. fetal distress
b. breech presentation
c. dystocia or failure to progress
d. prior cesarean delivery

23–4. In the United States what percentage of fetuses presenting as breech are delivered by cesarean?

a. 25
b. 38
c. 75
d. 83

23–5. What is the incidence of uterine rupture in women with prior classical cesareans?

a. 1 to 3%
b. 4 to 9%
c. 12 to 15%
d. 20 to 25%

23–6. Which of the following is an absolute contraindication to a trial of labor after a previous cesarean delivery?

a. two prior transverse cesarean births
b. oxytocin
c. prior classical cesarean delivery
d. prior dystocia

23–7. What is the likelihood of uterine rupture during trial of labor in women with 2 prior cesarean deliveries (Caughey and associates, 1999)?

a. 0.6%
b. 1.8%
c. 3.7%
d. 5.4%

23–8. What is the expected success rate for vaginal delivery in women with prior cesareans undergoing trial of labor?

a. 30%
b. 50%
c. 70%
d. 90%

23–9. If dystocia diagnosed during the second stage of labor was the indication for prior primary cesarean section, what is the vaginal birth after cesarean success rate?

a. 13%
b. 34%
c. 67%
d. 90%

23–10. What effect will labor induction have on the incidence of uterine rupture in woman with prior cesarean deliveries?

a. decreased
b. the same as spontaneous labor
c. increased
d. unknown since oxytocin is contraindicated in these women

23–11. Which of the following is an advantage of the transverse skin incision?

a. exposure of uterus and appendages
b. easy to extend incision rapidly
c. cosmetics
d. less hematoma formation subfascially

23–12. Which of the following is NOT an advantage of low transverse cesarean deliveries?

a. easier to repair
b. less blood loss
c. fewer problems with adhesions from bowel
d. ability to safely extend incision laterally

23–13. What type of incision divides the rectus muscles with scissors?

a. Maylard
b. Kerr
c. Krönig
d. Frank-Letzko

23–14. What is the least common type of cesarean operation?

a. low vertical
b. Kerr-Munro
c. Krönig
d. classical

23–15. What is a major side effect of oxytocin 10 U intravenously bolus given postpartum?

a. respiratory distress
b. hypertension
c. hypotension
d. seizures

23–16. Which of the following is true when the uterine incision is repaired with vicryl?

a. increased adhesion to bowel
b. increased scar separation
c. less blood loss
d. less infection

23–17. Which of the following is a benefit of not reapproximating the visceral and peritoneal peritoneum?

    a. decreased blood loss
    b. decreased return of bowel function
    c. decreased dehiscence
    d. decreased analgesia postoperatively

23–18. A decrease in which of the following is the major benefit of closing the subcutaneous layer?

    a. blood loss
    b. wound dehiscence
    c. fascial dehiscence
    d. wound infection

23–19. Which of the following is NOT an indication for a classical cesarean incision?

    a. cannot visualize the lower segment
    b. transverse lie
    c. premature breech
    d. term breech (frank)

23–20. What is the incidence of bladder injury at the time of cesarean delivery?

    a. 0.3 per 1000
    b. 0.7 per 1000
    c. 1.4 per 1000
    d. 2.8 per 1000

23–21. What is the average blood loss with an elective cesarean hysterectomy?

    a. 500 mL
    b. 1000 mL
    c. 1500 mL
    d. 3000 mL

23–22. Which of the following prophylactic antibiotics has been shown to decrease postpartum endometritis?

    a. metronidazole
    b. ampicillin
    c. tetracycline
    d. azithromycin

23–23. The cesarean delivery rate in the United States has stabilized at approximately what percentage?

    a. 10
    b. 25
    c. 33
    d. 50

24

Hypertensive Disorders in Pregnancy

24–1. What percentage of pregnancies are complicated by hypertension?

    a. <1
    b. 3 to 4
    c. 6 to 8
    d. 10 to 12

24–2. How is hypertension in pregnancy defined?

    a. blood pressure 160/100 or greater
    b. blood pressure 140/90 or greater
    c. increased systolic pressure by 30 mm Hg
    d. increased diastolic pressure by 15 mm Hg

24–3. Who of the following is MOST likely to develop true preeclampsia?

    a. a 16-year-old primigravida
    b. a 24-year-old gravida 4, para 3
    c. a 25-year-old primigravida
    d. a 35-year-old with essential hypertension

24–4. Which Korotkoff phase sound is used to diagnose pregnancy-induced hypertension?

    a. phase III
    b. phase IV
    c. phase V
    d. phase VI

24–5. What percentage of eclamptic women do not have proteinuria?

    a. 0
    b. 5
    c. 10
    d. 20

24–6. With regard to preeclampsia, proteinuria is defined as how much urinary excretion?

    a. >100 mg/24 hr
    b. >200 mg/24 hr
    c. >300 mg/24 hr
    d. >500 mg/24 hr

24–7. Which of the following is NOT diagnostic of severe preeclampsia?

    a. increased serum creatinine
    b. 1+ proteinuria
    c. thrombocytopenia
    d. elevated liver enzymes

24–8. Which of the following is considered an abnormal 24-hour urinary protein for the diagnosis of severe preeclampsia?

    a. >300 mg/24 hr
    b. >1 gm/24 hr
    c. >2 gm/24 hr
    d. >4 gm/24 hr

24–9. With preeclampsia, what is the significance of severe, right upper-quadrant pain?

    a. cholecystitis
    b. pancreatitis
    c. tension on Glisson's capsule
    d. Teitze syndrome

24–10. When is eclampsia least likely to occur?

   a. antepartum
   b. intrapartum
   c. immediately postpartum
   d. after 48 hr postpartum

24–11. How is the pathophysiology of preeclampsia characterized?

   a. vasodilatation
   b. vasospasm
   c. hemodilution
   d. hypervolemia

24–12. What is the incidence of pregnancy-induced hypertension most commonly cited to be?

   a. <1%
   b. 2 to 3%
   c. 5 to 7%
   d. >10%

24–13. Which of the following is associated with a decrease in hypertensive diseases in pregnancy?

   a. twins
   b. smoking
   c. obesity
   d. age >35

24–14. Which of the following is characteristic in preeclampsia?

   a. Cardiac output is decreased and peripheral resistance decreased.
   b. Cardiac output is decreased and peripheral resistance increased.
   c. Cardiac output is increased and peripheral resistance increased.
   d. As vascular resistance increases, so does cardiac output.

24–15. Which of the following is true concerning blood volume in eclampsia?

   a. similar to the nonpregnant state
   b. similar to the normal pregnant state
   c. lower than the nonpregnant state
   d. increased compared with the normal pregnant state

24–16. In women with preeclampsia, what is the usual cause of acute tubular necrosis?

   a. severe hypertension
   b. fragmentation hemolysis
   c. hemorrhage with inadequate replacement
   d. glomerular capillary endotheliosis

24–17. Which of the following characterizes thrombocytopenia in women with preeclampsia?

   a. platelet activation
   b. platelet consumption
   c. increased platelet production
   d. all of the above

24–18. Which of the following is NOT an abnormal erythrocyte finding in severe pregnancy-induced hypertension?

   a. discocytes
   b. schizocytes
   c. reticulocytosis
   d. echinocytes

24–19. Which of the following is relatively reduced in women with preeclampsia?

   a. renin
   b. angiotensin II
   c. aldosterone
   d. all of the above

24–20. How is the level of aldosterone affected by preeclampsia in pregnant women?

   a. increased
   b. decreased
   c. unchanged from normal pregnancy
   d. at the same level as in nonpregnancy

24–21. What is the effect of atrial natriuretic peptide?

   a. increased cardiac output
   b. increased vasospasm
   c. conservation of sodium
   d. conservation of water

24–22. What happens to renal plasma flow and glomerular filtration rate in preeclampsia?

   a. increase
   b. remain the same
   c. decrease
   d. vary greatly

24–23. Which of the following is the characteristic glomerular lesion of preeclampsia?

   a. endotheliosis
   b. capillary leaks
   c. burst cells
   d. clang cell

24–24. What characterizes hepatic artery resistance in preeclampsia?

   a. absent
   b. decreases
   c. remains the same
   d. increases

24–25. What percentage of women with right upper-quadrant pain have computed tomography scan evidence of hepatic hemorrhage?

   a. 5 to 7
   b. 20 to 25
   c. 50 to 55
   d. 70 to 75

24–26. What percentage of women with eclampsia have cerebral edema?

   a. 1
   b. 10
   c. 30
   d. 50

24–27. Which is true of blindness occurring in conjunction with severe preeclampsia?

   a. likely central in origin
   b. often permanent
   c. usually unilateral
   d. identified in the majority of severe preeclamptics

24–28. What is the mean diameter of the myometrial spiral arterioles in women with preeclampsia?

   a. 50 μm
   b. 100 μm
   c. 200 μm
   d. 500 μm

24–29. What is the mean diameter of the myometrial spiral arterioles in normal pregnant women?

   a. 50 μm
   b. 100 μm
   c. 200 μm
   d. 500 μm

24–30. Which of the following does NOT decrease placental blood flow?

   a. furosemide
   b. apresoline
   c. thiazide diuretics
   d. magnesium sulfate

24–31. Which of the following characterizes normotensive pregnant women?

   a. They are refractory to angiotensin II.
   b. They are sensitive to angiotensin II.
   c. They react to angiotensin II in a way similar to nonpregnant women.
   d. They react to angiotensin II in a way similar to men.

24–32. Which of the following best characterizes the effects of 81 mg of aspirin taken daily?

   a. $\uparrow$thromboxane A$_2$; $\uparrow$prostacyclin; $\uparrow$prostaglandin E$_2$
   b. $\uparrow$thromboxane A$_2$; $\downarrow$prostacyclin; $\uparrow$prostaglandin E$_2$
   c. $\downarrow$thromboxane A$_2$; $\downarrow$prostacyclin; $\downarrow$prostaglandin E$_2$
   d. $\downarrow$thromboxane A$_2$; $\uparrow$prostacyclin; $\downarrow$prostaglandin E$_2$

24–33. Low-dose aspirin given to pregnant women causes which of the following?

   a. decreases thromboxane
   b. increases prostacyclin
   c. increases prostaglandin E$_2$
   d. all of the above

24–34. Which of the following characterizes nitric oxide in severe preeclampsia?

   a. increased production
   b. decreased release
   c. decreased production
   d. no change

24–35. Of the following, which is NOT considered to be a predisposing factor to preeclampsia?

   a. family history of preeclampsia
   b. multiple fetuses
   c. vascular disease
   d. multiparity

24–36. Which of the following has been shown by meta-analysis (not confirmed by randomized trial) to prevent preeclampsia?

   a. salt-restricted diet
   b. calcium supplementation
   c. low-dose aspirin
   d. zinc supplementation

24–37. Which of the following is NOT an indication of severe pregnancy-induced hypertension?

   a. upper abdominal pain
   b. oliguria
   c. creatinine 0.6 mg/dL
   d. fetal growth restriction

24–38. Which of the following are increased in preeclamptic women treated with labetolol?

   a. fetal growth restriction
   b. eclampsia
   c. severe preeclampsia
   d. all of the above

24-39. Which of the following is contraindicated in the treatment of chronic hypertension and pregnancy?

    a. methyldopa
    b. hydralazine
    c. angiotensin-converting enzyme inhibitors
    d. labetolol

24-40. In most women with preeclampsia, proteinuria will resolve within what time frame (days)?

    a. 2
    b. 3
    c. 5
    d. 7

24-41. How long does fetal bradycardia associated with an eclamptic seizure usually last?

    a. 30 sec
    b. 3 to 5 min
    c. 10 min
    d. >20 min

24-42. How is magnesium excreted?

    a. lungs
    b. liver
    c. kidneys
    d. gastrointestinal tract

24-43. What plasma magnesium level most often prevents seizures?

    a. 3 to 4 mEq/L
    b. 4 to 7 mEq/L
    c. 7 to 10 mEq/L
    d. over 10 mEq/L

24-44. At what serum level of magnesium do patellar reflexes disappear?

    a. 6 mEq/L
    b. 8 mEq/L
    c. 10 mEq/L
    d. 12 mEq/L

24-45. How is magnesium toxicity treated?

    a. calcium gluconate 1 g intravenously
    b. calcium gluconate orally
    c. calcium gluconate 1 g intravenously and discontinue magnesium
    d. dialysis

24-46. With a serum creatinine of 1.3 mg/dL, what should the dose of $MgSO_4$ be?

    a. increased
    b. kept the same
    c. reduced by half
    d. discontinued

24-47. What is the initial dose of hydralazine used to treat severe hypertension?

    a. 100 mg orally
    b. 50 mg intramuscularly
    c. 5 to 10 mg intravenous bolus
    d. all can be safely used

24-48. What initial intravenous dose of labetolol is utilized to control severe hypertension?

    a. 5 mg
    b. 10 to 20 mg
    c. 40 to 80 mg
    d. 100 mg

24-49. In severe preeclampsia with pulmonary edema, what immediate treatment should be given?

    a. furosemide intravenously
    b. digoxin
    c. hydrochlorothiazide
    d. fluid restriction

24-50. In nulliparas with preeclampsia-eclampsia, what is the risk of developing chronic hypertension in the future?

    a. less than for the general population
    b. the same as for the general population
    c. double that of the general population
    d. four times that of the general population

24-51. Which of the following is associated with severe preeclampsia?

    a. HLA-DR4 histocompatibility antigen
    b. variant of angiotensinogen gene
    c. factor V Leiden mutation
    d. all of the above

24-52. What is the recurrence rate of HELLP syndrome?

    a. 2%
    b. 5%
    c. 17%
    d. 25%

25

Obstetrical Hemorrhage

25–1. What is the approximate proportion of direct non-abortion-related obstetrical death due to hemorrhage?

    a. 5%
    b. 15%
    c. 30%
    d. 65%

25–2. Which of the following is characteristic of mid-trimester bleeding?

    a. of little consequence
    b. related to early effacement and tearing of small vessels
    c. previa or abruption will be found in 25%
    d. requires hospitalization

25–3. What is the frequency of placental abruption?

    a. 1 in 50
    b. 1 in 100
    c. 1 in 150
    d. 1 in 200

25–4. What is the current incidence of abruption severe enough to kill the fetus?

    a. 1 in 420
    b. 1 in 830
    c. 1 in 1100
    d. 1 in 1550

25–5. What is the overall perinatal mortality rate associated with abruptio placentae?

    a. 5%
    b. 10%
    c. 25%
    d. 50%

25–6. Which of the following is most commonly associated with placental abruption?

    a. trauma
    b. short umbilical cord
    c. folic acid deficiency
    d. hypertension

25–7. Which of the following ethnic groups has the lowest risk (rate) of abruptio placentae?

    a. African Americans
    b. whites
    c. Asians
    d. Latin Americans

25–8. The risk for abruptio placentae is increased by how much in women who smoke?

    a. not increased
    b. twofold
    c. fourfold
    d. eightfold

25–9. What is the relationship between factor V, folate reductase, or prothrombin mutation and abruptio placentae?

    a. significantly increased risk
    b. slightly decreased risk
    c. significantly decreased risk
    d. no association

25–10. What is the approximate risk of recurrent abruption with a subsequent pregnancy?

    a. 4%
    b. 12%
    c. 20%
    d. 33%

25–11. What is the most common presenting sign in women with abruptio placentae?

    a. preterm labor
    b. uterine tenderness
    c. back pain
    d. bleeding

25–12. What percentage of the total pregnant blood volume is lost with an abruption severe enough to cause fetal demise?

   a. 5
   b. 10
   c. 25
   d. 50 or greater

25–13. Which compound is responsible for lysing fibrin?

   a. thromboplastin
   b. plasmin
   c. prostacyclin
   d. factor III

25–14. How can acute tubular necrosis following abruption be prevented?

   a. cryoprecipitate
   b. volume replacement
   c. furosemide
   d. Swan-Ganz catheter

25–15. Which of the following is characteristic of a Couvelaire uterus?

   a. requires hysterectomy
   b. contracts adequately with stimulation
   c. results from excessive oxytocin
   d. requires fibrinogen therapy

25–16. Which of the following is the most ideal method of delivery for severe abruption with fetal demise?

   a. vaginal delivery
   b. immediate cesarean section
   c. cesarean section after blood replacement
   d. cesarean section after 5 U of cryoprecipitate

25–17. What is the baseline intraamniotic pressure with extensive placental abruption?

   a. 0
   b. 5 to 10 mm Hg
   c. 50 mm Hg or more
   d. >100 mm Hg

25–18. What is the incidence of placenta previa at term?

   a. 1 in 50
   b. 1 in 200
   c. 1 in 400
   d. 1 in 800

25–19. Which of the following is LEAST likely to result in a patient having placenta previa?

   a. primiparity
   b. previous cesarean section
   c. multiparity
   d. advanced maternal age

25–20. What is the incidence of previa in a woman with 3 previous cesarean sections?

   a. 0.5%
   b. 1.9%
   c. 3.1%
   d. 4.1%

25–21. What cell type is found along the myometrial spiral arterioles in biopsies from placental beds in pregnancies complicated by previa?

   a. polymorphonuclear
   b. mast
   c. trophoblastic giant
   d. Burneske

25–22. What is the most common characteristic sign or symptom in women with placenta previa?

   a. nonreassuring fetal heart rate
   b. painful bleeding
   c. painless bleeding
   d. coagulopathy

25–23. What is the most common method for diagnosis of placenta previa?

   a. abdominal x-ray
   b. arteriography
   c. sonography
   d. computed tomographic scanning

25–24. Which of the following is the most common cause of postpartum hemorrhage mandating hysterectomy?

   a. previa
   b. atony
   c. irreparable tears
   d. placental accreta

25–25. Late postpartum hemorrhage is defined as occurring how many hours after delivery?

   a. 1 hr
   b. 2 hr
   c. 8 hr
   d. 24 hr

25–26. What is the most common cause of postpartum hemorrhage?

   a. uterine atony
   b. retained placenta
   c. lacerations
   d. chorioamnionitis

25–27. Which of the following is NOT a predisposing factor to postpartum hemorrhage?

    a. prolonged labor
    b. term twins
    c. rapid labor
    d. patient with 1500 g infant

25–28. Bright red bleeding that continues even in the presence of a firmly contracted uterus is most likely due to which of the following?

    a. thrombocytopenia
    b. retained placenta
    c. lacerations
    d. ruptured uterus

25–29. Which of the following is characteristic of Sheehan syndrome?

    a. profuse lactation
    b. amenorrhea
    c. hyperthyroidism
    d. renal insufficiency

25–30. Following delivery of the placenta, which of the following is contraindicated?

    a. methergine 0.2 mg intramuscularly
    b. 20 U of oxytocin in 1000 mL Ringer's lactate solution
    c. 20 U of oxytocin intravenous bolus
    d. uterine massage

25–31. Intravenous bolus oxytocin may cause which of the following?

    a. hypotension and cardiac arrhythmias
    b. hypertension and headache
    c. hypotension and headache
    d. hypertension and cardiac arrhythmias

25–32. Intramuscular prostaglandin (PG) is used to treat hemorrhage due to atony. What is the preferred PG and its dosage?

    a. 15-methyl $F_{2\alpha}$ 1.0 g
    b. 15-methyl $F_{2\alpha}$ 0.25 mg
    c. 15-methyl E_2 1.0 g
    d. 15-methyl E_2 0.25 mg

25–33. When using carboprost, what happens to the PO_2?

    a. rises
    b. decreases
    c. remains unchanged
    d. drops initially then levels off

25–34. Which of the following is characteristic of placenta accreta?

    a. absent decidua basalis
    b. villi invade the myometrium

    c. villi penetrate the myometrium
    d. villi invade the parietal peritoneum

25–35. Which of the following is a microscopic feature of placenta accreta?

    a. cicatrix
    b. imperfect development of Nitabuch layer
    c. hypertrophy of the decidua
    d. trophoblastic proliferation

25–36. A woman with which of the following is LEAST likely to have a placenta accreta?

    a. previous cesarean section
    b. previous metroplasty
    c. four previous curettages
    d. primigravida

25–37. Which of the following is the best management approach to placenta accreta?

    a. cutting the cord and using oxytocin
    b. observation
    c. hysterectomy
    d. hypogastric artery ligation

25–38. What anesthetic agent is most ideal for replacing an inverted uterus?

    a. spinal analgesia
    b. thiopental
    c. succinylcholine
    d. halothane

25–39. What is the incidence of puerperal hematoma?

    a. 1 in 50 to 1 in 100 deliveries
    b. 1 in 300 to 1 in 1000 deliveries
    c. 1 in 1500 to 1 in 2000 deliveries
    d. 1 in 3000 to 1 in 4000 deliveries

25–40. Which artery is most often associated with vulvar hematomas?

    a. uterine
    b. cervical
    c. femoral
    d. pudendal

25–41. What is the most common presenting complaint with vulvar hematomas?

    a. excruciating pain
    b. hemorrhage
    c. constipation
    d. urinary retention

25–42. What is the approximate incidence of spontaneous uterine rupture in an unscarred uterus?

a. 1 in 500
b. 1 in 1,000
c. 1 in 5,000
d. 1 in 15,000

25–43. What is the most common cause of uterine rupture?

a. previous uterine perforation
b. excessive oxytocin
c. manual manipulation
d. separation of a previous cesarean section scar

25–44. What proportion of classical scar ruptures occur before labor?

a. all
b. one-half
c. one-third
d. one-fourth

25–45. What is the incidence of separation of the previous low transverse uterine scar during trial of labor?

a. 1 in 20
b. 1 in 100
c. 1 in 200
d. 1 in 500

25–46. Which of the following is NOT a major risk factor for rupture of the unscarred uterus?

a. oxytocin infusion
b. parity
c. prostaglandin E_2 gel
d. age <15 years

25–47. What is the most common finding in uterine rupture?

a. increased vaginal bleeding
b. sharp shooting pain
c. sudden increase in uterine contraction
d. sudden severe fetal heart rate decelerations

25–48. What is the incidence of fetal mortality in the presence of uterine rupture?

a. 5 to 10%
b. 25 to 30%
c. 50 to 75%
d. >90%

25–49. Where is the ureter located in relation to the ligature in internal iliac artery ligation?

a. superior
b. inferior
c. medial
d. lateral

25–50. What is the important mechanism in the efficacy of internal iliac artery ligation?

a. ischemia
b. reduction in pulse pressure
c. block of collateral circulation
d. all of the above

25–51. The internal iliac artery originates from which of the following arteries?

a. ovarian
b. aorta
c. common iliac
d. external iliac

25–52. What percentage of blood volume is contained in venules?

a. 10
b. 30
c. 50
d. 70

25–53. One hour after an acute blood loss of 1000 mL, which of the following characterizes the hematocrit?

a. no change
b. decreased by 3 vol%
c. decreased by 6 vol%
d. decreased by 12 vol%

25–54. During hemorrhage, at what minimum rate should urine flow be maintained to prevent renal tubular acidosis?

a. 10 cc/hr
b. 30 cc/hr
c. 100 cc/hr
d. 200 cc/hr

25–55. What is the best way to replace fluid loss in hypovolemic shock?

a. crystalloid only
b. crystalloid plus albumin
c. colloid only
d. crystalloid and blood

25–56 At what hemoglobin concentration does cardiac output substantively increase?

a. 5.0 g/dL
b. 7.0 g/dL
c. 8.5 g/dL
d. 14.0 g/dL

25–57. What is the shelf life of whole blood?

a. 20 days
b. 40 days
c. 80 days
d. 120 days

25–58. What will the increase in hematocrit be after 1 U of whole blood?

a. 3 to 4%
b. 6 to 8%
c. 10 to 12%
d. 14 to 16%

25–59. What is the most frequent coagulation defect found in women with blood loss and multiple transfusions?

a. thrombocytopenia
b. prolonged prothrombin time
c. prolonged whole bleeding time
d. AT-III deficiency

25–60. At what fibrinogen level can you expect to see lack of coagulation?

a. 25 mg/dL
b. 50 mg/dL
c. 100 mg/dL
d. 150 mg/dL

25–61. What is the hematocrit in 1 U of packed red cells?

a. 35 vol%
b. 45 to 50 vol%
c. 60 to 70 vol%
d. 80 to 90 vol%

25–62. By how much will the hematocrit increase after 1 U of packed red blood cells?

a. <0.5 vol%
b. 1.0 to 2.0 vol%
c. 3.0 to 5.0 vol%
d. 6.0 to 8.0 vol%

25–63. Which of the following factors is NOT a component of cryoprecipitate?

a. factor VIII:C
b. fetal fibronectin
c. factor VIII: von Willebrand factor
d. fibrinogen

25–64. How much fibrinogen is supplied in cryoprecipitate?

a. 50 mg
b. 100 mg
c. 150 mg
d. 200 mg

25–65. What is the current risk of human immunodeficiency virus infection after 1 U of blood?

a. 1 in 50,000
b. 1 in 150,000
c. 1 in 500,000
d. 1 in 5,000,000

25–66. What is the high estimated risk of post-transfusion hepatitis C?

a. 1 in 3000
b. 1 in 6000
c. 1 in 12,000
d. 1 in 25,000

25–67. What is the most common cause of severe consumptive coagulopathy in pregnancy?

a. fetal death
b. placenta previa
c. placental abruption
d. sepsis

25–68. The activity of which coagulation factor is decreased during normal pregnancy?

a. fibrinogen
b. VII
c. VIII
d. plasmin

25–69. What is mechanical disruption of the erythrocyte membrane within small vessels called?

a. microangiopathic hemolysis
b. ischemia
c. nutritional coagulopathy
d. intravascular coagulation

25–70. Which of the following is NOT characteristic of amniotic fluid embolism?

a. chest pain
b. hypotension
c. hypoxia
d. consumptive coagulopathy

25–71. What is the incidence of amniotic fluid embolism?

a. 1 in 1000
b. 1 in 5000
c. 1 in 10,000
d. 1 in 20,000

25–72. Which of the following is characteristic of the secondary phase of amniotic fluid embolism?

a. pulmonary hypertension
b. decreased systemic vascular resistance
c. decreased left ventricular stroke index
d. lung injury and coagulopathy

25–73. By what mechanism does endotoxin (lipopolysaccharide) activate the extrinsic clotting scheme?

a. cytokine-induced tissue factor expression
b. blocks thrombotic activity
c. increases plasmin activity
d. inhibits thromboplastin

26

Puerperal Infection

26–1. What percentage of maternal deaths are due to infection?

    a. <1
    b. 4 to 6
    c. 10 to 13
    d. 20 to 25

26–2. What is the definition of puerperal morbidity?

    a. temperature of 38.0°C (100.4°F) or greater after day 1
    b. temperature of 38.0°C (100.4°F) or greater on day 1
    c. temperature of 37.5°C (99.5°F)or greater
    d. temperature of 39°C (102.2°F) on day 1

26–3. Which of the following organisms is associated with high fever in the first 24 hours after childbirth?

    a. group A streptococcus
    b. *Bacteroides bivius*
    c. *Peptostreptococcus*
    d. *B. fragilis*

26–4. How can atelectasis be prevented?

    a. coughing and deep breathing
    b. deep breathing and taking aspirin
    c. not using morphine for pain control postoperatively
    d. giving theophylline prophylactically

26–5. Fever due to breast engorgement is self-limited and generally does not last longer than what time interval?

    a. one temperature elevation
    b. 24 hr
    c. 48 hr
    d. 72 hr

26–6. What is the single most significant risk factor for postpartum metritis?

    a. number of pelvic exams
    b. duration of labor

    c. duration of amniorrhexis
    d. route of delivery

26–7. Which of the following is considered a high-risk factor for metritis?

    a. labor <4 hr
    b. rupture of membranes for 6 hours
    c. cephalopelvic disproportion
    d. preterm labor

26–8. Heavy colonization of the vaginal tract with which bacteria is associated with postpartum infection?

    a. *Strep. pyogenes*
    b. *Strep. pneumoniae*
    c. *Strep. agalactiae*
    d. *Gardnerella vaginalis*

26–9. Which of the following risk factors is NOT associated with postpartum endometritis?

    a. one course of betamethasone
    b. prolonged labor induction
    c. obesity
    d. young maternal age

26–10. Which of the following lower genital tract organisms is not associated with increased postpartum infection?

    a. *Trichomonas vaginalis*
    b. group B streptococcus
    c. *G. vaginalis*
    d. *Mycoplasma hominis*

26–11. Which of the following organisms has been associated with toxic shock-like syndrome?

    a. *Staphylococcus epidermidis*
    b. *Escherichia coli*
    c. group A β-hemolytic streptococcus
    d. *Klebsiella pneumoniae*

26–12. Which of the following bacteria is anaerobic?

    a. *Enterococcus* sp.
    b. group A streptococcus
    c. *Staph. aureus*
    d. *Fusobacterium*

26–13. Which of the following is characteristic of uterine infections?

    a. pure anaerobic
    b. pure aerobic
    c. monoetiology
    d. polymicrobial

26–14. Which of the following organisms is implicated as a cause of late postpartum infection?

    a. *Neisseria gonorrhoeae*
    b. *Chlamydia trachomatis*
    c. *T. vaginalis*
    d. *B. bivius*

26–15. Bacterial isolates taken from the lower uterine segment at cesarean delivery correlate with isolates taken when postpartum?

    a. 1 day
    b. 3 days
    c. 5 days
    d. 10 days

26–16. Blood cultures are positive in what percentage of women with postpartum metritis?

    a. <0.1
    b. 1.0 to 2.0
    c. 8.0 to 10.0
    d. >10.0

26–17. Which of the following puerperal infections is associated with scant, odorless lochia?

    a. *C. trachomatis*
    b. *N. gonorrhoeae*
    c. *Enterococcus* sp.
    d. group A β-hemolytic streptococci

26–18. What percentage of cases of puerperal metritis will respond to antimicrobials within 72 hours?

    a. 25
    b. 50
    c. 75
    d. 90

26–19. How long should women with puerperal metritis be treated with antimicrobials?

    a. until afebrile for 24 h
    b. 5-day course
    c. 10-day course
    d. 14-day course

26–20. Which of the following antibiotic regimens is considered the "gold standard" therapy for puerperal metritis?

    a. ampicillin plus gentamicin
    b. gentamicin plus clindamycin
    c. ampicillin plus clindamycin
    d. ampicillin plus gentamicin plus clindamycin

26–21. Which of the following antibiotics is NOT considered a β-lactam antimicrobial?

    a. erythromycin
    b. mezlocillin
    c. cefoxitin
    d. cefotetan

26–22. Which of the following is a β-lactamase inhibitor?

    a. sodium salt
    b. acetic acid
    c. clavulanic acid
    d. sodium citrate

26–23. Which of the following is a carbapenem?

    a. carbenicillin
    b. imipenem
    c. ticarcillin
    d. primaxin

26–24. Which of the following inhibits the renal metabolism of imipenem?

    a. clavulanic acid
    b. sulbactam
    c. aztreonam
    d. cilastatin

26–25. What is the incidence of abdominal incisional infection after cesarean delivery if prophylactic antibiotics are given?

    a. 5.0%
    b. 2.0%
    c. 1.0%
    d. <0.1%

26–26. Which is NOT a risk factor for wound infection?

    a. hematoma
    b. anemia
    c. diabetes
    d. hyperthyroidism

26–27. What is the most common etiology of fascial dehiscence?

    a. poor surgical technique
    b. infection
    c. obesity
    d. coughing

26–28. Which of the following is NOT a risk factor for necrotizing fasciitis?

    a. obesity
    b. hypertension
    c. diabetes
    d. young maternal age

26–29. What is the antibiotic treatment of choice for necrotizing fasciitis?

    a. cephalosporins plus gentamicin
    b. β-lactam agent plus clindamycin
    c. gentamicin and clindamycin
    d. ampicillin and gentamicin

26–30. When compared with surgical peritonitis, puerperal peritonitis has less of which of the following?

    a. bowel distention
    b. abdominal rigidity
    c. pain
    d. all of the above

26–31. What is a parametrial phlegmon?

    a. an ovarian abscess
    b. a pelvic abscess in the pouch of Douglas
    c. a tubal abscess
    d. an induration from cellulitis in the broad ligament

26–32. Which of the following characterizes the examination in a woman with a phlegmon?

    a. fixed uterus deviated contralateral to phlegmon
    b. fixed uterus deviated ipsilateral to phlegmon
    c. marked abdominal distention
    d. absent bowel sounds

26–33. What is the recommended treatment of a parametrial phlegmon?

    a. antibiotics alone
    b. heparin plus antibiotics
    c. hysterectomy
    d. percutaneous drainage

26–34. What percentage of women with refractory pelvic infections will have abnormal radiographic findings [i.e., computed tomography (CT)]?

    a. 5 to 10
    b. 20 to 25
    c. 50 to 60
    d. >75

26–35. Severe septic phlebitis of the left ovarian vein, unlike that involving the right, extends to what location?

    a. vena cava
    b. left renal vein
    c. common iliac veins
    d. internal iliac vein

26–36. What is the clinical pathognomonic feature of a woman with septic pelvic thrombophlebitis?

    a. enigmatic fever
    b. lower abdominal pain
    c. leg pain
    d. distended abdomen

26–37. What is the cardinal symptom of ovarian vein thrombophlebitis?

    a. fever
    b. lower abdominal pain
    c. leg pain
    d. asymptomatic

26–38. Which of the following is the best test for pelvic phlebitis?

    a. the heparin challenge test
    b. ultrasound
    c. pelvic CT
    d. abdominal x-ray

26–39. What is the approximate incidence of episiotomy breakdown?

    a. 0.1%
    b. 0.5%
    c. 1.0%
    d. 5.0%

26–40. What is the most common etiology of episiotomy breakdown?

    a. poor nutrition
    b. devascularization
    c. failure to reapproximate tissues adequately
    d. infection

26–41. Of the following which is NOT a clinical finding in episiotomy infection?

    a. red, brawny wound edges
    b. lymphangitis
    c. edema
    d. serosanguineous exudate

26–42. Early repair of episiotomy breakdown is successful in what percentage of patients?

    a. <15
    b. 20 to 30
    c. 50 to 60
    d. >90

26–43. What is NOT a predisposing factor for episiotomy breakdown?

   a. human papillomavirus infection
   b. smoking
   c. coagulation disorders
   d. gonorrhea

26–44. Which of the following organisms cause in necrotizing fasciitis?

   a. aerobic alone bacteria
   b. anaerobic and aerobic bacteria
   c. fungi
   d. chlamydia

26–45. Which of the following is NOT recommended for the immediate treatment of necrotizing fasciitis?

   a. broad-spectrum antibiotics
   b. aggressive surgical debridement

   c. split-thickness skin grafts
   d. fascial debridement

26–46. Which of the following organisms is responsible for toxic shock syndrome?

   a. *Staph. aureus*
   b. *Staph. epidermidis*
   c. *Strep. pyogenes*
   d. *Staph. toxi*

26–47. Which of the following toxins is responsible for the profound endothelial injury in toxic shock syndrome?

   a. endotoxin
   b. hypogenic exotoxin
   c. pyodermic toxin
   d. toxic shock syndrome toxin-1

27

Preterm Birth

27–1. Where does the United States rank in infant mortality?

   a. first
   b. tenth
   c. twenty-fifth
   d. forty-fourth

27–2. What is the World Health Organization definition of a premature infant?

   a. <2500 g
   b. 38 weeks or less
   c. 37 weeks or less
   d. 36 weeks or less

27–3. What is the definition of an extremely low-birthweight infant?

   a. <2500 g
   b. <1500 g

   c. <1000 g
   d. <500 g

27–4. In general, at what gestational age and weight are the majority of obstetricians willing to perform a cesarean section for a nonreassuring fetal heart rate pattern?

   a. 24 weeks and 500 g
   b. 24 weeks and 750 g
   c. 26 weeks or 500 g
   d. 26 weeks or 750 g

27–5. What percentage of infants born less than 750 g can be expected to have an IQ <70 (according to Hack and associates, 1994)?

   a. 20
   b. 40
   c. 60
   d. 80

27-6. At what birthweight does the incidence of morbidity due to prematurity equal term infants?

    a. 1000 to 1300 g
    b. 1300 to 1600 g
    c. 1600 to 1900 g
    d. >1900 g

27-7. What is the most common cause of indicated preterm birth?

    a. fetal distress
    b. preeclampsia
    c. fetal growth restriction
    d. abruptio placentae

27-8. Which of the following products is NOT found in the amniotic fluid of women with infection associated with preterm labor?

    a. thromboxane
    b. lipopolysaccharide
    c. interleukin-6
    d. tumor necrosis factor

27-9. Which of the following is the most specific test of amniotic fluid to exclude intra-amniotic infection?

    a. glucose
    b. interleukin-6
    c. white blood cell count
    d. gram stain

27-10. Which of these tests is most sensitive?

    a. glucose
    b. interleukin-6
    c. white blood cell count
    d. gram stain

27-11. Which of the following vaginal infections is positively associated with preterm birth?

    a. bacterial vaginosis
    b. trichomonal vaginalis
    c. candida vaginalis
    d. herpes simplex infections

27-12. Which of the following preterm birth risk-scoring systems is universally beneficial?

    a. Papiernik
    b. Creasy
    c. MacDonald
    d. none

27-13. Which risk factor has the strongest association with recurrent preterm birth?

    a. smoking
    b. gestational diabetes

    c. prior preeclampsia
    d. prior preterm birth

27-14. Prenatal serial cervical exams to assess preterm dilatation and effacement are associated with which of the following?

    a. neither beneficial or harmful
    b. increased preterm delivery
    c. increased ruptured membranes
    d. improved perinatal outcomes

27-15. What is fetal fibronectin?

    a. mucopolysaccharide
    b. glycoprotein
    c. sugar
    d. essential nutrient

27-16. Which of the following best describes home uterine activity monitoring?

    a. It is ineffective in the prevention of preterm birth.
    b. It is "standard of care."
    c. It delays preterm delivery.
    d. It is approved by the American College of Obstetricians and Gynecologists.

27-17. Measurment of which of the following for preterm labor prediction is investigational?

    a. cortisol
    b. Group B streptococcal antibody
    c. leukocyte esterase
    d. salivary estriol

27-18. How is preterm labor defined?

    a. regular uterine contractions 5 to 8 min apart
    b. progressive change in the cervix
    c. dilatation to 1 cm or more or 80% or more effacement
    d. all of the above

27-19. With preterm rupture of membranes, in what percentage of cases will delivery be delayed 48 hours or more?

    a. 2
    b. 7
    c. 25
    d. 50

27-20. What is the preferred management of preterm rupture of membranes?

    a. antibiotics for 10 days
    b. tocolytics until 36 weeks gestation
    c. steroids until 36 weeks gestation
    d. expectant

27–21. What is the threshold gestational age (weeks) for lung hypoplasia if the membranes rupture prematurely?

    a. 17
    b. 20
    c. 23
    d. 28

27–22. In pregnancies with premature rupture of the membranes and chorioamnionitis, infants in the chorioamnionitis group are more likely to have which of the following?

    a. seizures in the first 24 hr
    b. intraventricular hemorrhage
    c. periventricular leukomalacia
    d. all of the above

27–23. The National Institutes of Health Consensus Development Conference (1995) recommends that glucocorticoids be given to mothers to decrease which of the following?

    a. neonatal mortality
    b. respiratory distress syndrome
    c. intraventricular hemorrhage
    d. a and b

27–24. What is the mechanism by which betamethasone reduces respiratory distress syndrome?

    a. increased cytokine production
    b. increased prostaglandin production
    c. increased surfactant production
    d. increased latency period

27–25. Which of the following is a maternal effect of ritodrine?

    a. hypoglycemia
    b. hypokalemia
    c. bradycardia
    d. hypertension

27–26. What is the mechanism of action of β-adrenergic agents?

    a. block thymidine kinase
    b. activate adenylcyclase
    c. blocks conversion of adenosine triphosphate to cyclic adenosine monophosphate (AMP)
    d. increases intracellular calcium

27–27. With meta-analysis, what have tocolytics been confirmed to do?

    a. prevent preterm birth
    b. delay delivery <48 hr
    c. delay delivery <120 hr
    d. not to work

27–28. What is the proposed mechanism of action for magnesium sulfate when used for tocolysis?

    a. blocks cyclic AMP
    b. increases intracellular calcium
    c. calcium antagonist
    d. stimulates β receptors

27–29. Which of the following tocolytics is associated with premature closure of the fetal ductus arteriosus?

    a. ritodrine
    b. nifedipine
    c. magnesium sulfate
    d. indomethacin

27–30. Which tocolytic agent enhances the toxicity of magnesium to produce neuromuscular blockade?

    a. nifedipine
    b. ritodrine
    c. indomethacin
    d. ethanol

27–31. Which of the following tocolytics is a competitive oxytocin-vasopressin antagonist?

    a. magnesium
    b. ritodrine
    c. atosiban
    d. nifedipine

27–32. Which of the following is an endogenous smooth muscle relaxer?

    a. endorphin
    b. nitroglycerin
    c. indomethacin
    d. magnesium sulfate

28

Postterm Pregnancy

28–1. According to the American College of Obstetricians and Gynecologists, a prolonged or postterm pregnancy is one which extends beyond what gestational age?

a. 37 weeks
b. 40 weeks
c. 42 weeks
d. 44 weeks

28–2. Postterm pregnancy is defined as greater than or equal to how many days gestation?

a. 280
b. 287
c. 294
d. 300

28–3. What is the incidence of postterm pregnancy in the United States?

a. 1%
b. 8 to 10%
c. 16 to 18%
d. ~24%

28–4. What happens to perinatal mortality after 42 weeks gestation?

a. decreases
b. no change
c. slight increase
d. significant increase

28–5. What is the incidence of neonatal seizures in a postterm fetus?

a. 0.9 per 1000
b. 1.8 per 1000
c. 3.6 per 1000
d. 5.4 per 1000

28–6. What percentage of prolonged or postterm pregnancies have meconium-stained amniotic fluid?

a. <1%
b. 5 to 10%

c. 25 to 30%
d. ~50%

28–7. Which of the following is NOT a description associated with the postmature infant?

a. smooth skinned
b. patchy peeling skin
c. long, thin body
d. worried looking faces

28–8. What happens to placental apoptosis (programmed cell death) after 41 weeks gestation?

a. no change
b. decreases
c. increases
d. no one really knows

28–9. How do cord plasma erythropoietin levels at 41 weeks or greater compare with those at 37 to 38 weeks?

a. slightly decreased
b. significantly decreased
c. slightly increased
d. significantly increased

28–10. Which of the following is the principle reason for increased fetal risks in the postterm pregnancy?

a. placental insufficiency
b. cord compression with oligohydramnios
c. decreased umbilical cord diameter
d. meconium-stained amniotic fluid

28–11. In a woman with a favorable cervix and an estimated fetal weight of 3850 g, what is the appropriate management at 42 weeks gestation?

a. expectant management or induction
b. fetal surveillance started
c. amniocentesis performed for lung maturation studies
d. cesarean section scheduled

28–12. In a woman with an unfavorable cervix and an estimated fetal weight of 3800 g, what is the appropriate management at 42 weeks gestation?

   a. labor induction
   b. cesarean section
   c. fetal surveillance plus hospitalization
   d. cervical ripening, then induction

28–13. How does membrane stripping or sweeping at 38 to 40 weeks gestation affect the frequency of postterm pregnancy?

   a. decreases
   b. no change
   c. increases
   d. unknown

29

Fetal Growth Disorders

29–1. How is low birthweight defined?

   a. <1500 g
   b. <2000 g
   c. <2500 g
   d. <3000 g

29–2. How is macrosomia defined?

   a. >4000 g
   b. >4100 g
   c. >4500 g
   d. >5000 g

29–3. What is the incidence of macrosomia?

   a. <0.1%
   b. ~1.0%
   c. 10.0%
   d. 25.0%

29–4. Which of the following cell growth phases occurs during the first 16 weeks of gestation?

   a. cellular hyperplasia and hypertrophy
   b. cellular hyperplasia
   c. cellular hypertrophy
   d. apoptosis

29–5. What is characteristic of the third phase of fetal growth?

   a. cellular death
   b. cellular swelling

   c. cellular hyperplasia
   d. cellular hypertrophy

29–6. At 34 weeks, the fetus will gain how many grams per day?

   a. 5 to 10
   b. 15 to 20
   c. 30 to 35
   d. 45 to 50

29–7. Which of the following is related to fetal overgrowth (macrosomia)?

   a. insulin-like growth factor I (IGF-I)
   b. insulin-like growth factor II (IGF-II)
   c. insulin
   d. insulin growth factor binding protein

29–8. What is the incidence of fetal growth restriction?

   a. <1%
   b. 3 to 10%
   c. 15 to 20%
   d. ~25%

29–9. How are small-for-gestational-age infants defined?

   a. below 2500 g
   b. below 2000 g
   c. below the 10th percentile
   d. below the 20th percentile

29–10. Which of the following is NOT a determinant of an infant's birthweight?

    a. ethnicity
    b. parity
    c. maternal weight
    d. 30-lb maternal weight gain during pregnancy

29–11. Which of the following is associated with growth restricted fetuses?

    a. hyperinsulinemia
    b. hypertriglyceridemia
    c. hyperglycemia
    d. anemia

29–12. Which of the following compounds is elevated in the plasma of growth restricted fetuses?

    a. prostacyclin
    b. adenosine
    c. interleukin-1
    d. epidermal growth factor

29–13. Which of the following is NOT associated with fetal growth restriction?

    a. birth asphyxia
    b. sepsis
    c. hypoglycemia
    d. hypothermia

29–14. How is symmetrical growth restriction characterized?

    a. reduction in head size
    b. reduction in body size
    c. reduction in both body and head size
    d. reduction in body and femur length

29–15. What is the brain-to-liver weight ratio in a severely growth-restricted infant?

    a. 1 to 2
    b. 2 to 1
    c. 3 to 1
    d. 5 to 1

29–16. Which of the following is NOT a risk factor for severe fetal growth restriction?

    a. maternal weight <100 lb
    b. fetal infections
    c. trisomy 21
    d. smoking

29–17. Which of the following is NOT associated with fetal growth restriction?

    a. toxoplasmosis infection
    b. cytomegalovirus infection
    c. congenital rubella
    d. human papillomavirus

29–18. Which of the following chromosomal disorders is NOT associated with fetal growth restriction?

    a. 45,X
    b. trisomy 18
    c. trisomy 13
    d. fetal growth restriction with all of the above

29–19. Which trisomy is responsible for confirmed placental mosaicism and many cases of previously unexplained fetal growth restriction?

    a. 13
    b. 16
    c. 18
    d. 21

29–20. Which of the following placental abnormalities is NOT associated with growth restriction?

    a. circumvallate placenta
    b. placenta previa
    c. acute abruption
    d. velamentous cord insertion

29–21. Which of the following ultrasound measurements is the most reliable index of fetal size?

    a. biparietal diameter
    b. abdominal circumference
    c. femur length
    d. intrathoracic ratio

29–22. Which sonographic measurement in a growth restricted fetus correlates best with significant perinatal mortality?

    a. biparietal diameter
    b. abdominal circumference
    c. femur length
    d. oligohydramnios

29–23. Which test of fetal well-being correlates with fetal metabolic acidosis at birth?

    a. reactive nonstress test
    b. negative contraction stress test
    c. biophysical profile of 8/10
    d. reversed end-diastolic umbilical artery velocimetry

29–24. What is the birthweight threshold for macrosomia if defined as 2 standard deviations above the mean at 40 weeks?

    a. 4000 g
    b. 4250 g
    c. 4500 g
    d. 5000 g

29–25. Which of the following is NOT a risk factor for macrosomia?

    a. diabetes
    b. female fetus
    c. maternal obesity
    d. gestational age >42 weeks

29–26. How is fetal weight accurately assessed prior to delivery?

    a. ultrasound
    b. x-ray pelvimetry
    c. Leopold's maneuvers
    d. not possible

29–27. Which of the following is least likely to be associated with macrosomia?

    a. intraventricular hemorrhage
    b. brachial plexus injury
    c. shoulder dystocia
    d. cephalopelvic disproportion

29–28. A primary cesarean section may be justified in a diabetic pregnancy at what estimated fetal weight?

    a. >4000 g
    b. >4250 g
    c. >4500 g
    d. not justified on estimated weight alone

30

Multifetal Pregnancy

30–1. What percentage of pregnancies involve multiple gestation?

    a. 1
    b. 3
    c. 5
    d. 7

30–2. What percentage of twins are monozygous?

    a. 10
    b. 25
    c. 33
    d. 50

30–3. Regarding monozygotic twins, at what time does division result in dichorionic diamnionic membranes?

    a. ≤72 hr after fertilization
    b. 72 to 120 hr after fertilization
    c. >120 hr but <240 hr after fertilization
    d. >264 hr after fertilization

30–4. Division of the monozygote between 4 and 8 days yields which of the following?

    a. diamnionic dichorionic
    b. diamnionic monochorionic
    c. monoamnionic monochorionic
    d. conjoined twins

30–5. What is a chimera?

    a. an individual with multiple phenotypes
    b. an individual with a mixture of genotypes
    c. a hermaphrodite
    d. a consequence of nondisjunction

30–6. What is superfecundation?

    a. Multigestation due to ovulatory drugs.
    b. Fertilization of 1 ovum with subsequent division on day 5.
    c. Multiple fertilization of 1 ovum.
    d. Fertilization of 2 ova within a short time but not at same coitus.

30–7. What is the incidence of monozygotic twins?

    a. 1 in 250

    b. dependent upon race

    c. dependent upon age

    d. dependent upon parity

30–8. What is the incidence of vanishing twins?

    a. <5%

    b. ~10%

    c. 20 to 60%

    d. >80%

30–9. In what race does the highest incidence of twins occur?

    a. African ancestry

    b. Asians

    c. whites

    d. equal in all races

30–10. Preterm twins have a greater incidence of which of the following when compared with preterm singletons?

    a. respiratory distress

    b. intraventricular hemorrhage

    c. necrotizing enterocolitis

    d. none of the above

30–11. What is the association of ovulation induction for infertility with multiple births?

    a. decreases multiple pregnancies

    b. increases multiple pregnancies

    c. increases only dizygotic twins

    d. does not affect the incidence of twins

30–12. What do monochorionic diamnionic membranes imply?

    a. monozygosity

    b. dizygosity

    c. does not reveal zygosity

    d. none of the above

30–13. What happens to the incidence of male fetuses in multiple gestations?

    a. decreased for twins, increased for triplets or greater

    b. increased for twins, decreased for triplets or greater

    c. increased with increasing number of fetuses

    d. decreased with increasing number of fetuses

30–14. Which of the following most strongly suggests dichorionic diamnionic twin pregnancy?

    a. lack of discordance

    b. sonographic measurement of the dividing membranes <2 mm

    c. 2 separate placentae

    d. all of the above

30–15. Which of the following ultrasound characteristics most strongly indicates monochorionic twins?

    a. same gender

    b. dividing membrane thickness 1 mm

    c. two placentas

    d. concordancy

30–16. What is the best test to diagnose twins prenatally?

    a. x-ray

    b. magnetic resonance imaging

    c. computed tomography scan

    d. ultrasound

30–17. What is the mean increase in maternal blood volume in twin gestation?

    a. 10 to 20%

    b. 40 to 50%

    c. 50 to 60%

    d. 70 to 80%

30–18. What is the average blood loss for a twin gestation delivered vaginally?

    a. ~250 mL

    b. 500 mL

    c. 750 mL

    d. 1000 mL

30–19. What is the incidence of major malformations in twin gestations?

    a. <1%

    b. 2%

    c. 4%

    d. 8%

30–20. What percentage of twins have fetal growth restriction?

    a. 10

    b. 25

    c. 33

    d. 67

30–21. What is the mean duration of gestation in weeks for twins?

    a. 32

    b. 34

    c. 36

    d. 38

30–22. Which of the following is increased when twin pregnancies are compared with singletons?

  a. perinatal mortality
  b. structural abnormalities
  c. cerebral palsy
  d. all of the above

30–23. What is the best management at 32 weeks' gestation when one twin is noted to have died in utero?

  a. immediate oxytocin induction of labor
  b. immediate delivery by cesarean
  c. observation
  d. heparin immediately to prevent coagulopathy

30–24. Which of the following is NOT a specific complication of monoamnionic twins?

  a. cord entanglement
  b. discordancy
  c. conjoined twins
  d. preterm labor

30–25. Which of the following is the most common type of conjoined twins?

  a. thoracopagus
  b. craniopagus
  c. ischiopagus
  d. pyopagus

30–26. Which of the following may be involved in the pathophysiology of twin-twin transfusion?

  a. multiple superficial vascular anastomoses
  b. solitary deep arteriovenous channel
  c. venous-venous connection
  d. arterial-arterial connection

30–27. Which of the following is NOT a diagnostic criterion for twin-twin transfusion?

  a. hemoglobin differences >5 g/dL
  b. birthweight differences >20%
  c. oligohydramnios in large twin
  d. placental vascular connection

30–28. What management strategy for pregnancies complicated by twin-twin transfusion is least risky?

  a. serial amniocenteses for decompression
  b. decompression amniocentesis
  c. fetoscopic laser occlusion of vessels
  d. observation

30–29. How is discordance in twins best measured?

  a. biparietal diameter
  b. abdominal circumference

  c. femur length
  d. crown-rump length

30–30. When twin discordancy exceeds 30%, which of the following is true?

  a. increased neonatal deaths
  b. fewer congenital anomalies
  c. less growth restriction
  d. increase in fetal deaths

30–31. When comparing outcomes after the in utero death of one twin, monochorionic surviving twins are more likely to have which of the following when compared to dichorionic surviving twins?

  a. hydrops
  b. anemia
  c. kernicterus
  d. respiratory distress

30–32. What is the daily folic acid requirement or recommendation for twin pregnancy?

  a. 0.1 mg
  b. 0.4 mg
  c. 1 mg
  d. 4 mg

30–33. Which of the following antenatal fetal testing in twins has been shown to lower antepartum death rates?

  a. none lower death rates
  b. nonstress test
  c. twice weekly biophysical profiles
  d. doppler velocimetry

30–34. What is the best way to prevent preterm delivery in twins?

  a. bedrest
  b. β-mimetics
  c. cervical cerclage
  d. hospitalization for complications

30–35. Positive risk factors for preterm birth in twins include which of the following?

  a. short cervical length
  b. positive fetal fibronectin
  c. positive IL-6 in cervicovaginal secretions
  d. a and b only

30–36. What is the most common intrapartum presentation for twins?

  a. cephalic-cephalic
  b. cephalic-breech
  c. breech-breech
  d. breech-cephalic

30–37. Interlocking twins is associated with which of the following presentations?

    a. cephalic-cephalic
    b. cephalic-breech
    c. breech-breech
    d. breech-cephalic

30–38. When outcomes in triplets are compared with twins and singletons, triplets are at greater risk for which of the following?

    a. retinopathy of prematurity
    b. mild intraventricular hemorrhage
    c. perinatal mortality
    d. all of the above

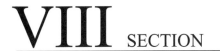

31

Abnormalities of the Fetal Membranes and Amnionic Fluid

31–1. What is the approximate incidence of meconium-stained amnionic fluid near term?

    a. 0.1%
    b. 1.0%
    c. 20.0%
    d. 50.0%

31–2. Before what gestational age (weeks) is meconium passage uncommon?

    a. 36
    b. 38
    c. 40
    d. 42

31–3. Which of the following is NOT associated with meconium-stained amniotic fluid?

    a. postterm pregnancy
    b. cesarean delivery
    c. fetal acidemia
    d. chorioamnionitis

31–4. The increased perinatal mortality associated with meconium-stained amniotic fluid is primarily due to which of the following?

    a. aspiration of thick meconium by fetus
    b. neonatal sepsis
    c. placental insufficiency
    d. hypoxic brain damage

31–5. What is the histological finding in chorioamnionitis?

    a. plasma cells and mononuclear cells
    b. plasma cells and polymorphonuclear leukocytes
    c. mononuclear cells and polymorphonuclear leukocytes
    d. mononuclear cells and lymphocytes

31–6. What is the composition of amnion nodosum (amnionic caruncles)?

    a. vernix and ectodermal debris
    b. mononuclear cells and macrophages
    c. lymphocytes and polymorphonucleocytes
    d. eosinophils and vernix

31–7. What congenital anomaly is associated with amnion nodosum?

    a. ventral septal defect
    b. spina bifida
    c. omphalocele
    d. renal agenesis

31–8. At what point in normal gestation (weeks) should the amnionic fluid volume be approximately 1000 mL?

    a. 16
    b. 28
    c. 36
    d. 40

31-9. Polyhydramnios is an amnionic fluid volume greater than which of the following?

   a. 1200 mL
   b. 1600 mL
   c. 2000 mL
   d. 2400 mL

31-10. Hydramnios is diagnosed by an amniotic fluid index greater than which of the following?

   a. 20 cm
   b. 24 cm
   c. 28 cm
   d. 32 cm

31-11. Which of the following has been shown to influence amniotic fluid volume?

   a. altitude
   b. maternal hydration
   c. maternal dehydration
   d. all of the above

31-12. What is the incidence of hydramnios?

   a. 0.2%
   b. 1.0%
   c. 12.0%
   d. 20.0%

31-13. What is the most common cause of hydramnios?

   a. fetal anomalies
   b. idiopathic
   c. maternal diabetes
   d. multifetal gestation

31-14. Which of the following anomalies are NOT associated with polyhydramnios?

   a. central nervous system abnormalities
   b. duodenal atresia
   c. esophageal atresia
   d. renal agenesis

31-15. Idiopathic hydramnios is associated with an increase in which of the following?

   a. amniotic fluid embolism
   b. cesarean delivery rate
   c. uterine rupture
   d. meconium aspiration

31-16. After the first trimester, amniotic fluid volume correlates most strongly with which of the following?

   a. fetal cardiac output
   b. maternal fluid status
   c. maternal rest in left lateral recumbent position
   d. fetal urine production and excretion

31-17. What is the most likely cause of increased amnionic fluid in cases of anencephaly?

   a. decreased swallowing
   b. increased transudation
   c. decreased urination
   d. increased fetal urine output

31-18. Which of the following labor complications is NOT associated with hydramnios?

   a. cord prolapse
   b. late fetal heart rate decelerations
   c. postpartum hemorrhage
   d. uterine dysfunction

31-19. Which of the following is NOT a maternal symptom associated with hydramnios?

   a. edema
   b. dyspnea
   c. ileus
   d. preterm labor

31-20. What is a frequent maternal complication of hydramnios?

   a. preeclampsia
   b. hypertonic uterine activity
   c. placental abruption
   d. postterm pregnancy

31-21. How much amniotic fluid should be removed per hour during therapeutic amniocentesis for hydramnios?

   a. 100 mL
   b. 250 mL
   c. 500 mL
   d. 1000 mL

31-22. Which drug, when given orally to mothers, decreases fetal urine output?

   a. aspirin
   b. cimetidine
   c. bromocriptine
   d. indomethacin

31-23. What is the side effect of using indomethacin for the management of hydramnios?

   a. altered neonatal bleeding times
   b. maternal hypotension
   c. partial constriction of the fetal ductus arteriosus
   d. premature separation of the placenta

31–24. Based on sonographic findings, how is oligohydramnios defined?

    a. 3 pockets of amnionic fluid <2 cm each
    b. amnionic fluid index of 5 cm or less
    c. amnionic fluid index <20th percentile
    d. none of the above

31–25. Oligohydramnios is NOT associated with which of the following conditions?

    a. neural tube defects
    b. premature rupture of membranes
    c. renal agenesis
    d. urinary tract obstruction

31–26. Which class of drugs is strongly associated with oligohydramnios?

    a. angiotensin-converting enzyme inhibitors
    b. α-adrenergic blockers
    c. calcium channel blocking agents
    d. hydralazine

31–27. Which of the following findings in the fetus is NOT associated with oligohydramnios?

    a. club foot
    b. adhesions of amnion to fetus
    c. decreased subcutaneous tissues
    d. pulmonary hypoplasia

31–28. Which of the following is most responsible for the increased rate of cesarean delivery when oligohydramnios is present?

    a. coexistent fetal anomalies
    b. fetal malpresentation
    c. nonreassuring fetal heart rate patterns
    d. uterine dysfunction during labor

31–29. Which of the following is true regarding amnioinfusion during labor to prevent the complications of oligohydramnios?

    a. high complication rate
    b. increased duration of labor
    c. low complication rate
    d. no benefits to fetal or maternal outcomes

32

Diseases and Abnormalities of the Placenta

32–1. What is the name for incomplete division of the placenta with fetal vessels extending from one lobe to the other?

    a. placenta bipartita
    b. placenta succenturiata
    c. placenta membranacea
    d. fenestrated placenta

32–2. What is the name for small accessory lobes that develop in the fetal membranes?

    a. fenestrated placenta
    b. placenta bilobata

    c. placenta succenturiata
    d. placenta membranacea

32–3. What is the incidence of placenta succenturiata?

    a. 0.3%
    b. 5.0%
    c. 10.0%
    d. 30.0%

32–4. Of the abnormal placentations, which is NOT associated with postpartum hemorrhage?

    a. placenta bipartita
    b. placenta succenturiata
    c. fenestrated placenta
    d. ring-shaped placenta

32–5. Of the abnormal placentas listed, which is associated with fetal growth retardation?

    a. placenta succenturiata
    b. placenta bilobata
    c. fenestrated placenta
    d. ring-shaped placenta

32–6. In which placental type is the chorionic plate smaller than the basal plate?

    a. membranaceous
    b. ring-shaped
    c. extrachorial
    d. fenestrated

32–7. Which of the following is the most common placental lesion?

    a. previa
    b. abruption
    c. infarcts
    d. deciduitis

32–8. What is the incidence of placental infarcts in term uncomplicated pregnancies?

    a. 10%
    b. 25%
    c. 50%
    d. 67%

32–9. What is the incidence of placental infarcts in pregnancies complicated by severe hypertension?

    a. 25%
    b. 33%
    c. 50%
    d. 67%

32–10. Which of the following is NOT a morphological indication of aging in a term placenta?

    a. syncytial degeneration
    b. villous stroma hyalinization
    c. clotting beneath the syncytium
    d. regeneration of trophoblast

32–11. At what point in pregnancy does one expect to see calcification in more than one-half of placentas examined?

    a. 21 weeks
    b. 25 weeks

    c. 29 weeks
    d. 33 weeks

32–12. Sonographic findings of placental calcifications correlate somewhat with which of the following?

    a. fetal lung maturity
    b. fetal growth restriction
    c. increased perinatal mortality
    d. maternal hyperparathyroidism

32–13. Villous (fetal) artery thrombosis is NOT associated with which of the conditions listed below?

    a. diabetes
    b. twins
    c. severe maternal hypertension
    d. stillbirth

32–14. Striking enlargement of the chorionic villi is associated with which of these conditions?

    a. fetal hydrops
    b. twins
    c. postdates pregnancy
    d. class A_1 diabetes

32–15. What is the mean length of the normal umbilical cord at term?

    a. 25 to 30 cm
    b. 35 to 40 cm
    c. 45 to 50 cm
    d. 55 to 60 cm

32–16. Which of the following is increased in pregnancies with long umbilical cords?

    a. abruptio placentae
    b. uterine inversion
    c. true knots
    d. furisitis

32–17. What percentage of infants missing one umbilical artery will have congenital anomalies?

    a. 3
    b. 10
    c. 30
    d. 50

32–18. Which of the following is NOT increased in fetuses with hypercoiled cords?

    a. postterm pregnancy
    b. meconium-stained amniotic fluid
    c. fetal distress
    d. preterm birth

32–19. What is insertion of the cord at the placental margin called?

   a. velamentous insertion
   b. vasa previa
   c. Battledore placenta
   d. true knot

32–20. In what type of placenta do the umbilical vessels separate in the membranes some distance from the placental margin?

   a. velamentous insertion
   b. vasa previa
   c. Battledore placenta
   d. true knot

32–21. Vasa previa is associated with which of the following?

   a. fetal exsanguination
   b. low-lying placenta
   c. succenturiate placenta
   d. all of the above

32–22. Which condition results from active fetal movements?

   a. vasa previa
   b. Battledore placenta
   c. true knots
   d. false knots

32–23. What is the rate of perinatal loss in the presence of true cord knots?

   a. 0.6%
   b. 6.0%
   c. 16.0%
   d. not increased

32–24. What is the incidence of single-loop nuchal cords?

   a. 0.2%
   b. 2.1%
   c. 12.0%
   d. 21.0%

32–25. Which of the following is true of nuchal cord loops?

   a. causes pathologic fetal acidemia
   b. increases perinatal mortality
   c. resolves as labor progresses
   d. increases variable fetal heart rate decelerations

32–26. Which of the following is associated with cord stricture?

   a. deficiency of Wharton's jelly
   b. hyperactive fetus

   c. twins
   d. cocaine use

32–27. What is the etiology of true cysts of the umbilical cord?

   a. intra-amniotic infection
   b. remnants of the allantois
   c. liquefaction of Wharton's jelly
   d. associated with congenital anomalies

32–28. What is the etiology of false cysts of the umbilical cord?

   a. intra-amniotic infection
   b. remnants of the allantois
   c. liquefaction of Wharton's jelly
   d. associated with congenital anomalies

32–29. For which situation is the pathologic examination of the placenta and umbilical cord considered the most cost-effective and informative?

   a. all obstetrical deliveries
   b. specific high-risk maternal conditions
   c. stillbirths
   d. all cases of chorioamnionitis

32–30. Which of the following is NOT considered a high-risk factor in the clinical classification of gestational trophoblastic tumors?

   a. pretherapy human chorionic gonadotropin level of 30,000
   b. liver metastases
   c. antecedent term pregnancy
   d. prior chemotherapy failure

32–31. Which of the following is typical of the karyotypes and chromosomal origin of complete hydatidiform moles?

   a. 46,XX or 46,XY; all paternal origin
   b. 69,XXX or 69,XXY; maternal and paternal origin
   c. 46,XX; all maternal origin
   d. 46,YY; all paternal origin

32–32. The majority of partial moles have which chromosomal complement?

   a. haploid
   b. diploid
   c. triploid
   d. tetraploid

32–33. What is the incidence of persistent trophoblastic diseases following a complete mole?

   a. 5%
   b. 10%
   c. 20%
   d. 30%

32–34. Which of the following is NOT true of a partial molar pregnancy?

   a. Hydatidiform changes are more focal and less advanced than complete moles.
   b. A fetus or fetal tissues may be present.
   c. Triploidy is common.
   d. Theca-lutein cysts are common.

32–35. What is the incidence of nonmetastatic gestational trophoblastic disease following a partial mole?

   a. 1 to 2%
   b. 4 to 8%
   c. 15 to 20%
   d. 40 to 50%

32–36. What is the etiology of theca-lutein cysts?

   a. abnormal karyotype
   b. increased prolactin receptors
   c. increased follicle-stimulating hormone
   d. increased chorionic gonadotropin

32–37. In which of the following clinical situations are theca-lutein cysts least likely to present?

   a. maternal hyperthyroidism
   b. hydatidiform mole
   c. fetal hydrops
   d. multifetal gestation

32–38. What is the incidence of molar pregnancy in the United States and Europe?

   a. 1 in 10,000
   b. 1 in 7,000
   c. 1 in 1,000
   d. 1 in 700

32–39. At what maternal age does the highest frequency of molar pregnancy occur?

   a. 15 to 20 years
   b. 25 to 30 years
   c. 35 to 40 years
   d. >45 years

32–40. What is the most universal sign or symptom of molar pregnancy?

   a. thyroid dysfunction
   b. increased uterine size
   c. bleeding
   d. hyperemesis

32–41. What causes the increase in plasma thyroxine in women with molar pregnancies?

   a. increased fetal thyroxine production
   b. estrogen-induced increased total thyroxine

   c. increased levels of human chorionic gonadotropin
   d. unknown

32–42. What imaging technique is most useful in diagnosing molar pregnancy?

   a. x-ray
   b. ultrasound
   c. computed tomographic pelvimetry
   d. magnetic resonance imaging

32–43. What is the treatment of choice for a 16-week-size hydatidiform mole?

   a. sharp curettage
   b. prostaglandin induction
   c. suction evacuation
   d. hysterotomy

32–44. In which case below is the incidence of malignant trophoblastic disease increased?

   a. partial molar pregnancies
   b. advanced maternal age (>40 years)
   c. teenager
   d. presence of a 14 cm, theca-lutein cyst

32–45. When used after molar pregnancy, oral contraceptives have been associated with which of the following?

   a. persistent or recurrent invasive disease
   b. facilitation of careful follow-up
   c. interference with the decline in serial chorionic gonadotropin
   d. increase in recurrence rate during next pregnancy

32–46. What percentage of gestational trophoblastic tumors follow normal pregnancy?

   a. 10
   b. 25
   c. 33
   d. 50

32–47. What is the key histological diagnostic feature of choriocarcinoma?

   a. an increase in cytotrophoblast
   b. a decrease in syncytial trophoblast
   c. absence of a villous pattern
   d. absence of cellular anaplasia

32–48. Which of the following are characteristic placental site trophoblastic tumors?

   a. many prolactin-producing cells
   b. predominantly syncytial trophoblast
   c. absent villous pattern
   d. increased gonadotropin-producing cells

32–49. What is the best drug choice for persistent gestational trophoblastic disease?

    a. doxorubicin
    b. cisplatin
    c. methotrexate
    d. bleomycin

32–50. What is the therapy of choice for high-risk metastatic disease?

    a. etoposide, methotrexate, actinomycin, cyclophosphamide, vinicristine
    b. methotrexate alone
    c. MAC (methotrexate, actinomycin, and cyclophosphamide)
    d. methotrexate and actinomycin

32–51. Which of the following is NOT a variable used to determine Brewer score for the prognosis of gestational trophoblastic tumor?

    a. length of time since diagnosis
    b. number of metastases
    c. prior chemotherapy
    d. sites of metastasis

32–52. Which of the following is the only benign placental tumor?

    a. chorioangioma
    b. fibroma
    c. mesenchymal rest cell
    d. placental site tumor

32–53. Which of the following pregnancy complications may be due to large chorioangiomas?

    a. oligohydramnios
    b. polyhydramnios
    c. abruption
    d. severe hypertension

32–54. Which of the following tumors is most likely to metastasize to the placenta?

    a. breast cancer
    b. melanoma
    c. lung cancer
    d. endometrial cancer

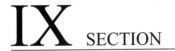
*Reproductive Success
and Failure*

33

Abortion

33–1. What is the term for no visible fetus in the sac?

    a. septic abortion
    b. miscarriage
    c. blighted ovum
    d. polar body

33–2. What is a fetus that becomes dry and compressed called?

    a. macerated
    b. fetus papyraceous
    c. fetus compressus
    d. Spalding sign

33–3. How many weeks after an abortion does ovulation usually occur?

    a. 2 to 3
    b. 4 to 5
    c. 5 to 6
    d. 6 to 7

33–4. In healthy fertile women over age 40, what is the percentage of abortion in clinically recognized pregnancies in the first trimester?

    a. 5 to 6
    b. 10 to 12
    c. 15 to 18
    d. 24 to 27

33–5. Which of the following is NOT associated with an increased abortion rate?

    a. advanced maternal age
    b. advanced paternal age
    c. pregnancy within 3 months of a live birth
    d. Class A_1 diabetes mellitus

33–6. In first-trimester abortions, what is the most common chromosomal anomaly?

    a. triploidy
    b. autosomal trisomy
    c. tetraploidy
    d. structural anomaly

33–7. Which of the following is associated with trisomies?

    a. isolated nondisjunction
    b. unbalanced translocation
    c. chromosome deletion
    d. polar body fertilization

33–8. What autosomal trisomy has not been found in abortuses?

    a. 1
    b. 13
    c. 16
    d. 18

33–9. Which of the following is associated with euploid abortions?

    a. 8 weeks gestation
    b. adolescence
    c. maternal disease
    d. paternal factors

33–10. Of the following, which is most likely to cause abortion?

    a. *Toxoplasma gondii*
    b. *Listeria monocytogenes*
    c. *Chlamydia trachomatis*
    d. Herpes simplex

33–11. What is the incidence of abortion in those with insulin-dependent diabetes compared to the general population?

   a. increased
   b. decreased
   c. the same
   d. not related to glucose control

33–12. Of the following, which is NOT associated with an increased abortion rate?

   a. tobacco
   b. oral contraceptives
   c. radiation over 5 rad
   d. coffee in excess of 4 cups per day

33–13. How much is the risk of abortion increased for every 10 cigarettes smoked per day?

   a. 0.3 times
   b. 0.6 times
   c. 1.2 times
   d. 2.4 times

33–14. At what level of coffee consumption might the abortion rate be increased?

   a. >2 cups
   b. >4 cups
   c. >6 cups
   d. >8 cups

33–15. Of the following, which is NOT associated with an increased risk of abortion?

   a. diagnostic x-ray
   b. lead
   c. benzene
   d. ethylene oxide

33–16. What causes pregnancy loss in women with antiphospholipid antibodies?

   a. placental thrombosis and infarction
   b. increased vascularization of decidual basalis
   c. increased prosatcyclin release
   d. protein C activation

33–17. Which of the following is the most common inherited thrombophilia found in women with two or more early pregnancy losses?

   a. protein S deficiency
   b. factor V Leiden mutation
   c. protein C resistance
   d. ATIII deficiency

33–18. Which of the following uterine abnormalities has the greatest likelihood of spontaneous abortions?

   a. uterine didelphys
   b. uterine septa

   c. bicornuate uterus
   d. leiomyomata

33–19. How is an incompetent cervix most frequently diagnosed?

   a. sonography
   b. passage of a #8 Hegar dilator through the internal os
   c. history
   d. hysterography

33–20. What is the approximate success rate following cerclage?

   a. 15%
   b. 30%
   c. 60%
   d. 90%

33–21. At 8 weeks' gestation if vaginal bleeding occurs, what is the risk of spontaneous abortion?

   a. 10%
   b. 30%
   c. 50%
   d. 70%

33–22. Which of the following is NOT associated with bleeding at 8 weeks' gestation?

   a. preterm labor
   b. low birthweight
   c. neonatal mortality
   d. malformations

33–23. At 8 weeks' gestation a woman has bleeding, and an intrauterine device "string" is visible at the external os. Because the woman desires to keep the pregnancy, what is the best plan of management?

   a. bed rest
   b. antibiotics
   c. progesterone
   d. removal of intrauterine device

33–24. At 8 weeks' gestation a woman has vaginal bleeding of supracervical origin. Which of the following is helpful in regard to prognosis?

   a. chorionic gonadotropin of 2400 mIU/mL
   b. plasma estriol
   c. serum progesterone of 18 ng/mL
   d. ultrasound with a fetus and fetal heart tones

33–25. Which of the following has been shown to be effective in termination of first-trimester missed abortions?

   a. methotrexate
   b. prostaglandin E_1
   c. prostacyclin
   d. oxytocin

33–26. In a woman with three or more recurrent spontaneous abortions, which of the following is true?

  a. Risk of abortion is about 80%.
  b. Rate of successful pregnancy is 20%.
  c. Parental karyotyping is recommended.
  d. Artificial insemination is needed.

33–27. What famous case established the legality of elective abortion in the United States?

  a. Jones vs. Smith
  b. Harris vs. Harper
  c. Roe vs. Wade
  d. Anonymous vs. United States

33–28. What percentage of D-negative women become sensitized after an abortion if prophylaxis is not given?

  a. 1
  b. 5
  c. 10
  d. 20

33–29. Which of the following is impregnated with anhydrous magnesium sulfate?

  a. Cervidil
  b. Dilapan
  c. laminaria
  d. Lamicel

33–30. Which of the following is true regarding RU-486 (mifepristone)?

  a. causes severe malformations
  b. is most effective prior to 6 weeks' gestation
  c. devoid of side effects
  d. almost 100% effective when used as an abortifacient

Ectopic Pregnancy

34–1. What is the approximate incidence of ectopic versus normal pregnancy in the United States?

  a. 1 in 100
  b. 1 in 500
  c. 1 in 1000
  d. 1 in 1500

34–2. In which of the following are tubal pregnancies NOT increased?

  a. history of salpingitis
  b. tubal anomalies
  c. previous ectopic pregnancy
  d. abnormal embryos

34–3. What is the chance of recurrent ectopic pregnancy after one previous ectopic pregnancy?

  a. 1 to 5%
  b. 7 to 15%
  c. 17 to 25%
  d. 17 to 35%

34–4. Which of the following is NOT a risk factor for ectopic pregnancy?

  a. medroxyprogesterone acetate use
  b. in utero exposure to diethylstilbestrol
  c. luteal phase defect
  d. assisted reproductive techniques

34–5. Which method of contraceptive failure has the highest ectopic rate?

  a. intrauterine device
  b. oral contraception
  c. tubal sterilization
  d. hysterectomy

34–6. Ectopic pregnancies account for what percentage of pregnancy-related deaths?

a. 5
b. 10
c. 20
d. 25

34–7. What is the most common ectopic tubal implantation site?

a. fimbria
b. ampulla
c. isthmus
d. cornua

34–8. What is the Arias-Stella reaction?

a. is specific for ectopic gestation
b. may be confused with a malignancy
c. is specific for intrauterine gestation
d. is the result of unopposed estrogen

34–9. Which of the following is true about interstitial pregnancy?

a. represents 3% of tubal pregnancies
b. frequently ruptures later (8 to 16 weeks)
c. is usually associated with massive hemorrhage if ruptured
d. all of the above

34–10. What is the most common symptom of ectopic pregnancy?

a. bleeding
b. pain
c. dizziness
d. gastrointestinal symptoms

34–11. Heterotopic pregnancy is most common with the use of which of the following?

a. assisted-reproductive techniques
b. intrauterine devices
c. progesterone-only contraceptives
d. tubal ligation

34–12. Which of the following signs or symptoms most strongly implies a ruptured ectopic pregnancy with sizable intraperitoneal hemorrhage?

a. heavy vaginal bleeding
b. lower abdominal pain, unilateral
c. nausea and vomiting
d. shoulder pain on inspiration

34–13. Use of enzyme-linked immunosorbent assays for chorionic gonadotropin are positive in what percentage of ectopic pregnancies?

a. 50
b. 75
c. 95
d. 100

34–14. Which is the most sensitive pregnancy test?

a. latex agglutination inhibition slide test
b. latex agglutination inhibition tube test
c. enzyme-linked immunosorbent assay (ELISA)
d. serum radioimmunoassay (β-hCG)

34–15. A patient with a positive pregnancy test and a serum progesterone of less than 5 ng/mL indicates which of the following?

a. an ectopic pregnancy
b. an intrauterine pregnancy
c. a nonviable pregnancy
d. a viable pregnancy

34–16. Using vaginal ultrasound, when can an intrauterine gestational sac be seen reliably?

a. 4 menstrual weeks
b. 6 menstrual weeks
c. 7 menstrual weeks
d. 8 menstrual weeks

34–17. Vaginal sonography can detect an intrauterine gestational sac when the serum β-hCG reaches what level?

a. 1000 mIU/mL
b. 1500 mIU/mL
c. 2000 mIU/mL
d. 2500 mIU/mL

34–18. What percentage of ectopic pregnancies are diagnosed prior to rupture?

a. 60
b. 70
c. 80
d. 90

34–19. What is the mean doubling time for β-hCG in early pregnancy?

a. 24 hr
b. 48 hr
c. 72 hr
d. 96 hr

34–20. What is the lowest normal increase for β-hCG in early pregnancy during a 48-hour interval?

a. 33%
b. 44%
c. 55%
d. 66%

34–21. What percentage of normal pregnancies will be incorrectly labeled as abnormal if the standard of showing at least a 66 percent rise in β-hCG level over 48 hours is applied?

a. 5
b. 10
c. 15
d. 20

34–22. Sonographic evidence of an ectopic pregnancy includes which of the following?

a. adnexal mass
b. fluid in the cul de sac
c. lack of intrauterine gestational sac
d. all of the above

34–23. By how many days following resection of an ectopic pregnancy does serum hCG decrease to 10 percent of preoperative levels?

a. 2 days
b. 4 days
c. 8 days
d. 12 days

34–24. Compared with salpingectomy, more conservative surgical approaches to ectopic pregnancy, such as salpingostomy, offer what advantage?

a. a lower risk of subsequent ectopic pregnancy
b. a higher rate of subsequent intrauterine pregnancy
c. a higher rate of subsequent fertility
d. lower cost and recovery time

34–25. Which of the following would make methotrexate therapy for ectopic pregnancy less likely to succeed?

a. pregnancy of 5 weeks' duration
b. tubal mass 3.5 cm
c. fetal heart motion
d. a primigravid patient

34–26. What is the failure rate of methotrexate therapy for an ectopic pregnancy?

a. 1 to 3%
b. 5 to 10%
c. 12 to 15%
d. 15 to 20%

34–27. Patients undergoing methotrxate therapy for ectopic pregnancy should be counseled to avoid which of the following?

a. alcohol
b. multivitamins with folic acid
c. sexual intercourse
d. all of the above

34–28. During the first week of successful single-dose methotrexate therapy for ectopic pregnancy, serum levels of β-hCG should decrease by how much?

a. 15%
b. 25%
c. 33%
d. 50%

34–29. Disadvantages of direct injection of drugs into ectopic pregnancy masses include which of the following?

a. lower success rates
b. need for laparoscopy or culdocentesis
c. worrisome side effects
d. all of the above

34–30. Abdominal pregnancy most commonly results from reimplantation after which of the following?

a. dehiscence of uterine scar
b. physical trauma
c. rupture of tubal pregnancy
d. induced abortion

34–31. Which is the preferred management of the placenta in abdominal pregnancies?

a. leave in situ
b. inject methotrexate into the placental mass
c. dissect off the implantation site
d. await spontaneous separation intraoperatively

34–32. Which of the following is a component of Spiegelberg criteria for ovarian pregnancy?

a. intact tube is on affected side
b. fetal sac occupies position of the ovary
c. ovarian ligament must connect uterus and ovary
d. all of the above

34–33. Which of the following has caused an increase in the incidence of cervical pregnancies?

a. high cesarean section rates
b. in vitro fertilization
c. advancing maternal age
d. increased use of cervical loop excision

34–34. What is the preferred method of therapy for a cervical pregnancy in a stable patient?

a. hysterectomy
b. cerclage
c. embolization
d. chemotherapy with methotrexate

35

Abnormalities of the Reproductive Tract

35–1. Which of the following is commonly associated with müllerian duct deformities?

    a. cardiac anomalies
    b. renal anomalies
    c. gastrointestinal tract abnormalities
    d. limb anomalies

35–2. The müllerian ducts fuse to form the uterus at what gestational age?

    a. 5 weeks
    b. 10 weeks
    c. 15 weeks
    d. 20 weeks

35–3. Dissolution of the uterine septum to form the uterine cavity is completed by what gestational age?

    a. 5 weeks
    b. 10 weeks
    c. 15 weeks
    d. 20 weeks

35–4. The vagina forms between the müllerian tubercle and which of the following?

    a. mesonephric ducts
    b. ureteral ducts
    c. urogenital sinus
    d. uterus

35–5. The fused müllerian ducts give rise to all EXCEPT which of the following structures?

    a. cervix
    b. upper vagina
    c. uterine body
    d. vulva

35–6. A transverse vaginal septum is thought to result from which of the following?

    a. defective canalization of the vagina
    b. lack of fusion of the müllerian ducts

    c. unilateral müllerian duct atresia
    d. in utero infection

35–7. What is the sensitivity of ultrasound screening for uterine anomalies?

    a. 5%
    b. 20%
    c. 40%
    d. 90%

35–8. What percentage of women with müllerian defects have associated auditory defects?

    a. <1
    b. 15
    c. 33
    d. 55

35–9. A noncommunicating rudimentary uterine horn commonly leads to what gynecologic problems?

    a. dysmenorrhea
    b. endometriosis
    c. infertility
    d. all of the above

35–10. Pregnancy outcome in the presence of a unicornuate uterus shows what rate of fetal wastage?

    a. 10%
    b. 20%
    c. 40%
    d. 80%

35–11. What is the rate of breech presentation in uterine didelphys?

    a. 10%
    b. 20%
    c. 40%
    d. 80%

35–12. What is the incidence of spontaneous abortion in septate uteri?

　a. 10 to 20%
　b. 20 to 30%
　c. 40 to 50%
　d. 80 to 90%

35–13. Prophylactic cervical cerclages are indicated for women with which condition?

　a. unicornuate uterus
　b. septate uterus
　c. transvaginal septum
　d. all of the above

35–14. Transabdominal metroplasty is used to repair which uterine anomaly?

　a. arcuate uterus
　b. bicornuate uterus
　c. septate uterus
　d. unicornuate uterus

35–15. Hysteroscopic therapy is best utilized for which uterine anomaly?

　a. bicornuate uterus
　b. septate uterus
　c. uterine didelphys
　d. unicornuate uterus

35–16. What percentage of women exposed to diethylstilbestrol (DES) in utero have identifiable structural variations in the cervix and vagina?

　a. <1
　b. 5 to 10
　c. 25 to 50
　d. 66 to 75

35–17. Which of the following is NOT increased in DES-exposed women?

　a. ectopic pregnancy
　b. multiple gestation
　c. preterm delivery
　d. spontaneous abortion

35–18. DES-exposed women are at increased risk of clear-cell adenocarcinoma of which of the following?

　a. breast
　b. cervix
　c. uterus
　d. vagina

35–19. During pregnancy, Bartholin abscesses are caused by *Neisseria gonorrhoeae* in what percentage of cases?

　a. 10
　b. 20

　c. 40
　d. 80

35–20. How many women worldwide have undergone a form of female genital mutilation?

　a. 80,000
　b. 800,000
　c. 8,000,000
　d. 80,000,000

35–21. What is the form of female genital mutilation which causes the most serious medical and obstetrical complications?

　a. complete clitoridectomy
　b. hymenectomy
　c. infibulation
　d. partial vulvectomy

35–22. What is the most common type of fistula formation after prolonged obstructed labor?

　a. cervicovaginal
　b. rectovaginal
　c. uterovaginal
　d. vesicovaginal

35–23. Cervical stenosis diagnosed during labor is most commonly the result of which of the following?

　a. congenital abnormalities
　b. female genital mutilation
　c. prior conization of the cervix
　d. trauma from prior delivery

35–24. Which of the following is NOT a symptom of an incarcerated uterus?

　a. inability to void
　b. lower abdominal pain
　c. involuntary urinary leakage
　d. fever or chills

35–25. In a woman at term and in labor, an elongated vagina passing above the level of the fetal head likely represents which of the following?

　a. Bandl's refraction ring
　b. rupture of the uterus
　c. sacculation
　d. the presence of a leiomyoma

35–26. During pregnancy, a 14-cm myoma is noted. It is followed throughout pregnancy and the size does not change. This is likely due to which of the following?

　a. carneous degeneration
　b. decreased estrogen receptors
　c. increased epidermal growth factor
　d. increased progesterone receptors

35–27. What percentage of myomas show a significant size change during pregnancy?

    a. 25
    b. 50
    c. 75
    d. 100

35–28. What is the best pregnancy management for a 35-year-old nullipara who undergoes a myomectomy in which the endometrial cavity was entered?

    a. labor allowed
    b. labor allowed, with low forceps to shorten second stage
    c. cesarean section near term prior to labor
    d. oxytocin induction at 38 weeks

35–29. What is the most frequent and serious complication of benign ovarian cysts during pregnancy?

    a. malignant transformation
    b. rupture
    c. torsion
    d. dystocia

35–30. Which of the following ovarian neoplasms is diagnosed most often during pregnancy?

    a. benign cystic teratoma
    b. endodermal sinus tumor
    c. follicular cyst
    d. serous cystadenocarcinoma

35–31. What is the best management for a patient with a simple cyst measuring 8 cm found on pelvic examination and sonography during the eighth week of pregnancy?

    a. immediate laparotomy
    b. laparotomy at 16 to 20 weeks
    c. observation and serial sonography
    d. laparoscopic evaluation with drainage of cyst

35–32. A fetal sonographic study and amniotic fluid alphafetoprotein are normal, but an elevated serum alphafetoprotein is noted at 16 weeks. What is the most likely diagnosis?

    a. benign cystic teratoma
    b. dysgerminoma
    c. endodermal sinus tumor
    d. mucinous cystadenoma

35–33. What is the best course of action for a complex 12-cm adnexal mass noted at 18 weeks' gestation?

    a. observation
    b. laparotomy after delivery
    c. immediate laparotomy
    d. sonographically directed aspiration

X SECTION

Fetal Abnormalities: Inherited and Acquired Disorders

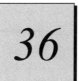

Genetics

36–1. What percentage of newborns have a structural anomaly?

    a. <1
    b. 2 to 3
    c. 7 to 8
    d. 10

36–2. How many genes comprise the haploid human genome?

    a. 20,000
    b. 40,000
    c. 80,000
    d. 120,000

36–3. Which of the following is NOT an associated anomaly in CHARGE?

    a. heart defects
    b. growth deficiency
    c. coloboma
    d. gonad anomalies

36–4. What is the approximate percentage of chromosomal abnormalities in live-born infants?

    a. 0.01
    b. 0.1
    c. 1.0
    d. 10

36–5. What is the frequency of chromosomal abnormalities among stillbirths and neonatal deaths?

    a. <1%
    b. 3%
    c. 6 to 11%
    d. 15 to 20%

36–6. What is the most common chromosomal abnormality in early spontaneous abortions?

    a. 45,X
    b. 47,XXY
    c. 47,XXX
    d. trisomy 16

36–7. Which of the following types of genetic disease is related to paternal age?

    a. trisomies
    b. multifactorial diseases
    c. translocations
    d. autosomal dominant disease

36–8. What is the frequency of new dominant mutations in newborns whose fathers are older than 40?

    a. 0.3%
    b. 1.0%
    c. 3.0%
    d. 10.0%

36–9. In a conception induced by intracytoplasmic sperm injection (ICSI), the fetuses are at risk for which of the following?

    a. monosomy X
    b. trisomy 16
    c. trisomy 21
    d. Y chromosome deletions

115

36–10. Which of the following is NOT a characteristic finding in newborns with Down syndrome?

   a. large head
   b. flattened occiput
   c. upslanting palpebral fissures
   d. clinodactyly

36–11. What is the recurrence risk of trisomy 21 in the subsequent children of young mothers?

   a. 1%
   b. 5%
   c. 12%
   d. 25%

36–12. What is the approximate risk of trisomy 21 in a 33-year-old woman?

   a. 1 in 70
   b. 1 in 150
   c. 1 in 500
   d. 1 in 1400

36–13. What is the approximate risk of trisomy 21 in a 40-year-old woman?

   a. 1 in 70
   b. 1 in 150
   c. 1 in 500
   d. 1 in 1200

36–14. What percentage of Down syndrome pregnancies in women 35 years and older will be lost by 16 weeks (time of amniocentesis)?

   a. <5
   b. 12
   c. 31
   d. 53

36–15. Trisomy 18 (Edwards syndrome) occurs in how many newborns?

   a. 1 in 1000
   b. 1 in 8000
   c. 1 in 16,000
   d. 1 in 24,000

36–16. Which of the following is NOT a facial feature in trisomy 18?

   a. prominent occiput
   b. malformed auricles
   c. short palpebral fissures
   d. large mouth

36–17. Which of the following is NOT an anomaly of trisomy 13 or Patau syndrome?

   a. cleft lip/palate
   b. omphalocele
   c. macrocephaly
   d. radial aplasia

36–18. Which of the following is usually NOT found in offspring with 47, XXY?

   a. small testicles
   b. gynecomastia
   c. short stature
   d. azoospermia

36–19. Which of the following traits is NOT characteristic of offspring with an extra Y chromosome (47,XYY)?

   a. tall
   b. severe acne
   c. learning disabilities
   d. severe mental retardation

36–20. Which of the following traits is usually NOT found in offspring with 45,X monosomy?

   a. short
   b. webbing of the neck
   c. coarctation of the aorta
   d. mental retardation

36–21. What deletion is responsible for the cri du chat syndrome?

   a. del (4p)
   b. del (5p)
   c. del (21p)
   d. del (Xp)

36–22. Which specific deletion is associated with Wolf-Hirschhorn syndrome?

   a. 2q
   b. 4p
   c. 6q
   d. 8p

36–23. Which of the following chromosomes is generally NOT involved in Robertsonian translocation?

   a. 1
   b. 13
   c. 14
   d. 21

36–24. What is the approximate recurrence risk of a translocation Down syndrome that occurred spontaneously (i.e., neither parent is a carrier)?

   a. 1%
   b. 5%
   c. 25%
   d. 50%

36–25. In the event of a 14/21 translocation in the father, what is the chance of having a child with Down syndrome?

    a. 1 to 2%
    b. 5%
    c. 15%
    d. 50%

36–26. Approximately what percentage of couples with recurrent pregnancy loss will have either a balanced Robertsonian or reciprocal translocation?

    a. <5
    b. 10
    c. 25
    d. 50

36–27. In which type of inversion is the inverted material from one arm and the centromere NOT within the inverted segment?

    a. pericentric
    b. paracentric
    c. unicentric
    d. monocentric

36–28. Mosaicism from which of the following chromosomes is NOT due to a partial conversion of a meiotic error?

    a. 2
    b. 9
    c. 16
    d. 22

36–29. Which of the following is NOT a characteristic of autosomal dominant inheritance?

    a. a single copy of the mutant gene is present
    b. horizontal transmission
    c. no skipped generations
    d. 50% chance of transmission to the offspring

36–30. What is the mechanism by which some autosomal dominant diseases appear to occur at earlier ages with subsequent generations?

    a. penetrance
    b. imprinting
    c. variable expressivity
    d. anticipation

36–31. Which of the following conditions is NOT inherited in an autosomal dominant fashion?

    a. achondroplasia
    b. adult polycystic kidney disease
    c. Marfan syndrome
    d. cystic fibrosis

36–32. Which of the following is NOT an autosomal recessive disease?

    a. Tay-Sachs disease
    b. congenital adrenal hyperplasia
    c. myotonic dystrophy
    d. sickle cell anemia

36–33. Which of the following is an X-linked disease?

    a. Von Willebrand disease
    b. neurofibromatosis
    c. Hunter syndrome
    d. Tay-Sachs disease

36–34. Mothers with phenylketonuria (PKU) are at increased risk of having a child with which of the following disorders?

    a. hydrocephaly
    b. spina bifida
    c. skeletal dysplasia
    d. mental retardation

36–35. What proportion of genes do second-degree relatives share?

    a. 1/2
    b. 1/4
    c. 1/8
    d. 1/16

36–36. What is the risk of having anomalous children resulting from incest (brother–sister or parent–child)?

    a. 1 to 5%
    b. 10 to 15%
    c. 25 to 30%
    d. 35 to 40%

36–37. Which of the following is an example of an X-linked dominant disorder?

    a. vitamin D-resistant rickets
    b. hemophilia A
    c. hemophilia B
    d. muscular dystrophy

36–38. Which of the following trinucleotide repeats is associated with the fragile X gene (FMR-1)?

    a. CGG
    b. CAG
    c. GCT
    d. GGG

36–39. What percentage of females with full mutations for fragile X syndrome will have some form of mental retardation?

    a. 5
    b. 25
    c. 50
    d. 100

36–40. Which of the following characteristics is NOT a usual manifestation of the fragile X syndrome in affected males?

    a. autism
    b. macro-orchidism
    c. mental retardation
    d. short stature

36–41. What is the best method for detection of both the size of the trinucleotide expansion and methylation of the fragile X gene?

    a. fluorescence in situ hybridization (FISH)
    b. cytogenetic techniques
    c. polymerase chain reaction (PCR)
    d. restriction endonuclease digestion and Southern blot

36–42. Which of the following X-linked conditions is an example of a trinucleotide repeat disorder?

    a. myotonic dystrophy
    b. hemophilia A
    c. hemophilia B
    d. Hunter syndrome

36–43. The gene containing the unstable trinucleotide repeat (ACG) and responsible for myotonic dystrophy is located on what chromosome?

    a. X
    b. Y
    c. 9
    d. 21

36–44. What is the mechanism by which the expression of a particular disease is dependent on whether the mutant gene was of paternal or maternal origin?

    a. penetrance
    b. imprinting
    c. uniparental disomy
    d. anticipation

36–45. Angleman and Prader-Willi syndromes are due to imprinting of which chromosome?

    a. 5
    b. 10
    c. 15
    d. 20

36–46. What is the mechanism by which both members of one pair of chromosomes are inherited from the same parent?

    a. imprinting
    b. variable expressivity
    c. uniparental disomy
    d. anticipation

36–47. Which of the following is NOT transmitted via multifactorial inheritance?

    a. ocular albinism
    b. pyloric stenosis
    c. clubfoot
    d. neural tube defect

36–48. Which of the following conditions may be prevented by preconceptional folic acid supplementation?

    a. congenital heart defects
    b. cleft lip
    c. fragile X syndrome
    d. neural tube defects

36–49. What is the term for the failure of the forebrain, meninges, vault of skull, and scalp to form?

    a. exencephaly
    b. anencephaly
    c. encephalocele
    d. iniencephaly

36–50. What is the number of base pairs in the human genome?

    a. 1 million
    b. 3 million
    c. 1 billion
    d. 3 billion

36–51. What percentage of the genome encodes genes?

    a. <1
    b. ~10
    c. ~25
    d. ~50

36–52. What are multiple coding sequences of a gene called?

    a. exons
    b. introns
    c. promoters
    d. demoters

36–53. Which of the following diseases is caused by a single mutation?

    a. cystic fibrosis
    b. myotonic dystrophy
    c. diabetes
    d. sickle cell anemia

36–54. Imprinting may be due to which of the following?

    a. polymorphism
    b. methylation
    c. new mutations
    d. replication

36–55. FISH is used to detect which of the following?

  a. new mutations
  b. aneuploidy
  c. polyploidy
  d. Fragile X

36–56. Southern blotting is a technique used to identify which of the following?

  a. histones
  b. deoxyribonucleic acid (DNA)
  c. ribonucleic acid (RNA)
  d. proteins

36–57. How many mutations have been shown to cause cystic fibrosis?

  a. 100
  b. 250
  c. 500
  d. 750

36–58. What is the in vitro technique in which large amounts of specific DNA sequences can be synthesized over a relatively short period of time?

  a. Southern blotting
  b. restriction endonuclease reaction
  c. polymerase chain reactions
  d. allele-specific oligonucleotide reaction

37

Prenatal Diagnosis and Fetal Therapy

37–1. What percentage of all pediatric hospital admissions result from genetic disorders?

  a. 1
  b. 5
  c. 10
  d. 25

37–2. What percentage of conceptions are aneuploid?

  a. 1
  b. 4
  c. 8
  d. 12

37–3. What percentage of first-trimester abortions are due to aneuploidy?

  a. 5
  b. 10
  c. 25
  d. 50

37–4. What percentage of stillbirths and neonatal deaths are attributable to chromosomal abnormalities?

  a. 1 to 3
  b. 5 to 7
  c. 10 to 12
  d. 15 to 20

37–5. What percentage of newborns have chromosomal abnormalities compatible with life?

  a. 0.15
  b. 0.65
  c. 1.15
  d. 6.5

37–6. Routine amniocentesis of all women over age 35 would detect what percentage of Down syndrome pregnancies?

  a. 10
  b. 20
  c. 40
  d. 80

37–7. At term, what is the risk of an aneuploid fetus in a 35-year-old woman?

    a. 1 in 50
    b. 1 in 100
    c. 1 in 200
    d. 1 in 300

37–8. What is the risk of recurrence of trisomy (same or different) in a young mother who has previously had a pregnancy complicated by an autosomal trisomy.

    a. 1%
    b. 3%
    c. 5%
    d. 10%

37–9. Which of the following is NOT an accepted indication for an invasive fetal diagnostic procedure?

    a. dizygotic twin pregnancy, maternal age over 31
    b. either parent has chromosomal inversion or translocation
    c. patient anxiety
    d. previous infant with autosomal trisomy

37–10. With regard to multifactorial or polygenic birth defects, what is the recurrence risk in first-degree relatives?

    a. 0.5%
    b. 1.0%
    c. 2.0 to 3.0%
    d. 10.0 to 15.0%

37–11. At what gestational age should a sonographic evaluation and fetal echocardiogram first be performed if the fetus is at risk for a cardiac malformation?

    a. 6 to 8 weeks
    b. 10 to 12 weeks
    c. 20 to 22 weeks
    d. 26 to 28 weeks

37–12. Which of the following is NOT an indication for targeted ultrasound and amniocentesis to evaluate for neural tube defects (NTDs)?

    a. family history of NTDs
    b. poorly controlled maternal diabetes
    c. high maternal fever early in gestation
    d. use of acetaminophen in first trimester

37–13. Exposure to which drugs is associated with increased risk of NTDs in the fetus?

    a. carbamazepine
    b. isotretinoin

    c. valproic acid
    d. all of the above

37–14. Individuals of Jewish ancestry are at increased risk for which of the following diseases?

    a. Canavan
    b. Gaucher
    c. Tay-Sachs
    d. all of the above

37–15. Cystic fibrosis (CF) is the most common monogenic disorder in persons of which ethnic background?

    a. African
    b. Asian
    c. Mediterranean
    d. Northern European

37–16. What percentage of children with neural tube defects are born into families with no prior history?

    a. 1
    b. 25
    c. 50
    d. 95

37–17. Which of the following structures is NOT involved in the synthesis of alpha-fetoprotein (AFP), a glycoprotein synthesized by the fetus?

    a. bone marrow
    b. yolk sac
    c. gastrointestinal tract
    d. liver

37–18. At what week of gestation is AFP concentration highest in both fetal serum and amniotic fluid?

    a. week 7
    b. week 11
    c. week 13
    d. week 17

37–19. Maternal serum AFP screening for NTDs is most sensitive at what gestational age?

    a. 8 to 10 weeks
    b. 12 to 14 weeks
    c. 16 to 18 weeks
    d. 20 to 22 weeks

37–20. Levels of maternal serum AFP are influenced by which of the following maternal factors?

    a. age
    b. race
    c. weight
    d. all of the above

37–21. How large an elevation (as measured in multiples of the median) of maternal serum AFP is considered abnormal for NTD screening purposes?

a. ≥0.5 to 1.5
b. ≥2.0 to 2.5
c. ≥3.0 to 3.5
d. ≥4.0 to 4.5

37–22. Which of the following accounts for the largest proportion of elevated maternal serum AFPs in the absence of a fetal anomaly?

a. incorrect gestational dating
b. undiagnosed fetal death
c. multiple gestation
d. maternal obesity

37–23. What percentage of elevated tests for maternal serum AFP represent a fetus with an NTD?

a. 2 to 6
b. 8 to 12
c. 12 to 16
d. 20 to 24

37–24. What percentage of maternal serum AFP tests are reported as abnormally elevated?

a. 0.5 to 2
b. 3 to 5
c. 7 to 9
d. 11 to 13

37–25. What is the most appropriate initial response to a maternal serum AFP that is less than 3 multiples of the median at 18 weeks' gestation?

a. amniocentesis
b. recommend pregnancy termination
c. repeat test in 4 weeks
d. targeted ultrasound

37–26. Which of the following cranial ultrasound findings is NOT associated with NTDs?

a. banana sign
b. cabbage sign
c. lemon sign
d. ventriculomegaly

37–27. What percentage of fetuses with spina bifida will have some type of cranial anomaly detected by ultrasound?

a. 99
b. 58
c. 25
d. 5

37–28. The likelihood of a neural tube defect associated with an elevated maternal serum AFP is decreased by approximately what percentage if the ultrasound screening is normal?

a. 65
b. 70
c. 95
d. 100

37–29. Which of the following fetal abnormalities is NOT a cause of elevated maternal serum AFP?

a. bladder exstrophy
b. cardiac malformation
c. cystic hygroma
d. oligohydramnios

37–30. What percentage of fetuses with isolated neural tube defects will have aneuploidy?

a. 2 to 7
b. 10 to 17
c. 25 to 30
d. 55 to 60

37–31. In a woman with elevated maternal serum AFP and normal amniotic fluid AFP, what further test should be done on the amniotic fluid?

a. acetylcholinesterase
b. C-reactive protein
c. fetal fibronectin
d. Δ OD 450

37–32. Unexplained elevated abnormal AFP levels are associated with which of the following?

a. fetal death
b. increased perinatal mortality
c. preterm delivery
d. all of the above

37–33. What percentage of Down syndrome fetuses are born to women under the age of 35?

a. 10
b. 30
c. 60
d. 80

37–34. Which of the following markers is NOT included in the "triple screen" for Down syndrome?

a. maternal serum AFP
b. placental lactogen
c. unconjugated estriol
d. chorionic gonadotropin

37–35. What percentage of fetuses with Down syndrome can be detected utilizing the triple screen?

    a. 25 to 30
    b. 60 to 70
    c. 80 to 90
    d. 100

37–36. What percentage of screen-positive multiple-marker tests actually represent a fetus with Down syndrome or other aneuploidy?

    a. 6
    b. 26
    c. 46
    d. 66

37–37. Fundamental problems of genetic testing for various diseases include which of the following?

    a. diagnosis unreliable
    b. treatments not available
    c. wide range of phenotypes
    d. all of the above

37–38. What is the most common cause of familial mental retardation?

    a. Down syndrome
    b. fragile X syndrome
    c. trisomy 13
    d. 47, XXY genotype

37–39. What is the carrier rate for the CF gene in whites of Northern European descent?

    a. 1 in 10
    b. 1 in 25
    c. 1 in 100
    d. 1 in 250

37–40. How many CF gene mutations have been described thus far, rendering tests for the CF gene imperfect?

    a. 10
    b. 75
    c. 100
    d. over 750

37–41. What is the most rational initial approach to major fetal malformations discovered by ultrasound?

    a. fetal karyotype
    b. maternal serum AFP
    c. parental karyotyping
    d. serial ultrasounds

37–42. According to the RADIUS trial, what percentage of major fetal anomalies may be detected prior to 24 weeks' gestation utilizing routine ultrasound of all pregnancies?

    a. 17
    b. 37
    c. 57
    d. 77

37–43. Which of the following early ultrasound findings is most strongly associated with Down syndrome?

    a. enlarged cardiac ventricles
    b. increased fetal muscular tone
    c. thickened nuchal fold
    d. vertebral anomalies

37–44. What is the fetal loss rate for genetic amniocentesis performed between 15 and 22 weeks' gestation?

    a. 1 in 50
    b. 1 in 100
    c. 1 in 200
    d. 1 in 500

37–45. Which of the following is a disadvantage of first-trimester amniocentesis compared with second-trimester amniocentesis?

    a. higher pregnancy loss rates
    b. increased foot deformities
    c. increased membrane rupture
    d. all of the above

37–46. Which of the following diagnostic procedures shows the highest fetal loss rate?

    a. second trimester amniocentesis
    b. transcervical chorionic villus sampling
    c. transabdominal chorionic villus sampling
    d. all have approximately equal loss rates

37–47. To minimize the risk of causing structural fetal defects, chorionic villus sampling is best done at what point in gestation?

    a. before 6 weeks
    b. before 9 weeks
    c. after 9 weeks
    d. after 12 weeks

37–48. In which of the following clinical situations would cordocentesis be appropriate?

    a. unexplained fetal hydrops
    b. red cell alloimmunization
    c. severe, unexplained fetal growth restriction
    d. all of the above

37–49. Procedure-related fetal loss from cordocentesis has been reported to be approximately what percentage?

    a. <0.5
    b. 1.0
    c. 3.0
    d. 5.0

37–50. What percentage of monozygotic twin pregnancies develop complications from twin-to-twin transfusion syndrome?

    a. <1
    b. 5
    c. 15
    d. 25

37–51. Currently, what is the most practical therapeutic intervention used to alleviate twin-to-twin transfusion syndrome?

    a. amniocentesis to decrease hydramnios of the recipient twin
    b. surgical joining of the two amniotic sacs

    c. feticide of donor twin
    d. laser ablation of vascular anastomoses

37–52. Fetal medical therapy is LEAST likely to show beneficial effects in which of the following fetal conditions?

    a. cardiac arrhythmias
    b. congenital adrenal hyperplasia
    c. maternal–fetal infections
    d. posterior urethral valves

37–53. In assessing the usefulness of fetal surgery to correct or ameliorate major malformations, which of the following should be considered?

    a. natural history and prognosis
    b. high incidence of genetic abnormalities
    c. maternal risks
    d. all of the above

38

Drugs and Medications

38–1. What percentage of children in the United States are born with a major birth defect?

    a. 1
    b. 3
    c. 5
    d. 7

38–2. What percentage of congenital anomalies (structural or functional) are caused by teratogens?

    a. 10
    b. 25
    c. 50
    d. 75

38–3. What is the average number of prescriptions, other than for vitamins, received by women during pregnancy in the United States?

    a. 1
    b. 3
    c. 5
    d. 7

38–4. What are identical defects with different etiologies called?

    a. hadegens
    b. parallel dysmorphisms
    c. phenocopies
    d. teratomas

38–5. Which of the following represents the preimplantation period?

   a. prefertilization
   b. fertilization to implantation
   c. fertilization through the 4 week
   d. fertilization through the 8 week

38–6. Which of the following represents the embryonic period?

   a. fertilization through week 6
   b. fertilization through week 10
   c. week 2 through 8
   d. week 1 through 12

38–7. Which of the following represents the fetal period?

   a. implantation through week 8
   b. implantation through week 12
   c. week 9 until term
   d. week 12 until term

38–8. Damage to a large number of cells during the embryonic period of development will likely result in which of the following?

   a. cell division to compensate for lost cells
   b. death of the embryo
   c. major structural malformations
   d. none of the above

38–9. Which of the following periods is most critical with regard to structural malformations?

   a. prefertilization
   b. zygote (ovum)
   c. embryonic
   d. fetal

38–10. By how many weeks of gestation is formation of the heart complete?

   a. 8
   b. 10
   c. 12
   d. 14

38–11. A relative risk greater than what value is generally needed to support an epidemiological link between a suspected teratogen and a birth defect?

   a. 1.5
   b. 2.0
   c. 3.0
   d. 4.0

38–12. What is the Federal Drug Administration (FDA) category for drugs for which controlled studies in humans have demonstrated no fetal risk?

   a. A
   b. B
   c. C
   d. D

38–13. What is the FDA category for drugs for which there are no adequate studies available?

   a. B
   b. C
   c. D
   d. X

38–14. Which of the following drugs is an FDA category X drug?

   a. coumarin
   b. isotretinoin
   c. acyclovir
   d. diazepam

38–15. What is the correlation between the FDA classification of drugs (i.e., A, B, C, D and X) and actual teratogenic risk?

   a. excellent
   b. good
   c. fair
   d. poor

38–16. What is the mechanism by which most teratogens act?

   a. alteration of tissue growth
   b. cell death
   c. errors in cellular differentiation
   d. unknown

38–17. Disturbance in folic acid metabolic pathways causes birth defects in all of the following structural areas EXCEPT which of the following?

   a. cardiac
   b. neural tube
   c. lip and palate
   d. reproductive tract

38–18. Periconceptual folate supplementation may be effective in preventing birth defects in mothers taking which type of medication?

   a. anticonvulsants
   b. corticosteroids
   c. hypoglycemics including insulin
   d. phenothiazines

38–19. Which of the following enzymes is needed to detoxify the oxidative intermediates of several potentially teratogenic drugs?

    a. areneoxidase
    b. aromatase
    c. epoxide hydrolase
    d. folate dehydrogenase

38–20. Which of the following women have an increased risk of birth defects?

    a. epileptic women on carbamazepine
    b. epileptic women on hydantoin
    c. untreated epileptic women
    d. all of the above

38–21. Special genes that play an essential role in the establishment of positional identity of structures along the body axis are known by which of the following terms?

    a. chronomorphic genes
    b. homeobox genes
    c. sequential transcription genes
    d. vertebrate morphometric genes

38–22. Paternal exposure to which of the following may cause an increase in early pregnancy losses?

    a. Agent Orange
    b. atomic radiation
    c. pesticides
    d. recreational drug use

38–23. Which of the following social or illicit substances is associated with mental retardation, cardiac defects, joint defects, and craniofacial anomalies?

    a. alcohol
    b. amphetamines
    c. lysergic acid
    d. heroin

38–24. How many drugs or substances are suspected or proven human teratogens?

    a. 12
    b. 22
    c. 220
    d. 1200

38–25. What is the safe daily threshold dose of absolute alcohol in pregnancy?

    a. 1 oz
    b. 3 oz
    c. 5 oz
    d. not established

38–26. Fetal alcohol syndrome is diagnosed prenatally by what method?

    a. amniocentesis
    b. cannot be diagnosed prenatally
    c. history of heavy alcohol consumption
    d. sonography

38–27. What percentage of infants born to epileptic mothers have malformations?

    a. 5
    b. 7
    c. 9
    d. 11

38–28. Which group of defects are seen in infants of epilepitic mothers at a rate almost 10 times that of the general population?

    a. facial clefts
    b. digital abnormalities
    c. cardiac anomalies
    d. gastrointestinal strictures

38–29. What percentage of exposed infants show recognizable features of fetal hydantoin syndrome?

    a. 1 to 3
    b. 7 to 10
    c. 13 to 17
    d. 21 to 27

38–30. What is the estimated risk of spina bifida from first-trimester valproic acid exposure?

    a. 1 to 2%
    b. 5 to 10%
    c. 20 to 25%
    d. 30 to 40%

38–31. Which of the following abnormalities is NOT part of the fetal warfarin syndrome?

    a. nasal hypoplasia
    b. stippled bone epiphyses
    c. ventral wall defects
    d. cerebral malformations

38–32. Which of the following antihypertensives has been reported to be associated with congenital hypocalvaria, renal tubular dysgenesis, oligohydramnios, and neonatal hypotension?

    a. sodium nitroprusside
    b. captopril
    c. clonidine
    d. labetalol

38-33. Which of the following is true of high doses of vitamin A ingested during pregnancy?

   a. It is a potent teratogen.
   b. Supplementation higher than recommended daily allowance is not advised.
   c. Causes slightly increased early pregnancy loss rate.
   d. Should be given at high doses only to treat related maternal diseases.

38-34. Which craniofacial defect is most strongly associated with use of isotretinoin?

   a. malformed or absent ears
   b. flattened nasal bridge
   c. hypoplastic upper lip
   d. microphthalmia

38-35. What percentage of infants exposed in utero to isotretinoin will have a major malformation?

   a. 5
   b. 20
   c. 33
   d. 50

38-36. Which of the following compounds is both highly teratogenic and has been detected in serum almost 3 years after cessation of therapy?

   a. isotretinoin
   b. etretinate
   c. tretinoin
   d. vitamin A

38-37. What is the relative risk of birth defects with use of topical tretinoin for acne?

   a. 1.0
   b. 2.0
   c. 3.5
   d. 4.5

38-38. During what period of gestation can exposure of a female fetus to exogenous androgens cause complete masculinization?

   a. 2 to 5 weeks
   b. 7 to 12 weeks
   c. 14 to 18 weeks
   d. 22 to 24 weeks

38-39. Which of the following hormones may cause virilization of the female fetus?

   a. clomid
   b. danazol
   c. prednisone
   d. all of the above

38-40. In utero exposure to diethylstilbestrol causes which of the following?

   a. male infertility
   b. testicular cancer
   c. uterine malformations
   d. vaginal adenocarcinoma

38-41. Which antineoplastic drug is most commonly associated with missing or hypoplastic digits on the hands and feet?

   a. aminopterin
   b. cyclophosphamide
   c. methotrexate
   d. platinum

38-42. Which antineoplastic agent is associated with severe cranial and limb abnormalities?

   a. bleomycin
   b. cyclophosphamide
   c. methotrexate
   d. platinum

38-43. What is the most typical problem seen with tetracycline ingestion during the fetal period of gestation?

   a. alopecia
   b. staining of the deciduous teeth
   c. hypoplastic fingernails and toenails
   d. peeling and discolored skin

38-44. Which of the following antimicrobials is known to cause fetal VIII nerve damage?

   a. ciprofloxacin
   b. erythromycin
   c. streptomycin
   d. tetracycline

38-45. Which of the following antibiotics given to the mother near delivery may result in significant hyperbilirubinemia in the newborn?

   a. penicillin
   b. cephalosporin
   c. clindamycin
   d. sulfonamides

38-46. Which of the following antibiotics is a folate antagonist?

   a. trimethoprim
   b. nitrofurantoin
   c. tetracycline
   d. erythromycin

38–47. Which of the following antifungal agents has been reported to be associated with conjoined twins in humans?

  a. nystatin
  b. clotrimazole
  c. amphotericin B
  d. griseofulvin

38–48. Which of the following antiviral drugs is used as an aerosol inhalation agent in intensive care nurseries and consistently produces hydrocephalus and limb abnormalities in rodents?

  a. acyclovir
  b. amantadine
  c. famciclovir
  d. ribavirin

38–49. There is a clear dose-dependent relation between tobacco smoking and which of the following?

  a. decreases in global intelligence scores
  b. fetal growth restriction
  c. degree of prematurity
  d. severity of pregnancy-induced hypertension

38–50. Fetuses carrying an allele for a rare polymorphism of transforming growth factor-alpha are at increased risk of which congenital malformations if their mothers smoke?

  a. cardiac anomalies
  b. cleft lip and/or palate
  c. limb deformities
  d. spina bifida

38–51. A large population-based U.S. study indicates what percentage of pregnancies involve cocaine exposure?

  a. 0.01
  b. 0.1
  c. 1.0
  d. 10.0

38–52. Which of the following complications is increased four-fold with maternal cocaine use?

  a. adult respiratory distress syndrome
  b. HELLP [hemolysis (H), elevated live enzymes (EL), and low platelets (LP)] syndrome
  c. placental abruption
  d. preeclampsia

38–53. The drug thalidomide, notorious for causing severe limb-reduction defects, and once again available, was originally used during what years?

  a. 1946 to 1950
  b. 1956 to 1960
  c. 1966 to 1970
  d. 1976 to 1980

38–54. Which of the following antibiotics has poor access to the fetus when given to the mother?

  a. penicillin
  b. erythromycin
  c. cephalosporins
  d. tetracyclines

38–55. Which of the following antibiotics is an alternative to an aminoglycoside?

  a. aztreonam
  b. azithromycin
  c. sulfonamide
  d. clindamycin

38–56. Which of the following antibiotics is the drug of choice for *Clostridium dificile* pseudomembranous colitis?

  a. ampicillin
  b. vancomycin
  c. aztreonam
  d. imipenem

38–57. Which of the following antibiotics has been reported to cause irreversible arthropathy in immature animals?

  a. fluoroquinolones
  b. vancomycin
  c. nitrofurantoin
  d. sulfonamides

38–58. Which of the following antibiotics is useful for the treatment of *Mycobacterium avium* complex (MAC) in patients with human immunodeficiency virus infection?

  a. streptomycin
  b. vancomycin
  c. isoniazid
  d. rifabutin

38–59. Acyclovir, used to treat herpes simplex and varicella infections, is ranked as what category for use in pregnancy?

  a. A
  b. B
  c. C
  d. X

38–60. Which of the following antiviral drugs is utilized to prevent or modify influenza infections and is a likely teratogen?

  a. acyclovir
  b. ganciclovir
  c. ribavirin
  d. amantadine

38–61. Which of the following antiparasitic agents has been shown to produce no adverse effects in over 1700 infants who were exposed to it in the first trimester?

   a. metronidazole
   b. lindane
   c. pyrimethamine
   d. spiramycin

38–62. Which of the following should NOT be used as first-line therapy for pediculosis pubis during pregnancy due to potential central nervous system toxicity in adults and, perhaps, fetuses?

   a. crotamiton
   b. lindane
   c. piperonyl butoxide
   d. pyrethrins

38–63. Which of the following antibiotics has been utilized for the treatment of toxoplasmosis without evidence of fetal effects?

   a. lindane
   b. chloroquine
   c. spiramycin
   d. metronidazole

38–64. Which antiarrhythmic drug should NOT be used in pregnancy due to the potential for fetal and neonatal hypothyroidism?

   a. amiodarone
   b. bretylium
   c. diltiazem
   d. procainamide

38–65. Which of the following antihypertensives could theoretically cause accumulation of cyanide in the fetal liver?

   a. methyldopa
   b. nitroprusside
   c. labetolol
   d. nifedipine

38–66. Formerly thought to cause new growth restriction and other adverse neonatal effects, which of the following antihypertensive drugs is probably safe for use in pregnancy and perhaps even beneficial?

   a. hydrochlorothiazide
   b. labetalol
   c. sodium nitroprusside
   d. verapamil

38–67. Calcium-channel antagonists, particularly verapamil, have been implicated as a cause of which of the following?

   a. anencephaly and spina bifida
   b. cardiac malformations
   c. limb defects
   d. unexplained fetal death

38–68. Which of the following diuretics has the theoretical potential for causing feminization of male fetuses?

   a. spironolactone
   b. ethacrynic acid
   c. acetazolamide
   d. hydrochlorothiazide

38–69. What is the incidence of deep vein thrombosis or pulmonary embolus in pregnancy, and therefore, fetal exposure to anticoagulants?

   a. 1 in 500
   b. 1 in 2500
   c. 1 in 5000
   d. 1 in 25,000

38–70. Which of the following antiasthmatic drugs has been shown to cause adverse fetal effects in humans?

   a. albuterol
   b. cromolyn
   c. corticosteroids
   d. none have shown adverse effects

38–71. What is the approximate molecular weight of enoxapanin (low-molecular-weight heparin)?

   a. 365
   b. 1000
   c. 4000
   d. 20,000

38–72. What FDA class drug is diazepam?

   a. category A
   b. category B
   c. category C
   d. category D

38–73. Which of the following anticonvulsant medications is NOT associated with the "anticonvulsant embryopathy" but is implicated in congenital cardiovascular defects and decreased cognitive function?

   a. phenytoin
   b. carbamazepine
   c. trimethadione
   d. phenobarbital

38–74. Which of the following antidepressants belongs to the selective serotonin re-uptake inhibitor (SSRI) class and appears safe for use in pregnancy?

    a. lithium
    b. nortriptyline
    c. monamine oxidase inhibitors
    d. fluoxetine

38–75. Which of the following psychotropic drugs has been associated with a slightly increased risk of fetal cardiovascular anomalies, especially Ebstein anomaly?

    a. amitriptyline
    b. imipramine
    c. lithium
    d. chlorpromazine

38–76. Which class of drugs is associated with hyperthermic crises with coincident administration of meperidine or certain anesthetic agents?

    a. benzodiazepines
    b. monoamine oxidase inhibitors
    c. SSRIs
    d. tricyclic antidepressants

38–77. For which indication are phenothiazines most often used in pregnancy?

    a. anxiety disorders
    b. depression
    c. hyperemesis
    d. psychosis

38–78. Which of the following analgesics has been associated with constriction of the fetus ductus arteriosus?

    a. meperidine
    b. indomethacin
    c. acetaminophen
    d. butorphanol

38–79. In what percentage of U.S. pregnancies are salicylates and/or acetaminophen used?

    a. 5
    b. 15
    c. 25
    d. 50

38–80. Which narcotic analgesic is most likely to be associated with a fetal sinusoidal heart rate pattern?

    a. butorphanol
    b. codeine
    c. meperidine
    d. morphine

38–81. Epidemiological studies of pregnancy loss and teratogenicity associated with occupational exposure to anesthetic inhalation agents show what association?

    a. weak increased risk
    b. definite increased risk
    c. no increased risk
    d. no studies have been done

38–82. What is the association between oral contraceptive use during the first trimester and congenital malformations?

    a. slightly increased risk
    b. greatly increased risk
    c. no increased risk
    d. insufficient information available

38–83. Which of the following statements regarding herbal remedies in pregnancy are true?

    a. The identity and quantity of ingredients are usually unknown.
    b. No human or animal studies of teratogenicity are available.
    c. Knowledge of complications is often limited to acute toxicities.
    d. All of the above.

38–84. What percentage of women are estimated to use illicit drugs, alcohol, and/or tobacco during pregnancy?

    a. 1 to 2
    b. 3 to 5
    c. 5 to 9
    d. 10 to 20

38–85. What percentage of women in the U.S. use marijuana or hashish?

    a. 2
    b. 5
    c. 10
    d. 15

38–86. Which of the following is seen more commonly in the infants and children of narcotic-addicted women?

    a. Children have smaller than average head circumference.
    b. There is increased risk of sudden infant death syndrome.
    c. Withdrawal symptoms are seen in neonates in the first 10 days.
    d. All of the above are seen.

39

Diseases and Injuries of the Fetus and Newborn

39–1. Which of the following is NOT a sign of hyaline membrane disease (respiratory distress syndrome, RDS)?

    a. increased respiratory rate
    b. chest wall retraction during inspiration
    c. grunting
    d. hypertension

39–2. A diffuse reticulogranular infiltrate and an air bronchogram on chest x-ray are most common in which of the following disorders of the newborn?

    a. hyaline membrane disease
    b. pneumonia
    c. meconium aspiration
    d. heart failure

39–3. Surfactant therapy is most efficacious for prevention or reduction of which of the following?

    a. persistent ductus arteriosus
    b. bronchopulmonary dysplasia
    c. intraventricular hemorrhage
    d. neonatal oxygen requirements

39–4. Which of the following is a complication of surfactant therapy?

    a. pulmonary hypertension
    b. intraventricular hemorrhage
    c. pneumonitis
    d. persistent ductus arteriosus

39–5. Which of the following is a complication of hyperoxia?

    a. pulmonary hemorrhage
    b. retinopathy
    c. pneumonitis
    d. intraventricular hemorrhage

39–6. At approximately what week does the concentration of lecithin relative to sphingomyelin begin to rise?

    a. week 28
    b. week 32
    c. week 34
    d. week 36

39–7. What is the lecithin–sphingomyelin (L/S) ratio of blood?

    a. 0.7
    b. 1.0
    c. 1.4
    d. 2.5

39–8. Which of the following tests is least likely to be affected by contaminants such as blood, meconium, or vaginal secretions?

    a. lecithin-sphingomyelin ratio
    b. phosphatidylglycerol measurement
    c. foam stability test
    d. fluorescent polarization

39–9. Which of the following tests is used to measure the surfactant-albumin ratio in uncentrifuged amnionic fluid?

    a. fluorescent polarization
    b. amnionic fluid absorbance at 650 nm
    c. dipalmitoylphosphatidylcholine (DPPC) test
    d. TDx-FLM

39–10. What lamellar body count would be indicative of fetal lung maturity?

    a. 4125/mL
    b. 8250/mL
    c. 17,500/mL
    d. 35,000/mL

39–11. Which of the following vitamins has been utilized in an attempt to prevent retrolental fibroplasia (retinopathy of prematurity)?

    a. A
    b. K
    c. E
    d. D

39–12. Which of the following therapies significantly improves term RDS?

    a. ECMO (extracorporeal membrane oxygenation)
    b. vitamin E
    c. high-dose surfactant
    d. nitric oxide

39–13. Approximately what percentage of pregnancies are complicated by meconium-stained fluid?

    a. 1
    b. 10
    c. 20
    d. 30

39–14. Which of the following mechanisms is felt to be responsible for the pathophysiological manifestations seen with meconium aspiration syndrome?

    a. mechanical blockage by meconium
    b. direct chemical damage by meconium
    c. meconium pneumonitis
    d. chronic fetal asphyxia

39–15. Which of the following markers is most likely to be abnormal in the umbilical cord blood of newborns with meconium-stained fluid?

    a. pH
    b. erythropoietin
    b. hypoxanthine
    c. lactate

39–16. Which of the following heart rate patterns is most likely to predict meconium aspiration?

    a. variable decelerations
    b. saltatory
    c. late decelerations
    d. none of the above

39–17. Most intraventricular hemorrhages of the preterm infant develop during which of the following time periods?

    a. first hour of birth
    b. first 24 h after birth
    c. first 72 h after birth
    d. first 7 days after birth

39–18. Which of the following factors best correlates with the presence of intraventricular hemorrhage?

    a. prematurity
    b. length of labor
    c. forceps delivery
    d. late decelerations

39–19. Approximately what percentage of all neonates born before 34 weeks will have evidence of intraventricular hemorrhage?

    a. 2
    b. 10
    c. 20
    d. 50

39–20. Approximately what percentage of asymptomatic term neonates have sonographic evidence of subependymal hemorrhage?

    a. <1
    b. 4
    c. 18
    d. 33

39–21. Which grade of intraventricular hemorrhage is associated with ventricular dilation?

    a. I
    b. II
    c. III
    d. IV

39–22. Which of the following has been proved to reduce the risk of intraventricular hemorrhage?

    a. vitamin K
    b. vitamin E
    c. phenobarbital
    d. corticosteroids

39–23. What is the most common form of cerebral palsy?

    a. diplegic
    b. hemiplegic
    c. quadriplegic
    d. extrapyramidal

39–24. What percentage of cerebral palsy cases are associated with mental retardation?

    a. 1
    b. 10
    c. 25
    d. 60

39–25. What is the approximate incidence of cerebral palsy in the United States?

    a. 1 to 2 per 100 live births
    b. 1 to 2 per 1000 live births
    c. 1 to 2 per 10,000 live births
    d. 3 to 5 per 10,000 live births

39–26. What is the incidence of cerebral palsy in low-birthweight (<2500 g) infants?

    a. 15 per 100 livebirths
    b. 15 per 1000 livebirths
    c. 15 per 10,000 livebirths
    d. 15 per 100,000 livebirths

39–27. What has happened to the incidence of cerebral palsy over the last 2 decades?

    a. slightly decreased
    b. markedly decreased
    c. markedly increased
    d. essentially unchanged

39–28. Which of the following factors is NOT strongly predictive of the presence of cerebral palsy in the newborn?

    a. forceps delivery
    b. maternal mental retardation
    c. birthweight less than 2000 g
    d. fetal malformations

39–29. What percentage of cerebral palsy can be attributed to asphyxia?

    a. 20
    b. 40
    c. 60
    d. 80

39–30. What fetal heart rate pattern is predictive of cerebral palsy?

    a. sinusoidal
    b. late decelerations
    c. severe variable decelerations
    d. none

39–31. What percentage of low-birthweight newborns with cerebral palsy had a grade III or IV intra-ventricular hemorrhage at birth?

    a. 5
    b. 28
    c. 40
    d. 94

39–32. What is the increased risk of cerebral palsy in low-birthweight newborns with grade III or IV intraventricular hemorrhage compared with controls or those with only a grade I or II hemorrhage?

    a. two fold
    b. eight fold
    c. sixteen fold
    d. hundred fold

39–33. Which of the following is the best predictor of cerebral palsy?

    a. Apgar score
    b. abnormal fetal heart rate pattern
    c. neonatal acidosis
    d. neonatal encephalopathy

39–34. What percentage of newborns with mild encephalopathy can be expected to have abnormal neurological development?

    a. 0
    b. 20
    c. 50
    d. 80

39–35. What percentage of newborns with moderate encephalopathy can be expected to develop normally neurologically?

    a. 0
    b. 20
    c. 50
    d. 80

39–36. What are the most common causes of cerebral palsy?

    a. prenatal factors
    b. perinatal factors
    c. postnatal factors
    d. unknown

39–37. What is the incidence of severe mental retardation?

    a. 3 per 100
    b. 3 per 1000
    c. 3 per 10,000
    d. 3 per 100,000

39–38. What is the approximate mean cord hemoglobin concentration at term?

    a. 10 g/dL
    b. 13 g/dL
    c. 17 g/dL
    d. 21 g/dL

39–39. Of the following, what is the most likely cause of fetal-to-maternal hemorrhage?

a. chorioangioma
b. placental abruption
c. placenta previa
d. oxytocin-induced labor

39–40. What fetal heart rate pattern is suggestive of severe fetal anemia?

a. sinusoidal
b. no beat-to-beat variability
c. repetitive late decelerations
d. hyperreactive

39–41. What is the chance that a D-negative woman, who delivered a D-positive but ABO-incompatible infant, will be D-isoimmunized by 6 months postpartum?

a. 2%
b. 12%
c. 20%
d. 42%

39–42. What is the chance that a D-negative woman, who delivered a D-positive but ABO-compatible infant, will be D-isoimmunized postpartum?

a. 1%
b. 5%
c. 16%
d. 33%

39–43. What percentage of newborns have ABO maternal blood group incompatibility?

a. 1
b. 10
c. 20
d. 50

39–44. The CDE (or rhesus) antigens are inherited independent of other blood group antigens and are located on which chromosome?

a. 1
b. 21
c. X
d. Y

39–45. Which of the following ethnic groups have the highest incidence of D-negativity?

a. blacks
b. whites
c. American Indians
d. Basques

39–46. Which of the following is NOT one of the criteria for confirming the diagnosis of ABO incompatibility?

a. mother is blood group O
b. fetus is blood group A or B
c. onset of jaundice after 7 days
d. varying degrees of anemia, reticulocytosis, and erythroblastosis

39–47. Which of the following red blood cell antigens does NOT cause hemolytic disease of the newborn?

a. CDE
b. Kell
c. Duffy
d. Lewis

39–48. What percentage of pregnant women will have atypical red blood cell antibodies?

a. 1
b. 5
c. 15
d. 20

39–49. What is the most common atypical red blood cell antibody encountered?

a. anti-Lewis
b. anti-Kell
c. anti-Duffy
d. anti-Kidd

39–50. How is detection of maternal antibodies that have been absorbed by fetal cells best accomplished?

a. indirect Coombs' test
b. direct Coombs' test
c. rosette test
d. enzyme-linked antiglobulin test

39–51. Which of the following is a Duffy antigen?

a. Jk^a
b. Jk^b
c. Fy^a
d. Du

39–52. The severity of ascites seen with hydrops fetalis is best correlated with which of the following?

a. portal hypertension
b. degree and severity of anemia
c. hypoproteinemia
d. decreased colloid oncotic pressure

39–53. What would the expected hemoglobin be in a fetus whose delta OD values from amniocentesis are in upper zone 2?

    a. 16 g/dL
    b. 14 to 16 g/dL
    c. 11.0 to 13.9 g/dL
    d. 8.0 to 10.9 g/dL

39–54. With D-isoimmunization, when the hemoglobin deficit obtained by fetal cord blood sampling exceeds 2 g/dL from the mean for normal fetuses of corresponding gestational age, what is the recommended next step?

    a. repeat sample in 1 week
    b. repeat sample in 2 weeks
    c. amniocentesis for optical density determination
    d. begin fetal transfusions

39–55. What type blood is utilized for initial exchange transfusion in the anemic newborn?

    a. O, D-negative
    b. O, D-positive
    c. maternal blood type, D-positive
    d. AB, D-negative

39–56. Approximately what percentage of D-negative women having early elective abortions become isoimmunized without D-immune globulin?

    a. <1
    b. 5
    c. 25
    d. 33

39–57. One dose of 300 μg of D-immunoglobulin will protect the mother against a bleed of approximately how much fetal blood?

    a. 5 mL
    b. 30 mL
    c. 90 mL
    d. 150 mL

39–58. In the otherwise uncomplicated newborn, what is the unconjugated bilirubin level above which kernicterus is likely to develop?

    a. 3 mg/dL
    b. 7 mg/dL
    c. 15 to 16 mg/dL
    d. 18 to 20 mg/dL

39–59. Which of the following compounds excreted into breast milk has been associated with jaundice of the newborn?

    a. 17α-hydroxylase
    b. pregnane 3α, 20 β-diol
    c. pregnenolone
    d. androstenedione

39–60. With physiological jaundice, what is the maximum level that serum bilirubin reaches?

    a. 2 mg/dL
    b. 5 mg/dL
    c. 10 mg/dL
    d. 18 mg/dL

39–61. Which of the following is most commonly used to lower the newborn serum level of bilirubin?

    a. phenobarbital
    b. fluorescent light
    c. vitamin K
    d. exchange transfusion

39–62. In approximately what percentage of fetuses with nonimmune hydrops is the cause idiopathic?

    a. 10
    b. 20
    c. 50
    d. 70

39–63. Which of the following intrinsic lesions is most commonly associated with nonimmune hydrops?

    a. cystic hygroma
    b. cardiac anomalies
    c. sacrococcygeal teratoma
    d. twin–twin transfusion

39–64. The mirror syndrome is a complication found in which of the following fetal conditions?

    a. duodenal atresia
    b. anal atresia
    c. hydrops
    d. twins

39–65. Which of the following fetal cardiac arrhythmias is most likely to be associated with nonimmune hydrops?

    a. supraventricular tachycardia (>200 bpm)
    b. bradycardia (<110 bpm)
    c. second-degree heart block
    d. ventricular extrasystole

39–66. What is the most likely cause of hemorrhagic disease of the newborn?

    a. autosomal dominant
    b. autosomal recessive
    c. maternal anticoagulation
    d. neonatal deficiency of vitamin K

39–67. What is the most likely diagnosis when the newborn has severe thrombocytopenia but the mother has a normal platelet count?

    a. immunological thrombocytopenia
    b. preeclampsia–eclampsia
    c. isoimmune thrombocytopenia
    d. maternal drug ingestion

39–68. Which of the following is NOT a common clinical finding in newborns with necrotizing enterocolitis (NEC)?

    a. pneumatosis intestinalis
    b. abdominal distention
    c. meconium stools
    d. ileus

39–69. What virus may be associated with NEC?

    a. picornavirus
    b. coronavirus
    c. herpes
    d. paramyxovirus

39–70. What is the most common type of intracranial hemorrhage encountered in the preterm newborn?

    a. intraventricular
    b. cortical
    c. periventricular
    d. subdural

39–71. What is the most common cause of intracranial hemorrhage?

    a. preterm birth
    b. birth trauma
    c. infection
    d. medication

39–72. Which is the focal swelling of the scalp from edema overlying the periosteum?

    a. cephalohematoma
    b. caput succedaneum

    c. periosteal hematoma
    d. caput periosteum

39–73. What is the approximate incidence in term births of brachial plexus injury?

    a. 1 in 12
    b. 1 in 100
    c. 1 in 500
    d. 1 in 3000

39–74. What percentage of brachial plexus injuries occur in macrosomic infants?

    a. 5
    b. 30
    c. 60
    d. 75

39–75. Approximately what percentage of facial paralysis injuries occur with spontaneous delivery?

    a. 1
    b. 11
    c. 22
    d. 33

39–76. What is the approximate incidence of clavicular fracture in live births?

    a. 0.3%
    b. 0.1 to 0.2%
    c. 1.0 to 2.0%
    d. 3.5%

39–77. Torticollis is more commonly associated with which of the following delivery modes?

    a. spontaneous vertex
    b. breech extraction
    c. forceps
    d. cesarean

XI SECTION

Techniques Used to Assess Fetal Health

Antepartum Assessment

40–1. What is the goal of antepartum fetal surveillance?

    a. prevent early deliveries
    b. delay delivery until lung maturity
    c. prevent fetal death
    d. increase fees for obstetricians

40–2. What is the negative predictive value of antenatal fetal tests?

    a. 10%
    b. 40%
    c. 70%
    d. ~100%

40–3. How early in gestation does passive unstimulated activity (movement) of the human fetus commence?

    a. 3 weeks
    b. 7 weeks
    c. 11 weeks
    d. 15 weeks

40–4. What is the longest time period during which fetal body movements are absent?

    a. 5 min
    b. 13 min
    c. 30 min
    d. 90 min

40–5. Continuous eye movements in the absence of body movements and no accelerations of the fetal heart is consistent with which of the following fetal behavioral states?

    a. 1F
    b. 2F
    c. 3F
    d. 4F

40–6. What is the mean length of the quiet or inactive state for term fetuses (i.e., "sleep cyclicity")?

    a. 11 min
    b. 23 min
    c. 75 min
    d. 105 min

40–7. What percentage of fetal body movements (recorded by Doppler device) will be perceived by the mother after 36 weeks?

    a. 16
    b. 38
    c. 65
    d. 90

40–8. What is the range of normal weekly counts of fetal movement?

    a. 20 to 600
    b. 20 to 950
    c. 50 to 600
    d. 50 to 950

40–9. In normal fetuses, what is the length of time that fetal breathing movements may be totally absent?

    a. 20 min
    b. 60 min
    c. 120 min
    d. 200 min

40–10. Irregular bursts of fetal breathing occur at which rate?

    a. 60 cycles/min
    b. 120 cycles/min
    c. 240 cycles/min
    d. 360 cycles/min

40–11. Which of the following variables is associated with absent fetal breathing movements?

    a. maternal meals
    b. decreased fetal heart rate
    c. sound stimuli
    d. labor

40–12. What controls fetal heart rate acceleration?

    a. autonomic function
    b. aortic baroreceptor reflexes
    c. carotid baroreceptor reflexes
    d. humeral factors such as atrial natriuretic peptide

40–13. What is the American College of Obstetricians and Gynecologists (ACOG) definition of a reactive nonstress test (NST)?

    a. 1 acceleration in 20 min
    b. 2 accelerations in 20 min
    c. 5 or more accelerations in 20 min
    d. 6 or more accelerations in 20 min

40–14. When fetal heart rate accelerations are insufficient, false-positive NSTs approach what level?

    a. 2%
    b. 10%
    c. 20%
    d. 90%

40–15. What did Hammacher call a fetal heart rate baseline that oscillates less than 5 bpm with no accelerations?

    a. silent oscillatory pattern
    b. terminal cardiotogram
    c. Parkland nonreassuring baseline
    d. normal

40–16. What is the associated perinatal pathology for the fetus with a nonreactive NST for 90 min?

    a. 10%
    b. 25%
    c. 50%
    d. 90%

40–17. What is the minimal level of sound necessary to evoke fetal movements?

    a. 50 dB
    b. 100 dB
    c. 500 dB
    d. 1000 dB

40–18. Which of the following is NOT a biophysical variable commonly used in the biophysical profile test?

    a. fetal heart rate acceleration
    b. fetal breathing
    c. fetal movement
    d. fetal urination

40–19. What is the false-normal rate for the biophysical profile test?

    a. 1 in 10
    b. 1 in 100
    c. 1 in 1000
    d. 1 in 10,000

40–20. Which of the following best describes a biophysical score of 6?

    a. normal score
    b. equivocal score
    c. abnormal score
    d. acidotic score

40–21. Doppler velocimetry may be useful in which of the following conditions?

    a. growth restriction
    b. diabetes
    c. preeclampsia
    d. lupus

40–22. What is the single best test of fetal well-being?

    a. CST
    b. NST
    c. Doppler velocimetry
    d. no single best test

40–23. What is the incidence of cerebral palsy in pregnancies managed with serial biophysical profiles compared to an untested group?

    a. 1/1000 versus 15/000
    b. 1/1000 versus 10/1000
    c. 1/1000 versus 5/1000
    d. both are the same

Ultrasound and Doppler

41–1. What do the transducers employed in real-time ultrasonography generate?

 a. single-pulse echo
 b. multiple-pulse echo activated at random
 c. multiple-pulse echo activated in sequence
 d. dual-pulse echo activated at random

41–2. What is the major biological hazard from fetal ultrasound?

 a. none
 b. early spontaneous abortions
 c. impaired neonatal hearing
 d. chromosomal breakage

41–3. Which of the following would NOT be a component of a "limited" ultrasound exam?

 a. amniotic fluid evaluation
 b. placental localization
 c. fetal heart motion
 d. fetal kidneys

41–4. In the RADIUS Trial, what was the major conclusion regarding routine ultrasound?

 a. Adverse perinatal outcomes were reduced.
 b. Preterm delivery was reduced.
 c. Fetal growth restriction was reduced.
 d. Perinatal outcome was not improved.

41–5. What is the major reason the RADIUS study is criticized?

 a. too many low-risk women
 b. detected too many anomalies
 c. done too late in gestation
 d. ineffective screening for eligible women

41–6. What would be the financial consequences of routine ultrasound to health care in the United States (DeVore and colleagues, 1996)?

 a. an increase of $280 million
 b. an increase of $1 billion

 c. a decrease of $280 million
 d. a decrease of $1 billion

41–7. What is the preferred fetal dimension for estimating gestational age at 8 to 10 weeks of pregnancy?

 a. femur length
 b. crown-rump length
 c. biparietal diameter
 d. humerus length

41–8. What is the easiest and most reproducible measurement to obtain in the eighteenth week of gestation?

 a. crown-rump length
 b. biparietal diameter
 c. abdominal circumference
 d. femur length

41–9. Using transabdominal sonography, when is the gestational sac reliably seen (weeks)?

 a. 4
 b. 6
 c. 8
 d. 9

41–10. Using transvaginal screening, when (in weeks) is the gestational sac usually seen?

 a. 3
 b. 5
 c. 7
 d. 8

41–11. What is the overall sensitivity of sonography in detecting fetal defects?

 a. 29%
 b. 53%
 c. 76%
 d. 99%

41–12. Which of the following sonographic views is used to measure the biparietal diameter and head circumference?

   a. transthalamic
   b. transventricular
   c. transcerebellar
   d. transhemispheric

41–13. What is the incidence of hydrocephalus?

   a. 0.3 to 0.8 per 100 births
   b. 0.3 to 0.8 per 1000 births
   c. 0.3 to 0.8 per 10,000 births
   d. 0.3 to 0.8 per 100,000 births

41–14. What is the average diameter of the lateral ventricular atrium between 15 and 35 weeks?

   a. 2 to 3 mm
   b. 5 to 7 mm
   c. 6 to 9 mm
   d. 12 to 15 mm

41–15. A free-floating or dangling choroid plexus is suggestive of which of the following diagnoses?

   a. hydrocephalus
   b. aqueductal stenosis
   c. choroid plexus cyst
   d. cerebral atrophy

41–16. What is the most common type of hydrocephalus?

   a. Dandy-Walker syndrome
   b. noncommunicating hydrocephalus
   c. communicating hydrocephalus
   d. aqueductal stenosis

41–17. What is the incidence of neural tube defects in the U.S.?

   a. 0.8 per 1000
   b. 1.6 per 1000
   c. 8 per 1000
   d. 16 per 1000

41–18. What is the accuracy of diagnosing anencephaly in the second trimester?

   a. 25%
   b. 50%
   c. 75%
   d. 100%

41–19. The presence of an encephalocele is an important feature of which of the following syndromes?

   a. Meckel-Gruber
   b. Hunter
   c. Hurler
   d. Edward

41–20. Which of the following signs describes frontal bone scalloping?

   a. lemon
   b. apple
   c. pear
   d. banana

41–21. What percentage of normal fetuses will have a choroid plexus cyst?

   a. 1 to 3
   b. 7 to 9
   c. 14 to 16
   d. 19 to 22

41–22. What is the most common chromosomal abnormality associated with a choroid plexus cyst?

   a. trisomy 21
   b. trisomy 13
   c. trisomy 18
   d. triploidy

41–23. What is the most common chromosomal anomaly associated with cystic hygromas in second- or third-trimester fetuses?

   a. trisomy 21
   b. trisomy 18
   c. monosomy X
   d. triploidy

41–24. What is the frequency of congenital diaphragmatic hernia?

   a. 1 in 200
   b. 1 in 1000
   c. 1 in 2000
   d. 1 in 10,000

41–25. What is the most specific sonographic finding in fetuses with diaphragmatic hernias?

   a. cystic structures behind the left atrium
   b. absence of intra-abdominal stomach bubble
   c. small abdominal circumference
   d. all of the above

41–26. What percentage of fetuses with a diaphragmatic hernia will have other associated major anomalies?

   a. 1
   b. 10
   c. 50
   d. 75

41–27. What is the incidence of congenital heart disease?

   a. 8 per 100
   b. 8 per 1000
   c. 8 per 10,000
   d. 8 per 30,000

41–28. What percentage of fetuses with congenital heart defects are due to multifactorial or polygenic factors?

    a. 1
    b. 10
    c. 50
    d. 90

41–29. What is the likelihood of aneuploidy in fetuses with an isolated cardiac malformation?

    a. 1%
    b. 15%
    c. 30%
    d. 50%

41–30. According to Lanouette and co-workers (1996) what is the positive predictive value of ultrasound for the detection of congenital heart defects?

    a. 25%
    b. 55%
    c. 75%
    d. 99%

41–31. In what percentage of fetuses is it possible to visualize the fetal stomach after 14 weeks?

    a. 5
    b. 25
    c. 76
    d. 98

41–32. What is the significance of hyperechogenic bowel?

    a. increased aneuploidy
    b. increased congenital infection
    c. associated with cystic fibrosis
    d. all of the above

41–33. Which of the following is more likely to be associated with aneuploidy?

    a. omphalocele
    b. gastroschisis
    c. esophageal atresia
    d. anal atresia

41–34. What percentage of fetuses with esophageal atresia or tracheoesophageal fistula will have associated anomalies?

    a. 5
    b. 25
    c. 50
    d. 78

41–35. What percentage of fetuses with the "double-bubble sign" (duodenal atresia) will have trisomy 21?

    a. 5
    b. 18

    c. 30
    d. 55

41–36. The fetal kidneys can routinely be visualized by what gestational age (weeks)?

    a. 8
    b. 12
    c. 18
    d. 22

41–37. What is the average urine output (per hour) in a fetus at term?

    a. 5 mL
    b. 20 mL
    c. 33 mL
    d. 50 mL

41–38. Which of the following characteristics is NOT associated with Potter syndrome?

    a. pulmonary hypoplasia
    b. limb deformities
    c. tight skin
    d. abnormal fascies

41–39. How is infantile polycystic kidney disease inherited?

    a. autosomal dominant
    b. autosomal recessive
    c. multifactorial
    d. sporadic

41–40. In which of the following arteries is the systolic-diastolic (S/D) ratio measured?

    a. fetal umbilical artery
    b. fetal carotid artery
    c. fetal aorta
    d. fetal vena cava

41–41. Doppler velocimetry has been shown to improve outcome of which of the following conditions?

    a. fetal growth restriction
    b. fetal hypoxia
    c. fetal distress
    d. none of the above

41–42. What is the Pourcelot index?

    a. pulsatility index
    b. resistance index
    c. S/D index
    d. reflectance index

41–43. What is the uterine blood flow at term?

    a. 50 mL per min
    b. 100 to 150 mL per min
    c. 300 to 425 mL per min
    d. 500 to 750 mL per min

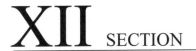

XII SECTION

Medical and Surgical Complications in Pregnancy

42

General Considerations and Maternal Evaluation

42–1. At which time during pregnancy are most nonobstetrical surgical procedures performed?

  a. first trimester
  b. second trimester
  c. third trimester
  d. postpartum

42–2. Which surgical procedure is most commonly performed in the second trimester?

  a. cholecystectomy
  b. ovarian cystectomy
  c. appendectomy
  d. tonsillectomy

42–3. In women exposed to general anesthesia during early gestation (4 to 5 weeks), what congenital anomaly is significantly increased?

  a. congenital heart defects
  b. hydrocephaly
  c. limb defects
  d. gastroschisis

42–4. What type of anesthesia is most commonly employed for nonobstetrical surgeries during pregnancy?

  a. epidural
  b. local infiltration
  c. general
  d. regional nerve blocks

42–5. Which of the following neonatal outcomes is affected by surgery (nonobstetrical)?

  a. stillborns
  b. birthweight <1500 g
  c. congenital malformations
  d. sepsis

42–6. What are the effects of laparoscopy on the human fetus?

  a. increased congenital anomalies
  b. increased spontaneous abortions
  c. fetal growth restriction
  d. currently unknown

42–7. Ultrasound is characterized by which of the following?

  a. short wavelength, low energy
  b. long wavelength, high energy
  c. long wavelength, low energy
  d. short wavelength, high energy

42–8. Which of the following is an example of radiation of short wavelength and high energy?

  a. x-ray
  b. microwaves
  c. ultrasound
  d. diathermy

42–9. During what period of development is ionizing radiation most likely to cause a lethal effect?

    a. preimplantation
    b. first trimester
    c. second trimester
    d. third trimester

42–10. What is the highest estimated risk of mental retardation when the embryo is exposed to radiation of 10 rad between 8 to 15 weeks' gestational age?

    a. 1 to 2%
    b. 4%
    c. 12%
    d. 20%

42–11. What is the risk of congenital malformations, growth retardation, or abortion from exposure to 1 to 5 rad of ionizing radiation at 8 to 15 weeks' gestation?

    a. 1 to 2%
    b. 5%
    c. 8%
    d. not increased

42–12. What is the most common type of anomaly seen in humans as a result of exposure to ionizing radiation (less than 20 rad)?

    a. central nervous system
    b. cardiac
    c. limb
    d. renal

42–13. What is the incidence of leukemia in children exposed to x-ray pelvimetry (1.5 to 2.0 rad)?

    a. 1 in 1000
    b. 1 in 2000
    c. 1 in 5000
    d. 1 in 10,000

42–14. Approximately how many exposed normal fetuses would have to be aborted to prevent one case of leukemia from a fetal radiation exposure of 1 to 2 rad?

    a. 100
    b. 1000
    c. 2000
    d. 20,000

42–15. What is the approximate fetal exposure from a maternal chest x-ray?

    a. <0.1 mrad
    b. 10 mrad
    c. 100 mrad
    d. 1 rad

42–16. What is the average fetal exposure from a single abdominal x-ray film?

    a. <0.1 mrad
    b. 10 mrad
    c. 100 mrad
    d. 1 rad

42–17. A single x-ray film for which of the following delivers the highest dose radiation to the fetus?

    a. chest
    b. abdomen
    c. rib
    d. hip

42–18. At term, to what dose of radiation is a fetus is exposed during a computed tomography scan of the abdomen?

    a. <0.05 rad
    b. 0.1 to 1.0 rad
    c. 1.5 to 2.0 rad
    d. 3.0 to 4.0 rad

42–19. What is the fetal risk from exposure to iodine[123] for diagnostic thyroid scanning?

    a. minimal perinatal morbidity
    b. moderate perinatal morbidity
    c. severe perinatal morbidity
    d. lethal perinatal morbidity

42–20. In magnetic resonance imaging (MRI), the strength of the magnetic field within the bore of the magnet is measured as which of the following?

    a. Gray (Gy)
    b. Tesla (T)
    c. Curie (Ci)
    d. rad

42–21. Which of the following is a clear indication for MRI during pregnancy?

    a. breech presentation in labor
    b. suspected appendicidal abscess
    c. lumbar disc evaluation
    d. evaluation of epilepsy

43

Critical Care and Trauma

43–1. Which of the following conditions is the least likely indication for invasive hemodynamic monitoring?

    a. unexplained pulmonary edema
    b. adult respiratory distress syndrome
    c. peripartum coronary artery disease
    d. asthma

43–2. Which vein is the best approach to use in women with coagulopathies that need pulmonary artery catheterization placement?

    a. antecubital
    b. internal jugular
    c. external jugular
    d. subclavian vein

43–3. Which of the following formulas represents systemic vascular resistance?

    a. stroke volume body surface area (BSA)
    b. mean systemic arterial pressure (mm Hg) − central venous pressure/cardiac output [(MAP − CVP)/CO] × 80
    c. mean pulmonary artery pressure (mm Hg) − mean pulmonary capillary wedge pressure (mm Hg)/cardiac output [(MPAP − PCWP)/CO] × 80
    d. CO/BSA

43–4. Intraventricular pressure and volume determine which of the following?

    a. afterload
    b. preload
    c. stroke index
    d. cardiac index

43–5. Which of the following parameters is used to assess left ventricular end-diastolic filling pressure (i.e., "preload")?

    a. central venous pressure
    b. pulmonary capillary wedge pressure

    c. cardiac index
    d. stroke volume

43–6. What two values are needed to construct a left ventricular function curve (i.e., Starling curve)?

    a. cardiac output and pulmonary capillary wedge pressure
    b. cardiac index and pulmonary vascular resistance
    c. stroke index and systemic vascular resistance
    d. left ventricular stroke work index and colloid oncotic pressure

43–7. What is ventricular wall tension during systole?

    a. preload
    b. afterload
    c. stroke index
    d. cardiac index

43–8. Which of the following is a commonly used agent for reduction of afterload in obstetrical patients?

    a. nitroglycerin
    b. hydralazine
    c. lasix
    d. propranolol

43–9. Which of the following agents is NOT utilized to improve myocardial contractility (i.e., inotropic state of the heart)?

    a. dopamine
    b. dobutamine
    c. propranolol
    d. isoproterenol

43–10. What is the most common complication from pulmonary artery catheterization?

    a. premature ventricular contractions
    b. arterial puncture
    c. pulmonary infarction
    d. pneumothorax

43–11. What percentage of patients have complications from indwelling arterial catheters?

    a. ~0.1
    b. <1.0
    c. 3.0 to 5.0
    d. 8.0 to 10.0

43–12. What is the mortality rate for acute respiratory failure in pregnant women?

    a. <1%
    b. 10%
    c. 25%
    d. 50%

43–13. Which of the following is a criterion for diagnosing the adult respiratory distress syndrome?

    a. partial pressure of O_2 (PO_2) > 50 mm Hg with fraction of inspired O_2 (FiO_2) > 0.6
    b. pulmonary capillary wedge pressure >12 mm Hg
    c. functional residual capacity increased
    d. arterial pressure of O_2 (PaO_2):FiO_2 < 250

43–14. How much oxygen is carried by each gram of hemoglobin at 90% saturation?

    a. 0.5 mL
    b. 1.25 mL
    c. 2.5 mL
    d. 5.0 mL

43–15. What is the minimum PO_2 necessary to maintain a 90% oxyhemoglobin saturation?

    a. 60 mm Hg
    b. 70 mm Hg
    c. 80 mm Hg
    d. 90 mm Hg

43–16. Which of the following is NOT associated with a rightward shift in the oxyhemoglobin dissociation curve (i.e., decreased hemoglobin affinity for oxygen and increased tissue-capillary interchange)?

    a. hypercapnea
    b. metabolic acidosis
    c. increased body temperature
    d. decreased 2,3-diphosphoglycerate

43–17. What is the normal $PaCO_2$ for pregnancy?

    a. 15 to 25 mm Hg
    b. 25 to 35 mm Hg
    c. 35 to 45 mm Hg
    d. 45 to 55 mm Hg

43–18. Which of the following colloid oncotic pressures is characteristic of severe preeclampsia during the antepartum period?

    a. 32 mm Hg
    b. 24 mm Hg
    c. 16 mm Hg
    d. 4 mm Hg

43–19. Under normal circumstances, what is the usual colloid oncotic pressure or wedge pressure gradient?

    a. 2 mm Hg
    b. 4 mm Hg
    c. 6 mm Hg
    d. ≥8 mm Hg

43–20. Which of the following group of bacteria is most likely to be associated with septic shock?

    a. *Enterobacteriaceae*
    b. anaerobic streptococci
    c. *Bacteroides* species
    d. *Clostridium* species

43–21. Which of the following organisms produces an endotoxin as opposed to an exotoxin?

    a. *Pseudomonas aeruginosa*
    b. *Staphylococcus aureus*
    c. group A streptococcus
    d. *Escherichia coli*

43–22. Which of the following is directly released upon lysis of the cell wall of gram-negative bacteria?

    a. complement
    b. kinins
    c. lipopolysaccharide
    d. tumor necrosis factor

43–23. What dose of dopamine causes β-receptor stimulation (i.e., increased vascular resistance and blood pressure)?

    a. <2 μg/kg
    b. 5 to 10 μg/kg
    c. 10 to 20 μg/kg
    d. 50 to 60 μg/kg

43–24. What is the incidence of physical trauma in pregnancy?

    a. 5%
    b. 8.5%
    c. 12.5%
    d. 25%

43–25. What percentage of minor maternal injuries are associated with traumatic placental abruptions?

    a. 1 to 6
    b. 10 to 16
    c. 20 to 26
    d. 30 to 36

43–26. Which of the following signs is most useful in predicting the absence of a placental abruption following trauma?

    a. absence of uterine contractions
    b. absence of bleeding
    c. presence of normal fetal heart tones
    d. absence of tense, painful uterus

43–27. What is the incidence of maternal visceral injuries with penetrating trauma?

    a. <5%
    b. 15 to 40%

    c. 50 to 70%
    d. nearly 100%

43–28. What is the best management of a pregnant woman at 30 weeks' gestation with burns over 60 percent of her body?

    a. continuous electronic monitoring of the fetus
    b. weekly biophysical profiles
    c. immediate delivery
    d. twice weekly contraction stress tests

43–29. What percentage of infants delivered 12 min after cardiopulmonary arrest will be neurologically intact?

    a. 10
    b. 33
    c. 83
    d. 98

Cardiovascular Diseases

44–1. What is the incidence of heart disease in pregnancy?

    a. 0.1%
    b. 1.0%
    c. 5.0%
    d. 10.0%

44–2. What causes at least one-half of heart disease in pregnancy?

    a. idiopathic cardiomyopathy
    b. constrictive pericarditis
    c. hypertension
    d. congenital heart lesions

44–3. Which of the following plays a role in the increased cardiac output in normal pregnancy?

    a. decreased peripheral vascular resistance
    b. increased stroke volume

    c. rise in resting pulse late in gestation
    d. all of the above

44–4. Most congenital heart defects are thought to be inherited by what genetic pattern?

    a. autosomal recessive
    b. autosomal dominant
    c. new point mutations
    d. polygenic inheritance

44–5. What is the incidence of fetal congenital heart disease in women born with cardiac anomalies?

    a. 3 to 10%
    b. 10 to 15%
    c. 20 to 35%
    d. 50 to 65%

44–6. Which of the following symptoms in pregnancy is most suggestive of heart disease?

　　a. tachycardia
　　b. tachypnea
　　c. syncope with exertion
　　d. peripheral edema

44–7. What is the fetal radiation dosage (maximum) expected with thallium^{201} studies?

　　a. 50 mrad
　　b. 250 mrad
　　c. 610 mrad
　　d. 1100 mrad

44–8. Which of the following is NOT an electrocardiographic change seen during normal pregnancy?

　　a. 15-degree left-axis deviation
　　b. altered voltage findings
　　c. mild ST changes in inferior leads
　　d. atrial or ventricular premature beats

44–9. Based on echocardiography, which of the following is a common pregnancy-induced finding?

　　a. tricuspid regurgitation
　　b. mitral valve prolapse
　　c. right atrial enlargement
　　d. aortic insufficiency

44–10. What is the New York Heart Association classification of a patient comfortable at rest but with dyspnea and fatigue slightly limiting normal activities?

　　a. I
　　b. II
　　c. III
　　d. IV

44–11. According to Siu and colleagues (1997), what was the observed incidence of congestive heart failure in 250 pregnant women with classes I or II heart disease?

　　a. 1%
　　b. 5%
　　c. 10%
　　d. 20%

44–12. According to the American College of Obstetricians and Gynecologists classification, which of the following heart lesions is associated with the greatest maternal mortality?

　　a. patent ductus arteriosus
　　b. aortic coarctation with valvar involvement
　　c. corrected tetralogy of Fallot
　　d. mitral stenosis with atrial fibrillation

44–13. In two studies totaling 726 pregnancies in women with classes I and II heart disease (Siu and co-workers, 1997, and McFaul and colleagues, 1988), what percentage of women died during pregnancy or the puerperium?

　　a. 0
　　b. 10
　　c. 50
　　d. 100

44–14. What is the first warning sign of cardiac failure?

　　a. persistent basilar rales and nocturnal cough
　　b. dyspnea on exertion
　　c. hemoptysis
　　d. progressive edema

44–15. Which of the following principles is advisable in managing labor and delivery in women with heart disease?

　　a. Tachycardia is managed with β-blockers.
　　b. Analgesia is minimized due to potential depressant effects on the myocardium.
　　c. Cesarean section is reserved for obstetrical indications.
　　d. All such patients should undergo pulmonary artery catheterization.

44–16. What is the preferred method of labor and delivery analgesia in most situations involving maternal heart disease?

　　a. oral analgesics
　　b. continuous epidural analgesia
　　c. spinal analgesia (saddle block)
　　d. paracervical block for second stage of labor and delivery

44–17. Which common complication of epidural analgesia is the most hazardous and potentially lethal in women with preload-sensitive cardiac lesions?

　　a. hypotension
　　b. arrhythmia
　　c. respiratory depression
　　d. cardiac ischemia

44–18. Which of the following anesthetic techniques is contraindicated in women with pulmonary hypertension?

　　a. intravenous analgesia
　　b. pudendal block
　　c. spinal block
　　d. general anesthesia

44–19. Which of these vital sign parameters (per minute) suggests early cardiac decompensation during labor?

    a. pulse <100, respirations <12
    b. pulse <100, BP >140/90
    c. pulse >100, respirations >24
    d. pulse >140, respirations >30

44–20. Which fetal complication is more common with warfarin use in pregnancy?

    a. malformations
    b. spontaneous abortion
    c. stillbirths
    d. all of the above

44–21. Which of the following prosthetic valve types is associated with less thromboembolic episodes?

    a. Bjork-Shiley prosthesis
    b. St. Jude medical prosthesis
    c. porcine xenografts
    d. no differences

44–22. What is the most serious disadvantage of switching from warfarin to heparin during pregnancy in women with mechanical valve prostheses?

    a. Risk of embryopathy is increased.
    b. Hemorrhage is more likely.
    c. Risk of thromboembolism is increased.
    d. Need for self-injection.

44–23. With respect to heparin anticoagulation during pregnancy, which of the following laboratory parameters should be maintained at a level of 1.5 to 2.5 times baseline value?

    a. bleeding time
    b. partial thromboplastin time
    c. prothrombin time
    d. thrombin time

44–24. If delivery occurs unexpectedly while the patient is fully anticoagulated on heparin and excessive bleeding occurs, what initial intervention is appropriate?

    a. ligation of hypogastric arteries
    b. infusion of fresh frozen plasma
    c. administration of protamine sulfate
    d. administration of vitamin K

44–25. What is the perinatal mortality rate associated with maternal pulmonary bypass (Weiss and colleagues, 1998)?

    a. 5%
    b. 30%
    c. 50%
    d. 90%

44–26. Which of the following is a common fetal response during cardiopulmonary bypass?

    a. persistent late decelerations
    b. bradycardia
    c. tachycardia
    d. repetitive variable decelerations

44–27. Which of the following is increased in pregnancies of women with prior mitral valvotomy?

    a. heart failure
    b. embolus
    c. atrial fibrillation
    d. all of the above

44–28. Which of the following is true during pregnancy of women with transplanted hearts?

    a. Maternal mortality exceeds 50%.
    b. The heart will show normal adaptation to pregnancy.
    c. The heart will show an increased response to normal physiological changes.
    d. There is no increased risk of cesarean delivery.

44–29. What is the most common cause of mitral valve disease in women in the United States at the present time?

    a. congenital valvar defects
    b. endocarditis sequelae
    c. mitral valve prolapse (acquired)
    d. rheumatic heart disease

44–30. What is the surface area of the normal mitral valve?

    a. $1.0 \ cm^2$
    b. $2.5 \ cm^2$
    c. $4.0 \ cm^2$
    d. $5.5 \ cm^2$

44–31. Symptoms develop when a stenotic mitral valve's surface area drops below what value?

    a. $1.0 \ cm^2$
    b. $2.5 \ cm^2$
    c. $4.0 \ cm^2$
    d. $5.5 \ cm^2$

44–32. Women with mitral stenosis are at great risk for which condition during labor?

    a. atrial rupture
    b. myocardial infarction
    c. ventricular tachycardia
    d. rate-related heart failure

44-33. Management of laboring women with mitral stenosis should NOT include which of the following?

 a. epidural analgesia
 b. endocarditis prophylaxis
 c. β-blockers to slow heart rate
 d. elective cesarean section

44-34. During pregnancy, what tends to happen to regurgitation associated with the mitral valve?

 a. decreases
 b. remains the same
 c. increases mildly
 d. increases significantly

44-35. What is the size of a normal aortic valve orifice?

 a. <0.5 cm^2
 b. 0.5 to 1.0 cm^2
 c. 2.0 to 3.0 cm^2
 d. >4.0 cm^2

44-36. What is the key functional problem that makes severe aortic stenosis a life-threatening condition for the pregnant patient?

 a. fixed cardiac output
 b. pulmonary edema
 c. valvar rupture
 d. ventricular arrhythmias

44-37. Management during labor in women with aortic stenoses should include which of the following?

 a. bacterial endocarditis prophylaxis
 b. narcotic epidural anesthesia
 c. treat infections and hemorrhage promptly
 d. all of the above

44-38. Past use of which drug increases the incidence of aortic valve and mitral valve insufficiency?

 a. cocaine
 b. steroids
 c. fenfluramine
 d. oral contraceptives

44-39. What is the incidence of congenital heart disease in the U.S.?

 a. 8 per 10,000 live births
 b. 8 per 1000 live births
 c. 18 per 1000 live births
 d. 28 per 1000 live births

44-40. Which of the following is the most common congenital heart defect identified in the newborn period?

 a. patent ductus arteriosus
 b. atrial septal defect (ASD)

 c. ventricular septal defect
 d. pulmonary stenosis

44-41. What is the most common ASD?

 a. ostium secundum type
 b. ovale type
 c. ostium primum type
 d. Roger type

44-42. What is the incidence of fetal atrial or ventricular septal defect if the mother has such a defect?

 a. 1 to 3%
 b. 5 to 10%
 c. 12 to 18%
 d. 20 to 25%

44-43. In which of the following maternal clinical situations is termination of pregnancy recommended?

 a. aortic regurgitation
 b. atrial septal defect
 c. tetralogy of Fallot, corrected
 d. Eisenmenger syndrome

44-44. Which of the following cardiac lesions is NOT associated with cyanosis?

 a. coarctation of the aorta
 b. tetralogy of Fallot
 c. Ebstein anomaly
 d. patent ductus arteriosus

44-45. Which of the following is NOT an associated finding in tetralogy of Fallot?

 a. ventricular septal defect
 b. overriding aorta
 c. right ventricular hypertrophy
 d. pulmonary stenosis

44-46. In women with tetralogy of Fallot, decreased peripheral vascular resistance in pregnancy leads to which of the following changes in cardiopulmonary hemodynamics?

 a. increased right-to-left shunting
 b. increased left-to-right shunting
 c. increased pulmonary hypertension
 d. decreased left-to-right shunting

44-47. What is the preferred mode of delivery in a woman with cyanotic heart disease?

 a. vaginal delivery with spinal analgesia
 b. elective cesarean section under general anesthesia
 c. vaginal delivery with narcotic epidural analgesia during labor
 d. elective cesarean section under epidural analgesia

44–48. Which of the following is associated with the development of Eisenmenger syndrome?

    a. right-to-left shunting occurs
    b. pulmonary hypertension occurs
    c. pulmonary vascular resistance greater than systemic vascular resistance
    d. all of the above

44–49. What is the usual etiology of maternal mortality in women with pulmonary hypertension?

    a. right ventricular overload
    b. diminished venous return
    c. pulmonary emboli
    d. mural thrombosis

44–50. According to recent community-based studies (Freed and colleagues, 1999), what is the incidence of mitral valve prolapse in the general female population?

    a. 2 to 3%
    b. 6 to 8%
    c. 10 to 12%
    d. 15 to 20%

44–51. During pregnancy, symptomatic mitral valve prolapse is best treated with which type of medication?

    a. anxiolytics
    b. β-blockers
    c. calcium-channel blockers
    d. digitalis

44–52. In which of the following situations should women with mitral valve prolapse receive intrapartum bacterial endocarditis prophylaxis?

    a. mitral valve regurgitation
    b. symptomatic
    c. cesarean section
    d. in all cases

44–53. Which of the following etiologic factors has been identified in women with peripartum cardiomyopathy?

    a. superimposed pregnancy-induced hypertension
    b. mitral stenosis
    c. viral myocarditis
    d. all of the above

44–54. What is the incidence of idiopathic cardiomyopathy during pregnancy?

    a. 1 in 3000
    b. 1 in 9000
    c. 1 in 15,000
    d. 1 in 30,000

44–55. What is the hallmark finding in idiopathic cardiomyopathy?

    a. rales
    b. peripheral edema
    c. diastolic murmur
    d. marked cardiomegaly

44–56. Which of the following is NOT recommended in the antepartum management of idiopathic cardiomyopathy?

    a. heparin
    b. digitalis
    c. angiotensin-converting enzyme inhibitor
    d. diuretics

44–57. What percentage of women with idiopathic peripartum cardiomyopathy show evidence of myocarditis if myocardial biopsy is performed?

    a. 10
    b. 25
    c. 50
    d. 75

44–58. Which of the following is a low-risk factor for bacterial endocarditis?

    a. aortic stenosis
    b. atrial septal defect
    c. ventricular septal defect
    d. aortic coarctation

44–59. What is the most common organism, particularly in parenteral drug abusers, with acute endocarditis?

    a. *Staphylococcus aureus,* coagulase-positive
    b. *Streptococcus pneumoniae*
    c. *Neisseria gonorrhoeae*
    d. group B streptococcus

44–60. Which of the following lesions secondary to bacterial endocarditis is most difficult to diagnose with echocardiography?

    a. 1.0-cm lesion on the aortic valve
    b. 0.5-cm lesion on the mitral valve
    c. 0.5-cm lesion on the aortic valve
    d. 1.0-cm lesion on the tricuspid valve

44–61. According to 1997 American Heart Association guidelines, during which obstetrical procedure is antibiotic prophylaxis recommended in individuals with high-risk cardiac lesions?

    a. chorionic villus sampling
    b. uncomplicated vaginal delivery
    c. cesarean delivery
    d. vaginal delivery with episiotomy

44-62. Which of the following tachyarrhythmias is most common in pregnancy?

    a. Wolff-Parkinson-White syndrome
    b. paroxysmal supraventricular tachycardia
    c. ventricular tachycardia
    d. panic attack

44-63. Which of the following treatments for supraventricular tachycardia is contraindicated in pregnancy?

    a. adenosine
    b. digoxin
    c. electrical cardioversion
    d. none of these are contraindicated

44-64. Which condition does NOT place pregnant women at increased risk for aortic dissection?

    a. Marfan syndrome
    b. coarctation of the aorta
    c. Noonan syndrome
    d. syphilitic aortitis

44-65. How is the definitive diagnosis of aortic dissection made?

    a. chest x-ray
    b. aortic angiography
    c. sonography
    d. magnetic resonance imaging

44-66. How is Marfan syndrome inherited?

    a. autosomal recessive
    b. autosomal dominant
    c. X-linked dominant
    d. polygenic

44-67. Which gene product is abnormal in Marfan syndrome?

    a. tubulin
    b. connexin
    c. fibrillin
    d. muscularium

44-68. Women are at increased risk for cardiovascular complications with aortic dilatation that is greater than which of the following?

    a. 20 mm in diameter
    b. 30 mm in diameter
    c. 40 mm in diameter
    d. 50 mm in diameter

44-69. With which of the following conditions is coarctation of the aorta associated?

    a. bicuspid aortic valve
    b. cerebral artery aneurysm
    c. Turner syndrome
    d. all of the above

44-70. What is the incidence of maternal mortality associated with aortic coarctation?

    a. 1%
    b. 3%
    c. 10%
    d. 30%

44-71. Concerning myocardial infarction in pregnancy, women are at greatest risk for mortality if the infarction occurs during which of the following periods?

    a. first trimester
    b. second trimester
    c. 2 weeks prior to labor
    d. 2 weeks after delivery

45

Chronic Hypertension

45–1. What is the increased likelihood of chronic hypertension in obese women compared to nonobese?

a. 2-fold
b. 4-fold
c. 10-fold
d. 20-fold

45–2. Treatment of mild-to-moderate hypertension in nonpregnant patients decreases which of the following?

a. mortality
b. stroke
c. cardiac events
d. all of the above

45–3. Nonpharmacological interventions to treat hypertension include all EXCEPT which of the following?

a. weight loss
b. physical activity
c. high-fat diet
d. smoking cessation

45–4. Evaluation of uncomplicated, long-standing, chronic hypertension early in pregnancy includes all EXCEPT which of the following?

a. serum creatinine
b. echocardiography
c. ophthalmologic evaluation
d. hepatic function

45–5. Women with chronic hypertension in pregnancy are at increased risk for which of the following?

a. placental abruption
b. placenta previa
c. spontaneous preterm birth
d acute fatty liver

45–6. Which of the following increases the risk of superimposed preeclampsia in women with hypertension?

a. family history of preeclampsia
b. hypertension for >5 years
c. prior pregnancy without preeclampsia
d. well-controlled blood pressure on a single medication

45–7. Low-dose aspirin in women with chronic hypertension is most likely to decrease which of the following?

a. preterm births
b. fetal growth restriction
c. preeclampsia
d. neonatal deaths

45–8. Which adverse pregnancy outcome is NOT increased in pregnancies complicated by chronic hypertension?

a. fetal growth restriction
b. preterm birth
c. spontaneous preterm rupture of membranes
d. perinatal death

45–9. When should antihypertensives be started in pregnancy to reduce blood pressure?

a. diastolic blood pressures >100 mm Hg
b. diastolic blood pressures >80 mm Hg with end-organ disease
c. systolics >140 mm Hg
d. immediately

45–10. Once antihypertensive agents are initiated, one can expect a decrease in which of the following?

a. adverse perinatal outcome
b. superimposed preeclampsia
c. proteinuria
d. maternal blood pressure

45–11. What is the mechanism of action of diuretics?

  a. increased peripheral vascular resistance
  b. increased sodium and water diuresis
  c. acts centrally to decrease sympathetic outflow or tone
  d. relaxes arterial smooth muscles

45–12. What is the mechanism of action of alpha-methyldopa?

  a. increased peripheral vascular resistance
  b. increased sodium and water diuresis
  c. acts centrally to decrease sympathetic outflow or tone
  d. relaxes arterial smooth muscles

45–13. What is the mechanism of action of hydralazine?

  a. increased peripheral vascular resistance
  b. increased sodium and water diuresis
  c. acts centrally to decrease sympathetic outflow or tone
  d. relaxes arterial smooth muscles

45–14. What antihypertensive has both alpha- and beta-adrenergic actions (blockade)?

  a. furosemide
  b. hydralazine
  c. propranolol
  d. labetalol

45–15. Which of the following agents is a calcium channel antagonist?

  a. verapamil
  b. metoprolol
  c. atenolol
  d. captopril

45–16. Which of the following inhibits the conversion of angiotensin I to angiotensin II?

  a. atenolol (β-blocker)
  b. nifedipine (calcium-channel blocker)

  c. captopril (ACE inhibitor)
  d. labetalol (α- and β-blocker)

45–17. What perinatal complication is seen with increased frequency in women with hypertension treated with antihypertensives (according to Sibai et al, 1983)?

  a. preterm labor
  b. fetal growth restriction
  c. respiratory distress
  d. pulmonary hypoplasia

45–18. Beta-blockers, in particular atenolol, are associated with which of the following perinatal morbidities?

  a. respiratory distress syndrome
  b. preterm birth
  c. hyperglycemia
  d. fetal growth restriction

45–19. Angiotensin-converting enzyme inhibitors are contraindicated in pregnancy due to what fetal effect?

  a. chromosomal anomaly
  b. fetal renal failure
  c. thrombocytopenia
  d. hydrocephalus

45–20. What is the incidence of superimposed pregnancy-induced hypertension with chronic hypertension?

  a. <1%
  b. 10%
  c. 25%
  d. 50%

46

Pulmonary Disorders

46–1. What is the incidence of asthma in pregnancy?

    a. 0.1 to 0.4%
    b. 1.0 to 4.0%
    c. 10.0 to 14.0%
    d. 20.0 to 24.0%

46–2. Which of the following cannot be measured directly?

    a. tidal volume
    b. residual volume
    c. minute ventilation
    d. expiratory reserve volume

46–3. Which of the following characterizes functional residual capacity during pregnancy?

    a. decreases by approximately 500 mL
    b. stays unchanged compared with nonpregnant values
    c. increases by approximately 500 mL
    d. increases by approximately 1 L

46–4. How much does basal oxygen consumption increase during the last one-half of pregnancy?

    a. 1 to 5 mL/min
    b. 10 to 15 mL/min
    c. 20 to 40 mL/min
    d. 60 to 80 mL/min

46–5. Dyspnea during pregnancy is attributed to which of the following?

    a. alveolar death
    b. alveolar growth
    c. hypoventilation and $\uparrow PaCO_2$
    d. hyperventilation and $\downarrow PaCO_2$

46–6. Which is inflammation of the lung parenchyma distal to the large airways and involving alveolar units?

    a. pneumonia
    b. asthma
    c. bronchopneumonia
    d. sarcoidosis

46–7. Which of the following organisms is the major cause of bacterial pneumonia in otherwise healthy patients?

    a. *Staphylococcus aureus*
    b. *Chlamydia trachomatis*
    c. *Mycoplasma pneumoniae*
    d. *Streptococcus pneumoniae*

46–8. Which of the following is a risk factor for lung colonization with *Legionella?*

    a. smoking
    b. diabetes
    c. acute viral pneumonia
    d. alcohol in moderation

46–9. What is the incidence of pneumonia complicating pregnancy at Parkland Hospital?

    a. 1 in 100
    b. 1 in 300
    c. 1 in 600
    d. 1 in 1000

46–10. A 27-year-old woman at 32 weeks' gestation presents complaining of cough, fever, chest pain, and dyspnea. Which of the following tests would be most helpful in making a diagnosis?

    a. complete blood cell count
    b. mycoplasma-specific immunoglobulin G
    c. urinalysis for pneumococcal antigen
    d. chest x-ray

46–11. Which of the following factors is NOT an indication for hospitalization of a woman with pneumonia?

    a. altered mental status
    b. hypertension
    c. hypothermia
    d. respiratory rate >30 breaths per min

46–12. What is first-line therapy in a pregnant woman with uncomplicated community-acquired pneumonia?

    a. dicloxicillin
    b. clindamycin
    c. ampicillin
    d. erythromycin

46–13. What is the approximate percentage of penicillin-resistant pneumococcus?

    a. 5
    b. 15
    c. 25
    d. 50

46–14. Pneumococcal vaccine should be given for which of the following conditions?

    a. sickle cell disease
    b. gestational diabetes
    c. pregnancy-induced hypertension
    d. all pregnancies

46–15. Which of the following perinatal complications is associated with bacterial pneumonia?

    a. fetal growth retardation
    b. preterm labor
    c. persistent fetal circulation
    d. cerebral palsy

46–16. Pregnant women with which finding should be vaccinated against influenza no matter what stage of pregnancy?

    a. sickle cell trait
    b. hyperthyroidism
    c. insulin-dependent diabetes
    d. asymptomatic bacteriuria

46–17. What are the current Center for Disease Control recommendations for influenza vaccine in pregnancy?

    a. vaccinate only high-risk women
    b. vaccinate only if epidemic is expected
    c. vaccinate only if a new virus is expected
    d. all should be vaccinated after the first trimester

46–18. What is the treatment of choice for early-onset influenza in pregnancy?

    a. oseltamivir
    b. amantadine
    c. acyclovir
    d. ganciclovir

46–19. Primary infection with varicella may lead to pneumonia in what percentage of adults?

    a. 10
    b. 20
    c. 30
    d. 40

46–20. In a seronegative individual who is exposed to active infection, what is the attack rate for varicella?

    a. 30%
    b. 50%
    c. 70%
    d. 90%

46–21. Which of the following agents lowers the mortality in varicella pneumonia?

    a. acyclovir
    b. varicella zoster immunoglobulin
    c. gamma globulin
    d. all of the above

46–22. What is the mortality rate of varicella pneumonia during pregnancy?

    a. 5%
    b. 15%
    c. 35%
    d. 90%

46–23. What is the best management for a susceptible pregnant woman exposed to varicella for less than 96 hours?

    a. varicella isoimmunization IM
    b. varivax
    c. varicella-zoster immunoglobulin
    d. expectant management or observation

46–24. Which of the following treatment regimens is effective for *Pneumocystis carinii* pneumonia?

    a. ampicillin
    b. erythromycin
    c. trimethoprim-sulfamethoxazole
    d. azithromycin

46–25. In which of the following human immunodeficiency virus (HIV)-positive patients is aerosolized pentamidine or oral trimethoprim-sulfamethoxazole recommended prophylactically to prevent pneumocystis infection?

    a. $CD4^+$ count T-lymphocyte $< 200/\mu L$
    b. $CD4^+$ count T-lymphocyte $< 500/\mu L$
    c. $CD4^+$ count T-lymphocyte $< 750/\mu L$
    d. All HIV-positive women

46–26. Which of the following fungal infections may have stimulatory effects on estradiol-17β?

    a. coccidioidomycosis
    b. histoplasmosis
    c. blastomycosis
    d. sarcoidosis

46–27. In pregnant women with coccidioidomycosis, what finding is associated with a better prognosis?

    a. acute infection
    b. hypotension
    c. erythema nodosum
    d. HIV coinfection

46–28. What percentage of the general population has asthma?

    a. 0.5 to 1.5
    b. 3.0 to 4.0
    c. 6.0 to 8.0
    d. 10.0 to 12.0

46–29. Airway responsiveness and inflammation in persons with asthma are linked to which of the following chromosomes?

    a. 11q13
    b. 5q
    c. 14q
    d. all of the above

46–30. What proportion of those with asthma can expect worsening of disease during pregnancy?

    a. none
    b. one-fourth
    c. one-third
    d. one-half

46–31. Which of the following pregnancy complications is NOT increased in those with asthma?

    a. preterm labor
    b. perinatal mortality
    c. low-birthweight infants
    d. congenital anomalies

46–32. Which of the following findings is associated with the "danger zone" stage of asthma?

    a. pO_2 normal; pCO_2 decreased; pH increased
    b. pO_2 normal; pCO_2 increased; pH normal
    c. pO_2 decreased; pCO_2 normal; pH normal
    d. pO_2 decreased; pCO_2 decreased; pH increased

46–33. Which of the FEV_1 presented, as percentage of predicted values, is associated with respiratory acidosis (stage 4 asthma)?

    a. <20
    b. 35 to 49

    c. 50 to 64
    d. 65 to 80

46–34. For which reason is the pregnant woman with asthma more likely to develop hypoxia?

    a. increased residual volume
    b. decreased functional residual capacity
    c. decreased tidal volume
    d. increased inspiratory capacity

46–35. Which signs point to a potentially fatal asthmatic attack?

    a. use of accessory muscles, labored breathing
    b. central cyanosis, labored breathing
    c. use of accessory muscles, prolonged expiration
    d. central cyanosis, altered consciousness

46–36. Which of the following tests is most useful in monitoring airway obstruction?

    a. chest x-ray
    b. arterial blood gas
    c. FEV_1 (forced expiratory volume in 1 sec)
    d. pulse oximeter

46–37. What is the first-line therapy for mild asthma?

    a. antibiotics
    b. β-adrenergic agonist
    c. methylxanthines
    d. cromolyn sodium

46–38. Which of the following agents is used to stabilize mast cell membranes?

    a. theophylline
    b. cromolyn sulfate
    c. corticosteroids
    d. epinephrine

46–39. Which of the following analgesics is a nonhistamine-releasing narcotic and therefore should be used for those with asthma?

    a. morphine
    b. meperidine
    c. fentanyl
    d. codeine

46–40. Which agent should be used to treat postpartum hemorrhage in women with asthma?

    a. prostaglandin E_2
    b. prostaglandin $F_{2\alpha}$
    c. 15-methyl $PGF_{2\alpha}$
    d. none of the above

46–41. In which of the following locations is a pulmonary embolus unlikely to have originated?

    a. superficial thigh veins
    b. deep veins: leg
    c. deep veins: thigh
    d. deep veins: pelvis

46–42. Which of the following deficiencies is NOT associated with increased incidence of thromboembolic complications?

    a. protein M
    b. protein S
    c. protein C
    d. antithrombin III

46–43. What is the treatment for superficial thrombophlebitis?

    a. analgesia and coumarin
    b. analgesia and rest
    c. "mini dose" heparin
    d. full anticoagulation

46–44. Phlegmasia alba dolens is clinically suspected in which of the following situations?

    a. There is abrupt onset of leg pain and edema.
    b. Edema of both lower extremities exists.
    c. Red hot lower extremity is noted.
    d. None of the above apply.

46–45. What is the procedure of choice to diagnose deep venous thrombosis?

    a. impedance plethysmography
    b. real-time ultrasonography
    c. real-time ultrasound plus Doppler
    d. color Doppler ultrasonography

46–46. Where does thrombosis associated with pulmonary embolism in pregnant women frequently originate?

    a. popliteal veins
    b. femoral veins
    c. iliac veins
    d. vena cava

46–47. What is the approximate incidence of pulmonary embolism associated with pregnancy?

    a. 1 in 70 deliveries
    b. 1 in 700 deliveries
    c. 1 in 7000 deliveries
    d. 1 in 70,000 deliveries

46–48. A negative ventilation-perfusion scan is associated with pulmonary embolism in what percentage of patients?

    a. <1
    b. 2 to 4
    c. 8 to 10
    d. >15

46–49. In giving heparin subcutaneously every 12 hours, when should the activated partial thromboplastin time be checked?

    a. 2 hr after last dose
    b. 4 hr after last dose
    c. 6 hr after last dose
    d. immediately prior to next dose

46–50. In general, for "full" anticoagulation, what should the total daily dose of heparin be?

    a. 2000 to 5000 U
    b. 10,000 to 12,000 U
    c. 15,000 to 20,000 U
    d. 24,000 to 40,000 U

46–51. A major side effect of heparin is osteoporosis. This is more likely to occur in which situation listed below?

    a. <20,000 U/d for a short time
    b. treatment exceeds 6 mon
    c. >20,000 U/d for 3 mon
    d. >20,000 U/d for 6 mon

46–52. What is the most serious complication with heparin?

    a. hemorrhage
    b. thrombosis
    c. osteoporosis
    d. thrombocytopenia

46–53. How should a woman with deep venous thrombosis in a previous pregnancy be managed in a current pregnancy?

    a. careful observation
    b. minidose of subcutaneous heparin
    c. full prophylactic subcutaneous heparin
    d. low-dose aspirin

46–54. Which of the following is a serious complication seen in one-third of women on low-molecular-weight heparin?

    a. deep vein thromboemboli
    b. osteopenia
    c. pulmonary emboli
    d. thrombocytopenia

46–55. Which of the following is given to reverse the anticoagulation effects of heparin?

    a. protamine sulfate intravenously
    b. vitamin D
    c. vitamin E
    d. vitamin K 10 mg intravenously

46–56. Which of the following groups is NOT particularly at risk for tuberculosis?

    a. those who are pregnant
    b. the elderly
    c. the urban poor
    d. minorities

46–57. How should a pregnant woman who is tuberculin-positive but x-ray negative be managed?

    a. rifampin 10 mg/kg daily for 12 mon
    b. isoniazid 300 mg daily for 12 mon
    c. ethambutol for 12 mon
    d. observation and treatment after delivery

46–58. How should nonpregnant patients under age 35 who are tuberculin-positive but x-ray negative be treated?

    a. rifampin 10 mg/kg daily for 4 mon
    b. streptomycin for 12 mon
    c. isoniazid 300 mg daily for 12 mon
    d. pyridoxine for 12 mon

46–59. Which of the following antituberculosis agents is associated with severe congenital deafness if given during pregnancy?

    a. streptomycin
    b. isoniazid
    c. rifampin
    d. ethambutol

46–60. Which of the following x-ray findings is the hallmark of sarcoidosis?

    a. mediastinal widening
    b. diffuse infiltrates
    c. patchy infiltrates
    d. interstitial pneumonitis

46–61. How is symptomatic severe pulmonary sarcoidosis treated?

    a. betamethasone 12 mg intramuscularly every day
    b. decadron 6 mg orally twice a day
    c. prednisone 1 mg/kg/d
    d. cyclophosphamide 1 mg/kg/d

46–62. The cystic fibrosis transmembrane conductance receptor regulator (CFTR) is associated with which chromosome?

    a. 3p
    b. 5q
    c. 7q
    d. 9p

46–63. Which of the following electrolyte patterns in sweat is associated with cystic fibrosis?

    a. ↑sodium   ↓potassium   ↑chloride
    b. ↑sodium   ↑potassium   ↓chloride
    c. ↑sodium   ↓potassium   ↓chloride
    d. ↑sodium   ↑potassium   ↑chloride

46–64. Lung function in women with cystic fibrosis is improved by using which of the following to decrease the viscosity of sputum?

    a. recombinant human deoxiribonuclease I
    b. acetylcysteine mist
    c. bronchodilators
    d. diuretics

46–65. Treatment of carbon monoxide poisoning in pregnancy includes which of the following?

    a. supportive
    b. 100% O_2
    c. hyperbaric O_2
    d. all of the above

Renal and Urinary Tract Disorders

47–1. What percentage of women have dilation of the renal calyces during pregnancy?

   a. 10
   b. 30
   c. 50
   d. 70

47–2. During pregnancy, effective renal plasma flow is increased by what percentage?

   a. 5 to 10
   b. 20 to 30
   c. 40 to 65
   d. 80 to 90

47–3. What is the cut-off for significant proteinuria during pregnancy?

   a. 50 mg/d
   b. 100 mg/d
   c. 200 mg/d
   d. 300 mg/d

47–4. What is the average daily excretion of albumin during pregnancy?

   a. <50 mg
   b. 100 mg
   c. 200 mg
   d. 500 mg

47–5. What is postural (orthostatic) proteinuria?

   a. protein when ambulatory
   b. protein secondary to mild renal disease
   c. protein due to bacteriuria
   d. protein at night time in a patient with hypertension

47–6. Which of the following enhances the virulence of *Escherichia coli?*

   a. glycoprotein receptors
   b. *P-fimbriae*

   c. exotoxins
   d. nuclear pili

47–7. What is the prevalence of asymptomatic bacteriuria in pregnancy?

   a. 4%
   b. 2 to 7%
   c. 10 to 12%
   d. 20%

47–8. Which of the following is most likely be associated with covert bacteriuria?

   a. age <20 years
   b. hypertension
   c. sickle cell trait
   d. lupus

47–9. Using multivariate analysis, what are the adverse pregnancy outcomes associated with asymptomatic bacteriuria?

   a. low-birthweight infants
   b. preterm delivery
   c. acute antepartum pyelonephritis
   d. all of the above

47–10. What is the most likely diagnosis in a woman with frequency, urgency, pyuria, dysuria, and a sterile urine culture?

   a. *Escherichia coli* cystitis
   b. group B streptococcus cystitis
   c. *Chlamydia trachomatis* urethritis
   d. *Neisseria gonorrhoeae* urethritis

47–11. What is the most common serious medical complication of pregnancy?

   a. thrombophlebitis
   b. pneumonia
   c. pancreatitis
   d. pyelonephritis

47–12. Of the bacteria that cause renal infection, what is the incidence of P-fimbriae?

a. 10%
b. 35%
c. 70%
d. >80%

47–13. What organism is associated with antepartum pyelonephritis?

a. *Listeria monocytogenes*
b. *Klebsiella pneumoniae*
c. *Pseudomonas*
d. *Peptostreptococcus*

47–14. What percentage of women with acute antepartum pyelonephritis have bacteremia?

a. 7.5
b. 15.0
c. 22.5
d. 30.0

47–15. Which of the following is NOT included in the differential diagnosis for pyelonephritis?

a. chorioamnionitis
b. labor
c. pneumonia
d. abruptio placentae

47–16. What causes the large temperature swings (i.e., "hypothalamic instability") in pyelonephritis?

a. cytokines
b. interferons
c. endorphins
d. exotoxins

47–17. Which of the following cause alveolar injury, and hence respiratory insufficiency, in women with pyelonephritis?

a. prostaglandins
b. cytokines
c. interferons
d. endotoxins

47–18. Anemia in women with pyelonephritis is due to which of the following?

a. hemolysis induced by endotoxin
b. dilution due to hydration
c. increased erythropoietin production
d. cytokine-induced thrombocytopenia

47–19. What is the initial drug of choice for the treatment of pyelonephritis in pregnancy?

a. ampicillin
b. cephalosporin

c. aminoglycoside
d. ureidopenicillin

47–20. What percentage of renal stones are radiopaque?

a. 60
b. 70
c. 80
d. 90

47–21. An 18-year-old nulliparous black woman has been taking antibiotics for 4 days for pyelonephritis. She continues to have fever ranging from 38.9 to 39.6°C. Work-up reveals a right ureteral obstruction secondary to calculi. What is the next most appropriate step in her management?

a. Change antibiotics.
b. Continue present antibiotics.
c. Pass a double-J ureteral stent.
d. Perform percutaneous nephrostomy.

47–22. What is the incidence of bacteriuria in women with renal scarring from childhood infections?

a. 10%
b. 30%
c. 50%
d. 70%

47–23. What is the composition of the majority of renal stones?

a. struvite
b. calcium salts
c. uric acid
d. magnesium salts

47–24. What is the most common presenting symptom of renal stones in pregnant women?

a. flank pain
b. abdominal discomfort
c. hematuria
d. infection

47–25. Which of the following is NOT one of the five major glomerulopathic syndromes?

a. rapidly progressive glomerulonephritis
b. chronic pyelonephritis
c. nephrotic syndrome
d. acute glomerulonephritis

47–26. Which of the following are signs and symptoms of acute glomerulonephritis?

a. hematuria, proteinuria, edema, and hypertension
b. proteinuria and hypertension but no edema
c. hematuria, hypotension, and proteinuria
d. proteinuria, hypotension, and edema

47–27. Which of the following is NOT a fetal effect of glomerulonephritis?

   a. fetal loss
   b. fetal growth retardation
   c. preterm birth
   d. fetal intraventricular hemorrhage

47–28. What is the incidence of hypertension in pregnancy in women with glomerulonephritis?

   a. 10%
   b. 25%
   c. 50%
   d. 75%

47–29. What percentage of women with primary glomerulonephritis have worsening proteinuria?

   a. 20
   b. 40
   c. 60
   d. 80

47–30. Which of the following is NOT associated with a poor perinatal prognosis in parturients with glomerulonephritis?

   a. impaired renal function
   b. severe hypertension
   c. anemia
   d. proteinuria greater than 5 g per 24 hr

47–31. Which of the following is suggestive of chronic glomerulopathy?

   a. creatinine 0.6 mg/dL
   b. hematocrit 40%
   c. proteinuria 480 mg per 24 hr
   d. kidneys 11 cm in length ultrasonographically

47–32. What are the characteristics of nephrotic syndrome?

   a. proteinuria >300 mg/d, hyperlipidemia, and edema
   b. proteinuria >300 mg/d and hypolipidemia
   c. proteinuria >3000 mg/d, hyperlipidemia, and edema
   d. proteinuria >3000 mg/d and hypolipidemia

47–33. Which of the following is the most common cause of nephrotic syndrome?

   a. membranous glomerulopathy
   b. minimal change disease
   c. poststreptococcal glomerulonephritis
   d. amyloidosis

47–34. Successful pregnancy outcomes can be anticipated in women with nephrosis in which of the following circumstances?

   a. Woman is normotensive.
   b. Renal insufficiency is moderate.
   c. Proteinuria is <5 g/d.
   d. Hypertension is controlled with blood pressure medications.

47–35. What is the significance of proteinuria if it antedates pregnancy?

   a. benign
   b. associated with anemia in 25%
   c. hypertension in 70%
   d. preterm delivery in 10%

47–36. What is the mechanism of inheritance in adult polycystic kidney disease?

   a. sporadic
   b. X-linked recessive
   c. autosomal recessive
   d. autosomal dominant

47–37. Polycystic kidney disease is linked to the α-hemoglobin gene complex on the short arm of which chromosome?

   a. 1
   b. 11
   c. 16
   d. X

47–38. Which of the following is NOT a symptom of polycystic kidney disease?

   a. flank pain
   b. nocturia
   c. fever
   d. malaise

47–39. Which of the following is associated with polycystic kidneys?

   a. hepatic cysts
   b. mitral stenosis
   c. diverticulosis
   d. uterine anomalies

47–40. What is the adverse effect of pregnancy on women with polycystic kidney disease?

   a. increased spontaneous abortion
   b. increased stillbirths
   c. increased symptomatic urinary infection
   d. no adverse perinatal effect

47–41. What is the least common cause of end-stage renal disease?

    a. diabetes
    b. hypertension
    c. glomerulonephritis
    d. polycystic kidney disease

47–42. What is the average blood volume expansion in pregnant women with mild renal insufficiency?

    a. 10%
    b. 30%
    c. 50%
    d. 70%

47–43. What is the average blood volume expansion in pregnant women with severe renal insufficiency?

    a. 10%
    b. 25%
    c. 35%
    d. 45%

47–44. Which of the following is NOT associated with pregnancies in women with chronic renal insufficiency?

    a. anemia
    b. hypertension
    c. hypercalcemia
    d. preeclampsia

47–45. Which of the following is a major side effect from recombinant erythropoietin use in pregnancy?

    a. hyperviscosity
    b. hypertension
    c. human immunodeficiency viral transmission
    d. worsening renal function

47–46. In pregnancies complicated by severe renal insufficiency, pregnancy itself causes which of the following?

    a. accelerated renal insufficiency
    b. complete resolution of renal insufficiency

    c. partial resolution of renal insufficiency
    d. no appreciable change in renal function

47–47. Which of the following is NOT included in the differential diagnosis of renal transplant rejection during pregnancy?

    a. pyelonephritis
    b. preeclampsia
    c. respiratory distress syndrome
    d. recurrent glomerulonephropathy

47–48. Which of the following is most helpful in making the diagnosis of renal transplant rejection during pregnancy?

    a. renal biopsy
    b. clinical symptoms
    c. urinalysis
    d. renal vein laboratory studies

47–49. What percentage of pregnancies in women on chronic hemodialysis have anemia?

    a. 5 to 10
    b. 25 to 30
    c. 50 to 60
    d. 90 to 95

47–50. What is the most common cause of acute renal failure in pregnancy?

    a. drug abuse
    b. systemic lupus erythematosus
    c. preeclampsia or eclampsia
    d. sickle cell disease

47–51. Which of the following pregnancy complications is NOT associated with renal cortical necrosis?

    a. eclampsia
    b. placental abruption
    c. endotoxin-induced shock
    d. placenta previa

Gastrointestinal Disorders

48–1. What is the incidence of laparotomy during pregnancy?

a. 1 in 240
b. 1 in 500
c. 1 in 1000
d. 1 in 5000

48–2. What is the incidence of nonobstetrical surgery in pregnancy?

a. 1 in 200
b. 1 in 400
c. 1 in 800
d. 1 in 1600

48–3. Why does total parenteral nutrition require catheterization of the jugular or subclavian vein?

a. Thromboembolism occurs if given in a smaller vein.
b. The solution is hyperosmolar and needs to be diluted in a high-flow system.
c. Essential fatty acids block smaller veins.
d. The potassium content causes sclerosis of the smaller veins.

48–4. What is the most common complication associated with central catheters for hyperalimentation?

a. osmotic diuresis
b. thrombosis
c. electrolyte imbalance
d. infection

48–5. Which of the following findings would be expected in women with hyperemesis gravidarum?

a. hematocrit <30 vol%
b. creatinine 0.3 mg/dL
c. ALT 86 IU/L
d. K^+ 5.8 mEq/L

48–6. Which of the following antiemetics is Food and Drug Administration category B drug?

a. metoclopramide
b. promethazine
c. chlorpromazine
d. prochlorperazine

48–7. What is the etiology of reflux esophagitis in pregnancy?

a. constriction of upper esophageal sphincter
b. relaxation of upper esophageal sphincter
c. constriction of lower esophageal sphincter
d. relaxation of lower esophageal sphincter

48–8. Diaphragmatic hernias are herniations of abdominal contents through which foramen?

a. Morgagni
b. oavale
c. magnum
d. Morgan

48–9. Which of the following is a motor disorder of esophageal smooth muscle?

a. diaphragmatic hernia
b. hiatal hernia
c. reflux esophagitis
d. achalasia

48–10. Which of the following treatments is NOT indicated in the management of achalasia?

a. soft foods
b. anticholinergic drugs
c. pneumatic dilation
d. hyperalimentation

48–11. What organism is associated with peptic ulcer disease?

a. *Heliobacter stomachi*
b. *Heliobacter pylori*
c. *Heliobacter acidi*
d. *Heliobacter gastrecti*

48–12. Which of the following is associated with normal pregnancy?

    a. decreased mucus secretion
    b. increased gastric secretion
    c. decreased gastric motility
    d. constriction of lower esophageal sphincter

48–13. The majority of pregnancies with upper gastrointestinal bleeding have which of the following?

    a. Boerhaave syndrome
    b. stomach cancer
    c. Mallory-Weiss tears
    d. peptic ulceration

48–14. Which of the following is a dangerous complication associated with ulcerative colitis?

    a. toxic megacolon
    b. bloody diarrhea
    c. arthritis
    d. erythema nodosum

48–15. Which of the following HLA haplotypes is associated with ulcerative colitis?

    a. HLA-BW 35
    b. HLA-A2
    c. HLA-B3
    d. HLA-A16

48–16. Which active metabolite of sulfasalazine inhibits prostaglandin synthase?

    a. sulfazine-a
    b. sulfazine-b
    c. 2 aminosalicylic acid
    d. 5 aminosalicylic acid

48–17. What is the most likely course for ulcerative colitis that is quiescent at the beginning of gestation?

    a. no activation of disease during pregnancy
    b. active disease during pregnancy in 33%
    c. active disease during pregnancy in 67%
    d. active disease during pregnancy in 100%

48–18. What is a common long-term complication in a woman who has had a colectomy with mucosal proctectomy and ileal pouch-anal anastomosis?

    a. pouchitis
    b. large bowel obstruction
    c. proctitis
    d. fistula formation

48–19. What is the most common cause of bowel obstruction in pregnancy?

    a. infection
    b. adhesions
    c. cancer
    d. mechanical compression from the uterus

48–20. What is the most common symptom associated with bowel obstruction?

    a. nausea
    b. vomiting
    c. abdominal pain
    d. diarrhea

48–21. What is the cause of pseudo-obstruction of the colon (Ogilvie syndrome)?

    a. pelvic adhesions
    b. impacted stool
    c. adynamic colonic ileus
    d. medications used postpartum

48–22. Which of the following is NOT in the differential diagnosis of appendicitis in pregnancy?

    a. Crohn's disease
    b. placental abruption
    c. pyelonephritis
    d. pneumonia

48–23. Which of the following complications is associated with ruptured appendix and peritonitis?

    a. fetal growth restriction
    b. oligohydramnios
    c. chorioamnionitis
    d. preterm birth

48–24. What is the major histological lesion of intrahepatic cholestasis?

    a. centrilobular bile staining
    b. mesenchymal proliferation
    c. periportal necrosis
    d. centrilobular necrosis

48–25. What is the suspected pathogenesis of intrahepatic cholestasis, as compared to controls?

    a. increased human placental lactogen
    b. increased human chorionic gonadotropin
    c. decreased plasma estrogen
    d. decreased progesterone

48–26. Which of the following is appropriate in the management of intrahepatic cholestasis?

    a. azathioprine
    b. antihistamines
    c. ampicillin
    d. vitamin A

48–27. Which of the following is NOT an adverse pregnancy outcome associated with intrahepatic cholestasis?

    a. abruptio placentae
    b. preterm birth
    c. stillbirth
    d. postpartum hemorrhage

48–28. What is the prominent histological abnormality associated with acute fatty liver of pregnancy?

    a. intranuclear fat
    b. microvesicular fat
    c. massive hepatocellular necrosis
    d. all of the above

48–29. What is the etiology of acute fatty liver of pregnancy?

    a. autosomal recessive
    b. mitochondrial inheritance
    c. X-linked recessive
    d. polygenic

48–30. What is the major symptom in pregnancy complicated by acute fatty liver?

    a. malaise
    b. anorexia
    c. epigastric pain
    d. vomiting

48–31. What is the etiology of diabetes insipidus in pregnancies complicated by acute fatty liver?

    a. excessive levels of oxytocin
    b. elevated vasopressinase concentrations
    c. fatty deposits in supraoptic nuclei
    d. decreased blood flow to posterior pituitary

48–32. What is the pathologic liver lesion in preeclampsia secondary to?

    a. edema
    b. infection
    c. ischemia
    d. toxins

48–33. What percentage of the liver's blood supply comes from the hepatic artery?

    a. 10
    b. 25
    c. 33
    d. 50

48–34. Where are liver hematomas secondary to preeclampsia generally located?

    a. abdominal surface of the right lobe
    b. abdominal surface of the left lobe
    c. diaphragmatic surface of the right lobe
    d. diaphragmatic surface of the left lobe

48–35. What is the most common serious liver disease in pregnancy?

    a. intrahepatic cholestasis
    b. hepatitis
    c. preeclampsia
    d. acute fatty liver

48–36. Which of the following are due to a deoxyribonucleic acid virus?

    a. hepatitis A
    b. hepatitis B
    c. hepatitis C
    d. delta hepatitis

48–37. What is the incubation period for hepatitis A?

    a. 3 to 5 days
    b. 2 to 7 weeks
    c. 10 to 12 weeks
    d. >20 weeks

48–38. Which of the following hepatitis panels is associated with acute hepatitis A and chronic hepatitis B?

	HBsAg	Anti-HAV IgM	Anti-HBc IgM
a.	−	+	−
b.	+	+	+
c.	+	+	−
d.	+	−	+

48–39. Which of the following is recommended for a pregnant woman exposed to hepatitis A?

    a. gamma globulin
    b. hepatitis A immunoglobulin
    c. hepatitis B immunoglobulin (HBIG)
    d. HBIG plus gamma globulin

48–40. What is the frequency of chronic hepatitis B following acute disease?

    a. <1%
    b. 5 to 10%
    c. 20 to 25%
    d. 40 to 50%

48–41. What percentage of hepatitis B infected infants develop chronic infection?

    a. <1
    b. 5 to 10
    c. 20 to 30
    d. 70 to 90

48–42. What is the first virological marker for hepatitis B?

   a. HBeAg
   b. HBcAg
   c. HBsAg
   d. HB dane Ag

48–43. What is the significance of the e antigen of hepatitis B virus?

   a. viral shedding in the feces
   b. associated with infectivity
   c. number of circulating virus particles
   d. chronic carrier state

48–44. How should infants delivered to chronic hepatitis B carriers be treated?

   a. isolated from their mothers
   b. treated with HBIG
   c. vaccinated with recombinant vaccine
   d. given HBIG and recombinant vaccine

48–45. When is the antibody first detected in the majority of patients with hepatitis C?

   a. at 3 weeks
   b. at 9 weeks
   c. at 15 weeks
   d. at 1 year

48–46. What is the incidence of persistent hepatitis C infection that progresses to cirrhosis within 10 years?

   a. 5%
   b. 10%
   c. 20%
   d. 50%

48–47. Which of the following agents may be effective or beneficial in producing remission in one-half of chronic hepatitis C carriers?

   a. corticosteroids
   b. azathioprine
   c. interferon-α
   d. interleukin-2

48–48. What is the most common cause of cirrhosis in young women?

   a. alcohol
   b. hepatitis
   c. illicit drug use
   d. prescribed drugs

48–49. What is the normal portal vein pressure?

   a. <5 mm Hg
   b. 10 to 15 mm Hg

   c. 30 to 40 mm Hg
   d. 60 to 80 mm Hg

48–50. What is the portal vein pressure associated with esophageal varices?

   a. >10 mm Hg
   b. >20 mm Hg
   c. >30 mm Hg
   d. >40 mm Hg

48–51. What is the treatment of choice for acetaminophen overdosage?

   a. *N*-acetylcysteine
   b. glutathione
   c. induce emesis with charcoal
   d. aggressive fluids containing sodium bicarbonate

48–52. What is the most common pregnancy complication in women with liver transplants?

   a. anemia
   b. hypertension
   c. preterm delivery
   d. psychosis

48–53. What is the major component of gallstones?

   a. cholesterol
   b. calcium
   c. bile acids
   d. struvite

48–54. What is the cause of decreased gallbladder motility in pregnancy?

   a. estrogen
   b. progesterone
   c. cholecystokinin
   d. relaxin

48–55. Which of the following is NOT an acceptable nonsurgical approach to gallstone disease?

   a. chenodeoxycholic acid
   b. dietary changes
   c. intragallbladder methyl terbutyl ether
   d. extracorporeal shock wave lithotripsy

48–56. Which of the following is relatively contraindicated in pregnancy for the management of gallstones?

   a. laparoscopic cholecystectomy
   b. endoscopic retrograde cholangiopancreatography
   c. laparotomy at 12 weeks' gestation
   d. none of the above

48–57. Which of the following is NOT a cause of pancreatitis in pregnancy?

   a. trauma
   b. hypotriglyceridemia
   c. alcoholism
   d. gallstones

48–58. Which of the following portends a bad prognosis in women with pancreatitis?

   a. twin gestation
   b. hypercalcemia
   c. shock
   d. dehydration

48–59. Which laboratory finding confirms the diagnosis of pancreatitis?

   a. leukocytosis
   b. serum amylase three times normal
   c. low serum lipase
   d. hypocalcemia

48–60. What percentage of adults are obese?

   a. 12
   b. 25
   c. 33
   d. 40

48–61. Which of the following is the most common pregnancy problem identified in obese women as compared to nonobese women?

   a. hypertension
   b. postterm pregnancy
   c. macrosomia
   d. shoulder dystocia

48–62. What is the formula for body mass index (BMI)?

   a. weight in pounds, height in inches
   b. weight in pounds, height in meters squared
   c. weight in kilograms, height in centimeters
   d. weight in kilograms, height in meters squared

48–63. Using BMI and a cutoff of less than 27.3 for obesity, what is the percentage of obese young women in the United States?

   a. 20
   b. 30
   c. 40
   d. 50

48–64. What congenital anomaly is increased in the offspring of obese women?

   a. congenital heart disease
   b. renal agenesis
   c. tracheoesophageal fistula
   d. neural tube defects

Hematological Disorders

49–1. How is anemia defined in terms of hemoglobin concentration during the third trimester of pregnancy?

   a. <9 g/dL
   b. <10 g/dL
   c. <11 g/dL
   d. <12 g/dL

49–2. What are the most common causes of anemia during pregnancy?

   a. iron deficiency; acute blood loss
   b. iron deficiency; sickle cell disease
   c. folate deficiency; acute blood loss
   d. folate deficiency; sickle cell disease

49–3. Which of the following may increase in pregnancies complicated by anemia in the second trimester?

    a. pregnancy-induced hypertension
    b. gestational diabetes
    c. preterm birth
    d. urinary tract infection

49–4. Which of the following is NOT associated with high hemoglobin concentrations (>13.2 g/dL)?

    a. diabetes
    b. perinatal mortality
    c. low-birthweight infants
    d. preterm delivery

49–5. What are the total iron requirements for the mother and fetus during a normal pregnancy?

    a. 100 mg
    b. 300 mg
    c. 1000 mg
    d. 3000 mg

49–6. Which of the following has the most influence on iron stores in the infant?

    a. maternal iron status
    b. timing of cord clamping
    c. maternal vitamin C intake
    d. blood loss at time of delivery

49–7. At what hemoglobin level would you first expect to see erythrocyte hypochromia and microcytosis?

    a. <6 g/dL
    b. <7 g/dL
    c. <8 g/dL
    d. <9 g/dL

49–8. A peripheral smear in a black woman with a hemoglobin concentration of 8 g/dL reveals hypochromia and microcytosis. What is the most likely diagnosis?

    a. sickle cell anemia
    b. folate deficiency
    c. iron deficiency
    d. β-thalassemia

49–9. In the patient in question 49-8, serum ferritin and iron-binding capacity are obtained. Which of the following confirm your diagnosis?

    a. low ferritin; decreased iron-binding capacity
    b. low ferritin; increased iron-binding capacity
    c. high ferritin; decreased iron-binding capacity
    d. high ferritin; increased iron-binding capacity

49–10. Which of the following excludes iron deficiency as a cause of anemia?

    a. elevated serum iron-binding capacity
    b. normal serum ferritin
    c. bone marrow normoblastic hyperplasia
    d. positive sickle cell preparation

49–11. How much elemental iron per day is needed for the treatment of iron-deficiency anemia during pregnancy?

    a. 50 mg
    b. 100 mg
    c. 200 mg
    d. 400 mg

49–12. Which of the following is NOT associated with anemia?

    a. inflammatory bowel disease
    b. chronic renal disease
    c. essential hypertension
    d. systemic lupus erythematosus

49–13. What is the cause of anemia in women with acute antepartum pyelonephritis?

    a. decreased erythropoietin production
    b. increased red blood cell destruction due to endotoxemia
    c. dilution secondary to intravenous hydration
    d. decreased iron stores

49–14. In women with chronic renal disease, which of the following characterizes the degree of red blood cell mass expansion during pregnancy?

    a. same as a woman with normal renal function
    b. increased compared with normal pregnancy
    c. decreased by the corresponding degree of renal impairment compared with normal pregnancy
    d. does not occur because of low levels of ferritin

49–15. What is a worrisome side effect of recombinant erythropoietin to treat chronic anemia?

    a. hypertension
    b. expanded red blood cell mass
    c. placenta previa
    d. allergic reaction

49–16. What is the earliest morphological evidence of folic acid deficiency?

    a. hypersegmentation of neutrophils
    b. microcytosis
    c. macrocytic erythrocytes
    d. nucleated red blood cells

49–17. What is the treatment for pregnancy-induced megaloblastic anemia?

    a. nutritious diet only
    b. 1000 μg vitamin B_{12} every month
    c. 200 mg/d iron (supplemental)
    d. 1 mg/d folic acid, nutritious diet, and iron

49–18. In which of the following circumstances is folate 4 mg/d indicated?

    a. multifetal pregnancy
    b. Crohn's disease
    c. iron-deficiency anemia
    d. previous infant with neural tube defect

49–19. Serum vitamin B_{12} levels are decreased in pregnancy secondary to which of the following?

    a. increased fibrinogen
    b. decreased fibrinogen
    c. increased transcobalamin
    d. decreased transcobalamin

49–20. What is the treatment for pregnant women who have undergone a total gastrectomy?

    a. 1 μg vitamin B_{12} daily
    b. 1000 μg vitamin B_{12} monthly
    c. 1 mg folic acid daily
    d. 4 mg folic acid daily

49–21. What is the most common cause of autoimmune hemolytic anemia?

    a. drug-induced cold autoantibodies
    b. chronic inflammatory disease
    c. warm, active autoantibodies
    d. connective tissue disease

49–22. Which of the following may induce cold-agglutinin disease?

    a. *Chlamydia trachomatis*
    b. *Neisseria gonorrhoeae*
    c. *Streptococcus agalactiae*
    d. *Mycoplasma pneumoniae*

49–23. What is effective therapy for autoimmune hemolytic anemia?

    a. corticosteroids (e.g., prednisone 1 mg/kg/d)
    b. supplemental iron 200 mg/d
    c. folate 1 mg/d
    d. corticosteroids plus vitamin B_{12}

49–24. Which of the following drugs may induce antierythrocyte antibodies?

    a. ibuprofen
    b. erythromycin

    c. methyldopa
    d. acetaminophen

49–25. Which of the following is a hemopoietic stem-cell disorder characterized by formation of defective platelets, granulocytes, and erythrocytes?

    a. pregnancy-induced hemolytic anemia
    b. paroxysmal nocturnal hemoglobinuria
    c. autoimmune hemolytic anemia
    d. Diamond-Blackfan syndrome

49–26. On which of the following chromosomes is the abnormal gene for paroxysmal nocturnal hemoglobinuria located?

    a. 6
    b. 11
    c. 16
    d. X

49–27. Which of the following is the mutated gene responsible for paroxysmal nocturnal hemoglobinuria?

    a. PNH-1
    b. PIG-A
    c. URE-3
    d. XPN-F

49–28. What is the treatment for paroxysmal nocturnal hemoglobinuria?

    a. iron
    b. corticosteroids
    c. heparin
    d. bone marrow transplantation

49–29. How are most cases of spherocytosis inherited?

    a. autosomal recessive
    b. autosomal dominant
    c. X-linked recessive
    d. X-linked dominant

49–30. Autosomal recessive spherocytosis is caused by a deficiency of which of the following?

    a. spectrin
    b. protein S
    c. ankyrin
    d. protein C

49–31. How is glucose-6-phosphate dehydrogenase deficiency inherited?

    a. autosomal recessive
    b. autosomal dominant
    c. X-linked recessive
    d. X-linked dominant

49–32. What is the most common cause of aplastic anemia?

    a. drug-induced
    b. infection
    c. immunological disorder
    d. idiopathic

49–33. What is the major risk to a pregnant woman with aplastic anemia?

    a. hemorrhage
    b. preterm labor
    c. pregnancy-induced hypertension
    d. anemia

49–34. Which of the following is the therapy of choice for aplastic anemia if a suitable bone marrow donor is not available?

    a. corticosteroids
    b. testosterone
    c. antithymocyte globulin
    d. cytoxan

49–35. Hemoglobin S is owing to a substitution of which of the following?

    a. valine for glutamic acid at position 6
    b. glutamic acid for valine at position 6
    c. lysine for glutamic acid at position 6
    d. glutamic acid for leucine at position 6

49–36. What is the theoretical incidence of sickle cell anemia among blacks?

    a. 1 in 12
    b. 1 in 144
    c. 1 in 576
    d. 1 in 2000

49–37. Approximately how many blacks have the gene for hemoglobin C?

    a. 1 in 12
    b. 1 in 40
    c. 1 in 100
    d. 1 in 200

49–38. What is the approximate perinatal mortality in pregnancies complicated by hemoglobin SC disease?

    a. 10 in 1000
    b. 100 in 1000
    c. 200 in 1000
    d. 500 in 1000

49–39. Which of the following is NOT associated with hemoglobin SC disease in pregnancy?

    a. severe bone pain
    b. pulmonary infarction
    c. placental abruption
    d. adult respiratory distress syndrome

49–40. Which of the following is NOT considered effective in the management of pain from intravascular sickling?

    a. intravenous hydration
    b. morphine
    c. prophylactic red blood cell transfusions
    d. therapeutic red blood cell transfusions

49–41. Prophylactic red blood cell transfusions in pregnant women with sickle cell anemia is most likely to decrease which of the following?

    a. perinatal mortality
    b. maternal morbidity
    c. fetal growth retardation
    d. preterm delivery

49–42. In patients with sickle cell disease, what is the incidence of isoimmunization per unit of blood transfused?

    a. 1%
    b. 3%
    c. 10%
    d. 30%

49–43. Which of the following increases in pregnancies complicated by sickle cell trait?

    a. perinatal mortality
    b. abortion (spontaneous)
    c. low birthweight
    d. urinary tract infection

49–44. Hemoglobin C results from substitution of glutamic acid by what amino acid at position 6 of the β-chain?

    a. valine
    b. leucine
    c. lysine
    d. phenylalanine

49–45. Which of the following adverse pregnancy outcomes is increased in women with hemoglobin C trait?

    a. preterm deliveries
    b. fetal growth retardation
    c. perinatal mortality
    d. none of the above

49–46. Which of the following peripheral blood smears would be expected in a patient with hemoglobin E?

    a. hypochromia; microcytosis; erythrocyte targeting

    b. hypochromia; macrocytosis; erythrocyte targeting

    c. hypochromia; microcytosis; hypersegmented neutrophils

    d. hypochromia; macrocytosis; hypersegmented neutrophils

49–47. Which chromosome contains the gene for α-globin chain synthesis?

    a. 6
    b. 11
    c. 16
    d. 21

49–48. Which of the following patterns characterizes hemoglobin Bart?

    a. - -, a a
    b. - a,- a
    c. $\beta 4$
    d. $\gamma 4$

49–49. Which of the following ethnic groups is most likely to have hemoglobin Bart?

    a. whites of Mediterranean descent
    b. Asians
    c. Africans
    d. Greeks

49–50. Which chromosome contains the gene for β-globin chain synthesis?

    a. 6
    b. 11
    c. 16
    d. 21

49–51. Which of the following characterizes thalassemias?

    a. impaired production of β-globin chains
    b. increased destruction of erythrocytes containing hemoglobin F
    c. increased production of globin chains
    d. decreased production of hemoglobin F

49–52. Which of the following is elevated with β-thalassemias?

    a. hemoglobin A
    b. hemoglobin A_2
    c. hemoglobin F
    d. hemoglobin H

49–53. Which of the following characterizes β-thalassemia?

    a. increased β-chain production; decreased α chains
    b. increased β-chain production; increased α chains
    c. decreased β-chain production; decreased α chains
    d. decreased β-chain production; increased α chains

49–54. Which of the following agents is used to chelate iron?

    a. iron-bind
    b. deferoxamine
    c. EDTA
    d. diferritin

49–55. Which of the following helps to differentiate polycythemia vera (PCV) from secondary polycythemia?

    a. low values of erythropoietin in PCV
    b. low values of erythropoietin in secondary polycythemia
    d. peripheral smear with nucleated red cells
    d. peripheral smear with hypersegmented neutrophils in PCV

49–56. Which of the following causes of thrombocytopenia is owing to a lack of platelet membrane glycoprotein?

    a. May-Hegglin anomaly
    b. Bernand-Soulier syndrome
    c. hemolytic uremic syndrome
    d. drug-induced thrombocytopenia

49–57. Which of the following is inherited in an autosomal dominant fashion?

    a. Bernard-Souiler
    b. sickle cell anemia
    c. May-Hegglin anomaly
    d. idiopathic thrombocytopenia purpura

49–58. What is the mechanism of action of corticosteroids in the therapy of immunological thrombocytopenia purpura?

    a. suppresses phagocytic activity in the spleen
    b. decreases removal of platelets by the spleen
    c. causes short-term reticuloendothelial blockade and diminishes platelet sequestration
    d. increases platelet production

49–59. What is the fetal or neonatal risk of maternal immune thrombocytopenia purpura?

a. increased abortion rate
b. thrombocytopenia
c. necrotizing enterocolitis
d. no risk

49–60. Which of the following findings in women with immune thrombocytopenia purpura correlate closely with fetal platelet counts?

a. maternal platelet count
b. circulating antiplatelet antibodies
c. indirect platelet antiglobulin
d. no correlation with maternal status

49–61. What is the risk of neonatal thrombocytopenia in women with chronic immunological thrombocytopenia?

a. 3%
b. 6%
c. 12%
d. 24%

49–62. What is the average platelet count in women with essential thrombocytosis?

a. 200,000
b. 400,000
c. 800,000
d. 1,000,000

49–63. Which of the following is used to treat thrombocytosis that is complicating pregnancy?

a. hydroxyurea
b. coumadin
c. heparin
d. γ-interferon

49–64. Which of the following is NOT part of the pentad of thrombotic thrombocytopenic purpura?

a. fever
b. neurological abnormalities
c. hemolytic anemia
d. liver abnormalities

49–65. What is the pathogenesis of thrombotic microangiopathies?

a. unknown
b. microthrombi of hyaline material and platelets producing fluctuating ischemia
c. microthrombi (multiple) of erythrocyte clumps causing multiple infarctions
d. intravascular neutrophil aggregation stimulating cytokine production leading to end-organ failure

49–66. What is the most common presenting symptom in women with thrombotic thrombocytopenic syndrome?

a. fever
b. fatigue
c. hemorrhage
d. neurological abnormalities

49–67. What is the most common laboratory finding in women with thrombotic thrombocytopenic syndrome?

a. anemia
b. erythrocyte fragmentation
c. leukocytes
d. fibrin-split products

49–68. What is the treatment for thrombotic thrombocytopenic syndromes?

a. heparin
b. aspirin and dipyridamole
c. glucocorticoids
d. exchange transfusion with donor plasma and plasmapheresis

49–69. What is the perinatal mortality in pregnancies complicated by thrombotic thrombocytopenic syndromes?

a. 20%
b. 40%
c. 60%
d. 80%

49–70. Which factor is deficient in individuals with hemophilia A?

a. von Willebrand factor
b. antithrombin III
c. factor VIII:C
d. factor IX

49–71. Which of the following stimulates factor VIII:C release?

a. prednisone
b. γ-globulin
c. desmopressin
d. plasmapheresis

49–72. What is the most commonly inherited bleeding disorder?

a. von Willebrand disease
b. antithrombin III deficiency
c. factor VIII:C deficiency
d. factor IX deficiency

49–73. What is the site of synthesis of von Willebrand factor?

    a. liver
    b. endothelium and megakaryocytes
    c. megakaryocytes only
    d. kidney

49–74. Control of the synthesis of von Willebrand factor is on autosomal genes on which chromosome?

    a. 3
    b. 6
    c. 9
    d. 12

49–75. Which of the following hematologic disorders is inherited in an autosomal dominant fashion?

    a. factor VII deficiency
    b. factor X (Stuart-Power) deficiency
    c. factor XII deficiency
    d. protein C deficiency

49–76. How is protein C deficiency inherited?

    a. X-linked recessive
    b. autosomal recessive

    c. autosomal dominant
    d. multifactorial

49–77. What is the frequency of activated protein C resistance?

    a. <0.1%
    b. 0.5 to 1.0%
    c. 3.0 to 7.0%
    d. 10.0 to 12.0%

49–78. Hyperchromocystinemia is associated with an increased risk for all EXCEPT which of the following?

    a. atherosclerosis
    b. thromboembolism
    c. fetal renal agenesis
    d. fetal neural tube defects

49–79. Which of the following is associated with an increased incidence of abruptio placentae, fetal growth restriction, and thromboembolism in pregnancy?

    a. protein S deficiency
    b. protein C deficiency
    c. antithrombin III deficiency
    d. prothrombin G20210A mutation

50

Endocrine Disorders

50–1. The autoimmune component of endocrinopathies may be induced by which of the following?

    a. environmental factors
    b. genetic predisposition
    c. viral infection
    d. all of the above

50–2. What is the frequency of nontoxic goiter?

    a. 0.5%
    b. 2.0%
    c. 5.0%
    d. 10.0%

50–3. The thyroid undergoes which of the following changes during pregnancy?

    a. enlarges
    b. decreases in size
    c. remains the same size
    d. becomes nodular

50–4. Which of the following remains unchanged during pregnancy?

    a. total T_3 concentration
    b. total T_4 concentration
    c. thyrotropin-releasing hormone
    d. thyroid-binding globulin

50–5. Which of the following is true of a thyroid-stimulating hormone or thyrotropin (TSH) in pregnancy?

    a. carrier protein increased
    b. does not cross placenta
    c. produced by placenta
    d. serum concentration decreases

50–6. What is the role of chorionic gonadotropin in thyroid stimulation?

    a. marked stimulation
    b. slight stimulation
    c. no effect
    d. unclear

50–7. During most of pregnancy, how do free T_3 and free T_4 levels compare to normal nonpregnant levels?

    a. markedly increased
    b. slightly decreased
    c. markedly decreased
    d. unchanged

50–8. What is the incidence of thyrotoxicosis during pregnancy?

    a. 1 in 100
    b. 1 in 850
    c. 1 in 2000
    d. 1 in 10,000

50–9. Thyrotoxicosis in pregnancy is usually associated with elevated levels of which of the following?

    a. autoantibodies
    b. iodine
    c. thyrotropin-releasing hormone (TRH)
    d. thyroid-stimulating hormone (TSH)

50–10. What is the primary treatment for thyrotoxicosis during pregnancy?

    a. medical
    b. surgical
    c. combination of medical and surgical
    d. no treatment necessary

50–11. Which of the following medications may cause aplasia cutis?

    a. propylthiouracil
    b. methimazole
    c. verapamil
    d. captopril

50–12. Which of the following is a rare but potentially serious maternal complication of thioamide therapy?

    a. agranulocytosis
    b. gastrointestinal bleeding
    c. polycythemia
    d. seizures

50–13. Following initiation of one of the thioamide drugs for hyperthyroidism, what is the median time to normalization of the free thyroxine index?

    a. 1 to 2 weeks
    b. 3 to 4 weeks
    c. 7 to 8 weeks
    d. 12 to 14 weeks

50–14. Which of the following maternal complications is NOT increased with untreated thyrotoxicosis?

    a. death
    b. deep vein thrombosis
    c. heart failure
    d. preeclampsia

50–15. Which of the following fetal complications is NOT increased with maternal thyrotoxicosis?

    a. growth restriction
    b. preterm delivery
    c. postdates pregnancy
    d. stillbirths

50–16. What is the reported perinatal mortality rate in women with uncontrolled thyrotoxicosis?

    a. 1 to 2%
    b. 8 to 12%
    c. 18 to 22%
    d. 25%

50–17. Drugs useful in the treatment of "uncomplicated" thyroid storm include all EXCEPT which of the following?

    a. dexamethasone
    b. magnesium sulfate
    c. propylthiouracil
    d. potassium iodide

50–18. Overtreatment of maternal hyperthyroidism with propylthyiouracil rarely can lead to what neonatal abnormality?

    a. hearing loss
    b. hypocalcemia
    c. goiter
    d. seizures

50–19. In one series of over 200 women treated with thiourea drugs, what was the incidence of adverse fetal effects?

    a. less than 2%
    b. 5 to 7%
    c. 12 to 15%
    d. 25%

50–20. In long-term studies of children born to thyrotoxic mothers treated with propylthiouracil during pregnancy, what were the findings regarding adverse effects?

    a. increase in adverse intellectual development
    b. increase in adverse physical development
    c. increase in adverse thyroid function
    d. no adverse effects

50–21. Which of the following complications is NOT increased in pregnant women with hypothyroidism?

    a. heart failure
    b. macrosomia
    c. placental abruption
    d. preeclampsia

50–22. Serum levels of which marker are monitored to assess thyroxine therapy of maternal hypothyroidism?

    a. thyroid-stimulating hormone or thyrotropin (TSH)
    b. thyroid-releasing hormone
    c. total T_4 plus total T_3
    d. thyroid antibodies

50–23. Which of the following is the current recommendation regarding the treatment of subclinical hypothyroidism in women?

    a. Treat when T_4 levels decrease to low-normal range.
    b. Treat when TSH >10 μU/mL.
    c. Treat prior to development of symptoms.
    d. Treatment is not recommended.

50–24. Women with which of the following medical complications have an increased risk of subclinical hypothyroidism?

    a. chronic hypertension
    b. renal disease
    c. lupus erythematosus
    d. type I diabetes

50–25. Untreated maternal subclinical hypothyroidism may increase the risk of which pregnancy complication?

    a. diminished intelligence quotients in children
    b. pregnancy-induced hypertension
    c. preterm delivery
    d. all of the above

50–26. What is the risk of fetal anomalies in fetuses of mothers who have previously been treated (prior to pregnancy) with therapeutic radioiodine?

    a. 6%
    b. 8%

    c. 12%
    d. not increased

50–27. Endemic cretinism is seen in countries with high incidences of which dietary problem?

    a. low protein intake
    b. iodide deficiency
    c. elevated lithium levels in water supply
    d. manganese deficiency

50–28. What percentage of states require biochemical screening of newborns for hypothyroidism?

    a. 25
    b. 50
    c. 75
    d. 100

50–29. What is the frequency of congenital hypothyroidism?

    a. 1 in 40 to 70 infants
    b. 1 in 400 to 700 infants
    c. 1 in 4000 to 7000 infants
    d. 1 in 40,000 to 70,000 infants

50–30. What is the most common cause of congenital hypothyroidism in the United States?

    a. idiopathic
    b. thyroid agenesis
    c. thyroid dyshormonogenesis
    d. transient hypothyroidism

50–31. What percentage of solitary thyroid nodules during pregnancy will be malignant?

    a. <5
    b. 5 to 30
    c. 40 to 65
    d. 70 to 85

50–32. What percentage of women will have either clinical or biochemical evidence of thyroid dysfunction during the postpartum period?

    a. 1 to 2
    b. 5 to 10
    c. 15 to 20
    d. 25 to 30

50–33. Transient postpartum thyroiditis is associated with which of the following?

    a. depression
    b. fatigue
    c. palpitations
    d. all of the above

50–34. What is the role of calcitonin?

   a. increases serum calcium
   b. decreases serum calcium
   c. keeps calcium at a steady level
   d. has no effect on calcium

50–35. What happens to parathyroid hormone during pregnancy?

   a. increases
   b. decreases
   c. stays the same
   d. unclear

50–36. Which of the following is NOT a complication of hyperparathyroidism in pregnancy?

   a. generalized weakness
   b. hyperemesis
   c. pancreatitis
   d. thyrotoxicosis

50–37. Which of the following is generally NOT utilized for the treatment of hypercalcemic crisis?

   a. furosemide
   b. mithramycin
   c. oral phosphorus
   d. propranolol

50–38. What is the preferred treatment of hypoparathyroidism during pregnancy?

   a. vitamin D
   b. vitamin K
   c. phosphorus
   d. calcitonin

50–39. Which of the following hormones is probably NOT increased during pregnancy?

   a. cortisol
   b. renin
   c. aldosterone
   d. adrenal medullary hormone

50–40. What percentage of pheochromocytomas are extra-adrenal?

   a. 1
   b. 10
   c. 20
   d. 40

50–41. Urine levels of which of the following are NOT useful for the diagnosis of pheochromocytomas?

   a. cortisol
   b. vanillylmandelic acid
   c. metanephrines
   d. unconjugated catecholamines

50–42. Which of the following drugs is most useful for the treatment of pheochromocytoma?

   a. α-methyldopa
   b. phenoxybenzamine
   c. captopril
   d. verapamil

50–43. What is the most common etiology of Cushing syndrome in the general population?

   a. iatrogenic
   b. benign adrenal tumors
   c. adrenal carcinomas
   d. trophoblastic disease

50–44. What is the most common cause of Addison's disease today?

   a. tuberculosis
   b. histoplasmosis
   c. nonspecific granulomatous disease
   d. idiopathic autoimmune adrenalitis

50–45. Enlargement of the pituitary in pregnancy is due primarily to what process?

   a. generalized pituitary edema
   b. lactotropic cellular hyperplasia
   c. thyrotropic cellular hypertrophy
   d. increased vascular supply

50–46. Bromocriptine has proven efficacious for which of the following conditions during pregnancy?

   a. Graves' disease
   b. Addison's disease
   c. primary aldosteronism
   d. pituitary prolactinomas

50–47. What is the cutoff size used to distinguish a pituitary microadenoma from a macroadenoma?

   a. 5 mm
   b. 10 mm
   c. 15 mm
   d. 20 mm

50–48. What is an adverse fetal effects of bromocriptine?

   a. increase in stillbirths
   b. increase in growth retardation
   c. increase in microcephaly
   d. no adverse effect

50–49. What is the specific drug used to treat diabetes insipidus during pregnancy?

   a. 1-deamino-8-D-arginine vasopressin (DDAVP)
   b. renin
   c. oxytocin
   d. angiotensin

50–50. Transient diabetes insipidus is most likely encountered in pregnant women with which of the following complications?

    a. acute fatty liver
    b. severe preeclampsia
    c. HELLP syndrome
    d. hemolytic uremic syndrome

50–51. Which of the following syndromes is caused by pituitary ischemia and necrosis secondary to obstetrical blood loss?

    a. Budd-Chiari syndrome
    b. Kalman syndrome
    c. Sheehan syndrome
    d. multiple endocrinopathy syndrome

51

Diabetes

51–1. In what year did insulin become available?

    a. 1906
    b. 1922
    c. 1932
    d. 1948

51–2. White's classification for diabetes in pregnancy (1949) related which of the following to severity of maternal disease?

    a. maternal complications
    b. postpartum infections
    c. maternal death
    d. fetal risk

51–3. Type 1 diabetes is associated with HLA-D histocompatibility complex located on which chromosome?

    a. chromosome 3
    b. chromosome 6
    c. chromosome 21
    d. chromosome 22

51–4. What is the concordance rate for type 1 diabetes in monozygotic twins?

    a. 100%
    b. 80%
    c. 60%
    d. <50%

51–5. What is the concordance rate for type 2 diabetes in monozygotic twins?

    a. 100%
    b. 80%
    c. 60%
    d. >50%

51–6. Which of the following is the pathophysiology of type 2 diabetes?

    a. absence of the islet cells
    b. destruction of the islet cells
    c. insulin resistance in target tissues
    d. develops ketoacidosis if untreated

51–7. What is the overall percentage of pregnancies complicated by diabetes?

    a. <1
    b. 2 to 3
    c. 6 to 8
    d. >10

51–8. In general, what does glycosuria in pregnancy mean?

    a. represents lactose
    b. indicates diabetes
    c. lowered renal threshold
    d. treated with insulin

51–9. Which of the following is NOT a risk factor for gestational diabetes?

a. age <25 years
b. prior macrosomic infant
c. prior stillborn infant
d. sister with gestational diabetes

51–10. Screening for diabetes is recommended for all EXCEPT which of the following?

a. age >30
b. obesity
c. prior macrosomia
d. prior postterm pregnancy

51–11. What cut-off for the 50-g glucose screen would improve its sensitivity to >90% for detection of gestational diabetes?

a. 130 mg/dL
b. 135 mg/dL
c. 140 mg/dL
d. 145 mg/dL

51–12. How is gestational diabetes diagnosed?

a. 1 hr value after 50-g glucose load is elevated (exceeds 140 mg/dL)
b. elevated fasting value with a 100-g load of glucose
c. elevated 1 hr value with a 100-g load of glucose
d. 2 abnormal values are noted with a 100-g glucose tolerance test

51–13. What percentage of gestational diabetes will eventually develop into overt diabetes?

a. none
b. 10
c. 25
d. 50

51–14. Which class of those with gestational diabetes is NOT at increased risk for unexplained stillbirth?

a. A_1
b. A_2
c. B
d. C

51–15. In diabetes, which fetal organ is unaffected by fetal macrosomia?

a. heart
b. kidney
c. liver
d. brain

51–16. Which of the following is true concerning gestational diabetes?

a. increased with obesity
b. has a prevalence of 1 to 3%
c. normal perinatal mortality rate with appropriate treatment
d. all of the above

51–17. Which of the following factors is found in increased levels in large-for-gestational-age infants?

a. insulin-like growth factor I
b. insulin-like growth factor II
c. C peptide insulin
d. all of the above

51–18. What is the caloric requirement per ideal body weight of a woman with gestational diabetes?

a. 20 to 25 kcal/kg
b. 30 to 35 kcal/kg
c. 40 to 45 kcal/kg
d. 50 to 55 kcal/kg

51–19. What are the benefits of postprandial glucose surveillance?

a. better glucose control
b. less neonatal hypoglycemia
c. less macrosomia
d. all of the above

51–20. What is the recurrence rate for gestational diabetes in subsequent pregnancies?

a. 33%
b. 50%
c. 67%
d. 90%

51–21. With overt diabetes, what is the most common fetal malformation?

a. congenital heart defects
b. neural tube defects
c. caudal regression
d. renal agenesis

51–22. What is the prevalence of preeclampsia or eclampsia in type 1 diabetic pregnancies as compared with normal pregnancies?

a. less likely
b. increased twofold
c. increased threefold
d. increased fourfold

51–23. Which factor increases a diabetic woman's risk for spontaneous abortion?

    a. HgA₁C = 6.3%
    b. poor glycemic control in general
    c. preprandial glucose 115 mg/dL
    d. postprandial glucose 125 mg/dL

51–24. Which of the following is true concerning preconceptional glycemic control in overt diabetic women?

    a. may reduce congenital anomalies
    b. may reduce spontaneous abortions
    c. still has a greater congenital anomaly rate than in those who do not have diabetes
    d. all of the above

51–25. In general, what is true of "unexplained" fetal demise in overt diabetics?

    a. usually occurs before 30 weeks gestation
    b. fetus usually small for gestational age
    c. oligohydromnios is usually present
    d. likely due to chronic metabolic aberrations

51–26. What is the incidence of ketoacidosis in diabetic pregnancies?

    a. 0.5%
    b. 1.0%

    c. 3.0%
    d. 5.0%

51–27. Ideally, when should delivery of the overt diabetic pregnant woman occur?

    a. 34 weeks
    b. 36 weeks
    c. 38 weeks
    d. 40 weeks

51–28. What is the LEAST problematic, most effective method of contraception for diabetic patients?

    a. abstinence
    b. oral contraceptives
    c. intrauterine device
    d. sterilization

51–29. For which diabetic complication may pregnancy have a detrimental effect?

    a. proliferative retinopathy
    b. nephropathy
    c. hypertension
    d. nonproliferative retinopathy

Connective-Tissue Disorders

52–1. Which of the following is an inherited noninflammatory disorder of collagen metabolism?

    a. systemic lupus erythematosus (SLE)
    b. scleroderma
    c. Ehlers-Danlos syndrome
    d. rheumatoid arthritis

52–2. With which of the following are the seronegative spondyloarthropathies most strongly associated?

    a. antiphospholipid antibodies
    b. HLA-B27
    c. rheumatoid factor
    d. substance abuse

52–3. On which chromosome is the human leukocyte-associated (HLA) complex located?

a. 6p
b. 11p
c. 14q
d. 17q

52–4. Which of the following is decreased or depressed during pregnancy?

a. cell-mediated immunity
b. complement levels
c. immunoglobulin-secreting cells
d. circulating immune complexes

52–5. What happens to serum levels of autoantibodies during pregnancy?

a. increase
b. decrease
c. remain the same
d. unknown

52–6. What percentage of SLE occurs in women?

a. 30
b. 50
c. 70
d. 90

52–7. What is the overall 10-year survival for women with SLE?

a. 50%
b. 65%
c. 75%
d. 90%

52–8. What is the 20-year survival rate of SLE?

a. 20%
b. 50%
c. 70%
d. 90%

52–9. What is the frequency of SLE in women with one affected family member?

a. 1%
b. 2 to 3%
c. 10%
d. 25%

52–10. How many women with SLE have renal involvement?

a. 10%
b. 25%
c. 50%
d. 75%

52–11. Which of the following is a common clinical manifestation of SLE?

a. arthralgias
b. seizures
c. gastrointestinal lesions
d. venous thrombosis

52–12. Which is the best screening test for SLE?

a. anti-SM antibodies
b. cardiolipin antibodies
c. antiplatelet antibodies
d. antinuclear antibodies

52–13. Which of the following autoantibodies is specific for SLE?

a. anti-ribonucleic-acid (RNA)
b. antinuclear
c. anti-ds deoxyribonucleic acid (DNA)
d. anti-ribonucleoprotein

52–14. How many of the 11 criteria of the American Rheumatism Association must be present serially or simultaneously to make the diagnosis of SLE?

a. 2
b. 4
c. 8
d. 10

52–15. Which of the following drugs is NOT known to induce a lupus-like syndrome?

a. hydralazine
b. methyldopa
c. phenytoin
d. verapamil

52–16. What is the rate of major morbidity seen in pregnant patients with SLE?

a. 1%
b. 3%
c. 5%
d. 7%

52–17. What is the most common complication in pregnant women with lupus nephritis?

a. renal failure
b. hypertension
c. abruption
d. fetal demise

52–18. Which of the following is the usual first-line therapy for severe manifestations of SLE in pregnancy?

a. steroids
b. nonsteroidal anti-inflammatory drugs (NSAIDs)
c. azathioprine
d. cyclophosphamide

52–19. In the management of SLE, azathioprine should be used in the presence of which of the following?

  a. seizures
  b. steroid-resistant nephropathy
  c. lupus activation
  d. thrombocytopenia

52–20. Which of the following forms of reversible contraception is probably the most advantageous and safest for women with SLE?

  a. combination oral contraceptives
  b. intrauterine device
  c. progesterone-only implants or injections
  d. vaginal spermicides

52–21. What is the incidence of neonatal lupus?

  a. 1 to 3%
  b. 5 to 10%
  c. 15 to 20%
  d. 10 to 30%

52–22. Which of the following maternal antibodies is or are associated with congenital heart block in the newborn?

  a. anti-SSA(Ro) and anti-SSB(La)
  b. anti-ds DNA
  c. nuclear antibody (ANA)
  d. anti-RNA

52–23. What is the incidence of congenital heart block in the presence of the associated antibodies?

  a. 3%
  b. 7%
  c. 10%
  d. 15%

52–24. On average, how long does congenital or neonatal heart block secondary to maternal lupus last?

  a. 6 days
  b. 6 weeks
  c. 6 months
  d. permanent lesion requiring pacemaker

52–25. What percentage of infants with congenital heart block secondary to SLE will die within the first 3 years of life?

  a. 5
  b. 15
  c. 33
  d. 50

52–26. Antibodies of which class are antiphospholipid antibodies?

  a. IgG
  b. IgM
  c. IgA
  d. all three

52–27. Which of the following is associated with antiphospholipid antibody syndrome?

  a. arterial thromboses
  b. fetal losses
  c. venous thromboses
  d. all of these

52–28. Which of the following is thought to be bound by antiphospholipid antibodies, causing venous, arterial, or decidual thrombosis?

  a. annexin V
  b. β_2-glycoprotein I
  c. protein S
  d. all of these

52–29. Approximately what percentage of women with SLE will have the lupus anticoagulant?

  a. 5
  b. 25
  c. 33
  d. 75

52–30. What percentage of women with anticardiolipin antibodies will have the lupus anticoagulant?

  a. 5
  b. 20
  c. 50
  d. 90

52–31. Approximately what percentage of normal pregnant women will have nonspecific antiphospholipid antibodies in low titers?

  a. <1
  b. 5
  c. 15
  d. 25

52–32. Which clotting test is most specific for identifying the lupus anticoagulant?

  a. platelet neutralization procedure
  b. bleeding time
  c. prothrombin time
  d. partial thromboplastin time

52–33. What is the most commonly used test for identifying anticardiolipin antibodies?

   a. polymerase chain reaction (PCR)
   b. prothrombin time
   c. enzyme-linked immunosorbent assay (ELISA)
   d. monoclonal antibody test

52–34. Which of the following treatment protocols appears to result in the best pregnancy outcome for women with antiphospholipid antibodies and a history of fetal loss?

   a. corticosteroids plus low-dose aspirin
   b. corticosteroids plus heparin
   c. heparin plus low-dose aspirin
   d. aspirin alone

52–35. Which of the following HLA-haplotypes is associated with rheumatoid arthritis?

   a. HLA-DQ
   b. HLA-DR4
   c. HLA-DP
   d. HLA-DR2

52–36. What is the cornerstone of therapy for rheumatoid arthritis?

   a. NSAIDs
   b. corticosteroids
   c. sulfasalazine
   d. cyclosporine

52–37. What is the usual course of rheumatoid arthritis in pregnancy?

   a. not changed
   b. gradual deterioration
   c. rapid deterioration
   d. marked improvement

52–38. Which of the following proteins or hormones is likely to be responsible for the improvement in rheumatoid arthritis during pregnancy?

   a. cortisol
   b. estrogens
   c. pregnancy associated α_2-glycoprotein
   d. human placental lactogen

52–39. What adverse perinatal outcome is associated with rheumatoid arthritis?

   a. stillbirths
   b. fetal growth retardation
   c. preterm birth
   d. none of the above

52–40. What is the hallmark of systemic sclerosis?

   a. increased production of fibrin
   b. increased production of collagen
   c. decreased macrophage activity
   d. increased autoantibody production

52–41. What percentage of women with scleroderma will have antinuclear antibodies?

   a. 5
   b. 20
   c. 50
   d. 95

52–42. What is the 5-year survival rate of systemic sclerosis if there is renal or pulmonary involvement?

   a. >90%
   b. 75 to 80%
   c. <50%
   d. 25%

52–43. Which of the following is NOT a characteristic of the CREST syndrome?

   a. calcinosis
   b. Raynaud phenomenon
   c. seizures
   d. telangectasia

52–44. What is the treatment for systemic sclerosis?

   a. aspirin
   b. cortisol
   c. sulfasalazine
   d. no effective treatment

52–45. Which of the following vasculitis syndromes is associated with hepatitis B antigenemia?

   a. polyarthritis nodosa
   b. Wegener granulomatosis
   c. Grant-cell arteritis
   d. dermatomyositis

52–46. What percentage of adults developing dermatomyositis will have an associated malignant tumor?

   a. 1 to 2
   b. 15
   c. 33
   d. 50

52–47. Which of the following syndromes is inherited by an autosomal dominant gene?

   a. polymyositis
   b. polyarteritis nodosa
   c. Marfan syndrome
   d. dermatomyositis

52–48. Which of the following is characterized by hyperelasticity of the skin?

    a. dermatomyositis
    b. polyarteritis nodosa
    c. Marfan syndrome
    d. Ehlers-Danlos syndrome

52–49. Which of the following complications is increased in Ehlers-Danlos syndrome?

    a. preterm rupture of membranes
    b. hypertension
    c. eclampsia
    d. twinning

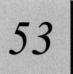

53

Neurological and Psychiatric Disorders

53–1. Which of the following is true of cranial computed tomography scanning during pregnancy?

    a. safe during pregnancy
    b. unsafe amounts of radiation exposure to the fetus
    c. should be replaced by magnetic resonance imaging (MRI)
    d. inferior to MRI for diagnosis of hemorrhagic lesions

53–2. What percentage of women will, at some time, suffer from migraine headaches?

    a. 6
    b. 12
    c. 18
    d. 24

53–3. What is the usual course of migraine headaches during pregnancy?

    a. minimal improvement
    b. dramatic improvement
    c. minimal worsening
    d. dramatic worsening

53–4. Which of the following drugs should NOT be utilized for the treatment of migraine headaches during pregnancy?

    a. meperidine
    b. propranolol
    c. ergonovine
    d. amitriptyline

53–5. What percentage of migraine headaches present for the first time during pregnancy?

    a. <5
    b. 5
    c. 10
    d. 15

53–6. How often is pregnancy complicated by maternal epilepsy?

    a. 1 in 200
    b. 1 in 500
    c. 1 in 2000
    d. 1 in 5000

53–7. What type of seizures involve a brief loss of consciousness without muscle activity and immediate recovery of consciousness?

    a. absence or petit mal
    b. temporal lobe
    c. complex partial
    d. simple

53–8. New-onset seizures during pregnancy should prompt what response by the health-care provider?

a. defer anticonvulsants to after first trimester
b. immediate complete evaluation
c. initiate antiseizure medications
d. perform arteriography

53–9. What is the frequency of congenital malformations in children of mothers with epilepsy compared to those of the general population?

a. increased
b. decreased
c. unchanged
d. unknown

53–10. Epidemiological data show an increase in which of the following obstetrical complications among epileptic women?

a. cerebral palsy
b. cesarean delivery
c. mean birthweight
d. perinatal mortality

53–11. Which of the following is depleted by most anticonvulsants and should, therefore, be supplemented in pregnancy?

a. cobalt
b. folic acid
c. pyridoxine
d. zinc

53–12. Parenteral administration of which of the following is recommended in newborns whose mothers take anticonvulsants?

a. vitamin A
b. vitamin D
c. vitamin E
d. vitamin K

53–13. Which of the following is the most reasonable approach to monitoring of pregnancy when the mother is epileptic in the absence of other complications?

a. anticonvulsant levels every 7 to 14 days
b. hospitalization in the third trimester
c. targeted midtrimester ultrasound exam
d. regular nonstress testing in the third trimester

53–14. What percentage of direct maternal deaths are caused by stroke?

a. 1
b. 10

c. 18
d. 29

53–15. During what period of time is there the highest risk of pregnancy-associated stroke?

a. second trimester
b. third trimester
c. labor
d. puerperium

53–16. What percentage of ischemic strokes are caused by antiphospholipid antibodies?

a. 5
b. 10
c. 33
d. 55

53–17. Cerebral venous thrombosis is NOT associated with which of the following?

a. hemorrhage or shock
b. preeclampsia
c. sepsis
d. thrombophilias

53–18. Which of the following conditions may be associated with sagittal venous sinus thrombosis?

a. antithrombin III deficiency
b. protein C deficiency
c. protein S deficiency
d. all of the above

53–19. When is venous thrombosis of the cerebral circulation most common?

a. first trimester
b. second trimester
c. labor
d. puerperium

53–20. What is the most common source of cerebral artery embolism in pregnancy?

a. carotid artery
b. aorta
c. subclavian artery
d. heart

53–21. Intracerebral hemorrhage in pregnancy is NOT associated with which of the following?

a. chronic hypertension
b. cocaine use
c. preeclampsia
d. atrial fibrillation

53–22. What is the most common cause of subarachnoid hemorrhage during pregnancy?

    a. circulating anticoagulant
    b. chronic hypertension
    c. preeclampsia
    d. rupture of a vascular malformation

53–23. Bleeding from a ruptured aneurysm is most common during what part of pregnancy?

    a. first half
    b. second half
    c. labor
    d. puerperium

53–24. What percentage of unresected arteriovenous malformations will bleed again within the first year?

    a. 5
    b. 15
    c. 25
    d. 50

53–25. What percentage of women with multiple sclerosis will have an exacerbation during the first few months postpartum?

    a. 5 to 10
    b. 30 to 40
    c. 50 to 60
    d. 80 to 90

53–26. How is Huntington's disease inherited?

    a. autosomal dominant
    b. autosomal recessive
    c. X-linked recessive
    d. multifactorial

53–27. Which of the following drugs is used in the treatment of myasthenia gravis?

    a. pyridostigmine
    b. propranolol
    c. indomethacin
    d. nifedipine

53–28. Women with myasthenia gravis frequently have hyperplasia of which of the following organs?

    a. liver
    b. thymus
    c. adrenal
    d. pituitary

53–29. Which of the following antibiotics should be utilized with caution in pregnant women with myasthenia gravis?

    a. penicillin
    b. cefalosporins
    c. aminoglycosides
    d. sulfonamides

53–30. What percentage of newborns will develop neonatal myasthenia gravis?

    a. 5
    b. 10 to 20
    c. 30 to 40
    d. 65

53–31. What percentage of Guillain-Barré syndrome follows a viral infection?

    a. 10
    b. 33
    c. 66
    d. 90

53–32. What percentage of persons with Guillain-Barré syndrome will have full recovery?

    a. 50
    b. 66
    c. 85
    d. 99

53–33. What is the incidence of Bell palsy in pregnant women compared with nonpregnant women?

    a. decreased
    b. the same
    c. increased
    d. has not been studied

53–34. Which of the following is an indicator of poor prognosis for Bell palsy during pregnancy?

    a. bilateral disease
    b. denervation by electromyography extends beyond 10 days
    c. recurrence in subsequent pregnancy
    d. all of the above

53–35. What percentage of pregnant women experience some symptoms of carpal tunnel syndrome?

    a. <1
    b. 3
    c. 5
    d. 25

53–36. What percentage of pregnant women with carpal tunnel syndrome will experience sufficient relief of pain with use of wrist splints during sleep?

    a. 10
    b. 25
    c. 50
    d. 80

53–37. Which of the following is NOT a complication of spinal cord injury?

   a. anemia
   b. urinary infection
   c. pressure necrosis of the skin
   d. diarrhea

53–38. Autonomic hyperreflexia is generally associated with a spinal cord injury above what level?

   a. T_5-T_6
   b. T_7
   c. T_{10}
   d. T_{12}

53–39. Which of the following is NOT typically associated with autonomic hyperreflexia?

   a. headache
   b. facial flushing
   c. hypertension
   d. loss of consciousness

53–40. Which of the following is utilized to decrease the frequency of autonomic hyperreflexia?

   a. nifedipine
   b. propranolol
   c. general anesthesia
   d. epidural or spinal analgesia

53–41. What is the most likely explanation for the high cesarean delivery rate for women with spinal cord injuries?

   a. dysfunctional uterine contraction pattern
   b. decreased expulsive forces
   c. inexperience of providers
   d. inability to detect labor

53–42. What is the preferred route of delivery for women with ventricular shunting for hydrocephalus?

   a. cesarean
   b. forceps
   c. vaginal delivery
   d. not known

53–43. Which of the following is NOT a symptom of pseudotumor cerebri?

   a. hyperacusis
   b. visual disturbances
   c. headaches
   d. stiff neck

53–44. Pregnancy complications seen in women with pseudotumor cerebri are likely due to its association with which of these conditions?

   a. diabetes
   b. obesity
   c. systemic hypertension
   d. thyroid disorders

53–45. Which of the following drugs is utilized for the treatment of pseudotumor cerebri?

   a. propranolol
   b. acetazolamide
   c. captopril
   d. nifedipine

53–46. Chorea gravidarum is seen in 2% of patients with what disease?

   a. Huntington's disease
   b. Guillan-Barré syndrome
   c. pseudotumor cerebri
   d. systemic lupus

53–47. What percentage of women will have a nonpsychotic postpartum depressive disorder?

   a. 10 to 15
   b. 20 to 25
   c. 45 to 50
   d. 65 to 70

53–48. In what percentage of suicides are major mood disorders a predisposing factor?

   a. 10
   b. 25
   c. 50
   d. 66

53–49. If one parent is schizophrenic, what is the empirical risk to their offspring of such a disorder?

   a. 1 to 2%
   b. 5 to 10%
   c. 65%
   d. 89%

53–50. What percentage of schizophrenics show social recovery with treatment over a 5-year period?

   a. 20
   b. 40
   c. 60
   d. 80

53–51. What percentage of people with personality disorders recognize their condition and seek therapy?

   a. 5
   b. 20
   c. 50
   d. 70

53–52. What percentage of pregnant women exhibit diagnostic criteria for major depression?

    a. 3
    b. 10
    c. 15
    d. 20

53–53. Which of the following has NOT been associated with pregnancy-related depression?

    a. hyperemesis gravidarum
    b. low socioeconomic status
    c. married over 10 years
    d. substance abuse

53–54. What percentage of pregnant women will experience postpartum blues?

    a. 5
    b. 15
    c. 30
    d. 50

53–55. How many days postpartum do postpartum blues usually develop?

    a. 3 to 6
    b. 14 to 21
    c. 30 to 60
    d. >60

53–56. Postpartum blues are common and thought to be due to withdrawal of which of the following?

    a. cortisol
    b. estrogen
    c. progesterone
    d. oxytocin

53–57. Depression is considered postpartum if it begins within what time interval post-delivery?

    a. 6 weeks
    b. 6 months
    c. 12 months
    d. 18 months

53–58. What is the recurrence risk of postpartum depression?

    a. 5%
    b. 20%
    c. 70%
    d. 95%

53–59. According to recent data, what percentage of women never recover completely from their postpartum depression?

    a. 2
    b. 10
    c. 20
    d. 40

53–60. What is the recurrence risk of postpartum psychosis?

    a. 5%
    b. 25%
    c. 50%
    d. 75%

53–61. How does the risk of psychosis during the postpartum period compare with the risk during other times of a woman's life?

    a. decreased slightly
    b. decreased markedly
    c. increased markedly
    d. no difference

53–62. What is currently considered the primary treatment for depression during pregnancy?

    a. electroconvulsive therapy
    b. monamine oxidase inhibitors
    c. selective serotomin reuptake inhibitors (SSRIs)
    d. tricyclic antidepressants

53–63. What is the complication rate of electroconvulsive therapy during pregnancy?

    a. 10%
    b. 25%
    c. 50%
    d. 75%

54

Dermatological Disorders

54–1. Hyperpigmentation of pregnancy is related to which of the following?

    a. cortisol
    b. aldosterone
    c. melanocyte-stimulating hormone
    d. unknown

54–2. What percentage of pregnant women demonstrate some skin darkening?

    a. 10
    b. 25
    c. 50
    d. 90

54–3. Severe or persistent chloasma can be treated postpartum with which of the following?

    a. hydrocortisone
    b. oral contraceptive pills
    c. tretinoin ointment
    d. ultraviolet light

54–4. Chloasma is a pigmentation of which of the following?

    a. areolae
    b. linea alba
    c. face
    d. inner thigh

54–5. Chloasma is seen in what percentage of pregnant women?

    a. 10
    b. 25
    c. 50
    d. 75

54–6. Which of the following is the most common behavior of nevi during pregnancy?

    a. decreased size
    b. increased size

    c. malignant transformation
    d. no size change

54–7. Which of the following best describes telogen effluvium?

    a. caused by high levels of melanocyte-stimulating hormone
    b. self-limiting and is resolved in 6 to 12 months
    c. associated with oral contraceptives
    d. all of the above

54–8. Which of the following hormones most likely causes spider angiomas during pregnancy?

    a. estrogen
    b. progesterone
    c. cortisol
    d. chorionic gonadotropin

54–9. Which of the following conditions results from a mild form of cholestatic jaundice?

    a. pruritis gravidarum
    b. capillary hemangiomas
    c. palmar erythema
    d. pruritic urticarial papules and plaques of pregnancy (PUPPP)

54–10. Cholestasis of pregnancy is caused by the dermal deposition of which of the following?

    a. bile acids
    b. bile salts
    c. bilirubin
    d. biliverdin

54–11. Lesions of PUPPP usually first appear in which of the following?

    a. abdomen
    b. buttocks
    c. extremities
    d. face

54–12. The pathophysiology of PUPPP is best described as which of the following?

    a. allergic
    b. autoimmune
    c. infectious
    d. uncertain

54–13. What effect does PUPPP have on perinatal morbidity?

    a. decreased
    b. increased in primigravidas
    c. increased in all gravidas
    d. no effect

54–14. Which of the following is characteristic of prurigo of pregnancy?

    a. adversely affects perinatal outcome
    b. develops early in pregnancy
    c. nonpruritic
    d. treated with antihistamines and topical steroids

54–15. Herpes gestationis is occasionally associated with which of the following?

    a. chorioangioma
    b. trophoblastic disease
    c. preeclampsia
    d. herpes zoster

54–16. Herpes gestationis typically shows which of the following behaviors in subsequent pregnancies?

    a. always recurs
    b. milder course
    c. never recurs
    d. presents later in gestation

54–17. What is the pathophysiology of herpes gestationis?

    a. allergic
    b. autoimmune
    c. infectious
    d. unknown

54–18. Of the following, which is most likely associated with Graves' disease?

    a. pruritus gravidarum
    b. pruritic urticarial papules and plaques of pregnancy
    c. herpes gestationis
    d. impetigo herpetiformis

54–19. Herpes gestationis usually responds to which of the following therapies?

    a. antihistamines
    b. high-dose oral contraceptives
    c. topical steroids
    d. ultraviolet light therapy

54–20. What is the effect of herpes gestationis on perinatal morbidity?

    a. increased
    b. decreased if on steroids
    c. no effect
    d. unclear

54–21. Which of the following is accompanied by constitutional symptoms and increased fetal morbidity and mortality?

    a. hydradentis suppurativa
    b. impetigo herpetiformis
    c. melanosis gravidarum
    d. pruritis gravidarum

54–22. Which of the following is a Food and Drug Administration category C drug for the treatment of acne?

    a. isotretinoin
    b. etretinate
    c. topical tretinoin
    d. benzoyl peroxide

55

Neoplastic Diseases

55–1. What is the approximate incidence of cancer in pregnancy?

    a. 1 in 600
    b. 1 in 6000
    c. 1 in 60,000
    d. 1 in 600,000

55–2. What are the most common malignancies in pregnancy?

    a. genital tract, melanoma
    b. melanoma, lung cancer
    c. lung cancer, genital tract
    d. stomach cancer, breast cancer

55–3. What is the earliest gestational age (weeks) the ovaries may be removed safely because placental progesterone production is adequate?

    a. 4
    b. 6
    c. 8
    d. 12

55–4. What is the characteristic adverse effect of high-dose radiation in pregnancy?

    a. leukemia and cardiac defects
    b. radiation nephritis and anal atresia
    c. microcephaly and mental retardation
    d. fetal cardiac defects and hydrocephalus

55–5. Which of the following doses provides a negligible risk from radiation for major malformations?

    a. <5 rad
    b. <10 rad
    c. <15 rad
    d. <20 rad

55–6. What is the calculated radiation exposure to a term fetus during radiotherapy to the breast?

    a. 20 rad
    b. 50 rad

    c. 100 rad
    d. 500 rad

55–7. Antineoplastic drugs are most hazardous when given at what gestational age?

    a. first trimester
    b. second trimester
    c. just before delivery
    d. postpartum breast feeding

55–8. What is the major risk from multidrug regimens for Hodgkin's lymphoma?

    a. ovarian fibrosis
    b. abortion
    c. fetal chromosomal damage
    d. fetal anomalies

55–9. How common is breast cancer during pregnancy?

    a. most common
    b. one of the top three
    c. tenth most common
    d. rare

55–10. Stage for stage, what influence does pregnancy have on the course of breast cancer?

    a. decreases survival
    b. increases survival
    c. no influence
    d. unknown

55–11. Pregnant women with breast cancer are more likely to have what stage disease?

    a. stage 0
    b. stage 1
    c. stage 2
    d. stages 3 and 4

55–12. Approximately what percentage of pregnant women with breast cancer will have nodal involvement?

a. 25
b. 50
c. 75
d. 90

55–13. What is the radiation exposure to the fetus from mammography?

a. <100 mrad
b. 250 mrad
c. 500 mrad
d. 750 mrad

55–14. Metastatic workup for breast cancer during pregnancy should include all EXCEPT which of the following?

a. chest x-ray
b. liver scan
c. magnetic resonance imaging
d. ultrasonography

55–15. Which of the following is NOT a recommended therapy for breast cancer during pregnancy?

a. mastectomy
b. mastectomy and node dissection
c. chemotherapy
d. radiotherapy

55–16. What is the recommended delay for future pregnancies following treatment of breast cancer?

a. 6 months to 1 year
b. 2 to 3 years
c. 5 years
d. 7 to 8 years

55–17. What is the most common presenting finding of Hodgkin's disease in pregnancy?

a. mediastinal adenopathy
b. peripheral adenopathy
c. rash
d. fever

55–18. Pregnant women with Hodgkin's disease are inordinately susceptible to which of the following complications?

a. infection
b. renal failure
c. breast cancer
d. ovarian cancer

55–19. Approximately what percentage of women treated for Hodgkin's disease with chemotherapy will resume normal menses?

a. 10
b. 20
c. 50
d. 90

55–20. What percentage of women with Hodgkin's disease will develop leukemia within 15 years?

a. 5
b. 20
c. 39
d. 55

55–21. What is the incidence of lymphoma in a woman with human immunodeficiency virus?

a. the same as for the general population
b. 1%
c. 5 to 10%
d. 15 to 20%

55–22. Myocardial damage and infarction is a complication in which of the following neoplasms?

a. breast
b. leukemia
c. melanoma
d. Hodgkin's disease

55–23. What is the incidence of leukemia in pregnancy?

a. 1 per 1000
b. 1 per 10,000
c. 1 per 100,000
d. 1 per 1,000,000

55–24. What percentage of pregnant women with acute leukemia will have a remission with chemotherapy?

a. 10
b. 25
c. 40
d. 75

55–25. How long should pregnancy be avoided following treatment for melanoma?

a. 1 to 2 years
b. 3 to 5 years
c. 8 to 10 years
d. should not become pregnant

55–26. What is the most common form of cancer encountered during pregnancy?

    a. breast
    b. melanoma
    c. hematologic
    d. genital

55–27. What is the diagnostic accuracy of colposcopically directed biopsy during pregnancy?

    a. 20%
    b. 66%
    c. 84%
    d. 99%

55–28. Which of the following is true regarding grade I and II cervical neoplasia in pregnancy?

    a. 35% progress to invasive cancer
    b. 70% progress to invasive cancer
    c. 35% regress postpartum
    d. 70% regress postpartum

55–29. How does pregnancy affect the survival rate for invasive carcinoma of the cervix?

    a. increases
    b. decreases
    c. no effect
    d. unknown

55–30. What effect does vaginal delivery through a cancerous cervix have on the prognosis?

    a. better than cesarean delivery
    b. worse than cesarean delivery

    c. no different from cesarean delivery
    d. unknown

55–31. What percentage of adnexal neoplasms during pregnancy are malignant?

    a. <1
    b. 5
    c. 20
    d. 38

55–32. Which is the most common ovarian neoplasm associated with pregnancy?

    a. epithelial
    b. germ cell
    c. stromal
    d. miscellaneous

55–33. What percentage of colon cancers are palpable by rectal examination?

    a. 20 to 25
    b. 25 to 40
    c. 60 to 70
    d. 88 to 95

55–34. What is the most common presenting symptom in a pregnant women with renal cell carcinoma?

    a. hematuria
    b. pain
    c. fever
    d. abdominal mass

56

Infections

56–1. At what stage of gestation (weeks) does fetal humoral immunity begin to develop?

    a. 4 to 8
    b. 9 to 15
    c. 17 to 24
    d. 36 to 40

56–2. What is the primary fetal response to infection?

    a. IgA production
    b. IgE production
    c. IgG production
    d. IgM production

56–3. What percentage of pregnant women with primary varicella infection develop pneumonitis?

    a. <1
    b. 10
    c. 25
    d. 40

56–4. In varicella-exposed susceptible immunocompromised individuals, the Centers for Disease Control and Prevention recommends prophylaxis with which of the following?

    a. varicella vaccine
    b. varicella-zoster immunoglobulin
    c. immunoglobulin
    d. gamma globulin

56–5. What is the absolute risk of varicella embryopathy if the mother has varicella prior to 20 weeks' gestation?

    a. <1%
    b. 2%
    c. 10%
    d. 20%

56–6. Which of the following is NOT part of the varicella embryopathy?

    a. chorioretinitis
    b. multicystic kidneys

    c. limb atrophy
    d. cortical atrophy

56–7. When should varicella-zoster immunoglobulin be administered to the newborn?

    a. delivery within 21 days of maternal disease
    b. delivery within 10 days of maternal disease
    c. delivery within 5 days of maternal disease
    d. maternal disease occurs at 7 days of newborn age

56–8. Which of the following agents has specific activity against influenza A?

    a. amantadine
    b. acyclovir
    c. ganciclovir
    d. adenosine araboside

56–9. Which of the following adult psychiatric diseases may be related to fetal exposure to influenza A?

    a. schizophrenia
    b. bipolar disorder
    c. depression
    d. acute psychosis

56–10. Which of the following infections is due to a ribonucleic acid (RNA) paramyxovirus?

    a. herpes
    b. mumps
    c. influenza
    d. varicella

56–11. What associated pregnancy complications are increased in women with measles?

    a. stillbirths
    b. abortions
    c. fetal anomalies
    d. abruptio placentae

56–12. Which of the following is likely to produce a cough and lower respiratory infection (i.e., pneumonia)?

　　a. rhinovirus
　　b. coronavirus
　　c. echovirus
　　d. adenovirus

56–13. What is the case fatality rate from the hantavirus?

　　a. <10%
　　b. 10%
　　c. 35%
　　d. 60%

56–14. Which of the following is associated with Coxsackievirus viremia in the fetus?

　　a. pancreatitis
　　b. cholecystitis
　　c. cystitis
　　d. encephalomyelitis

56–15. Which of the following tests is used to confirm the diagnosis of erythema infectiosum?

　　a. antistreptolysis titer
　　b. parvovirus IgM titer
　　c. rubella IgM titer
　　d. coxsackievirus IgM

56–16. In which of the following situations might parvovirus be associated with aplastic crisis?

　　a. iron-deficiency anemia
　　b. thalassemia minor
　　c. Gaucher disease
　　d. sickle cell anemia

56–17. "Mirror syndrome," or maternal hydrops syndrome, is associated with which of the following viruses?

　　a. polio
　　b. parvovirus
　　c. rubella
　　d. cytomegalovirus

56–18. Which of the following adverse fetal effects has been reported to be caused by maternal parvovirus infection?

　　a. microcephaly
　　b. hydrocephaly
　　c. hydrops
　　d. cardiac defects

56–19. By how many days does rubella viremia precede clinically evident disease?

　　a. 1
　　b. 4
　　c. 7
　　d. 21

56–20. How long after appearance of rash does rubella IgM persist?

　　a. 14 days
　　b. 28 days
　　c. 14 weeks
　　d. 28 weeks

56–21. Congenital rubella syndrome is more common during which weeks of gestation?

　　a. 8 to 10
　　b. 12 to 14
　　c. 16 to 18
　　d. 36 to 38

56–22. Which of the following is a handicap associated with cytomegalovirus infection?

　　a. deafness
　　b. diabetes
　　c. cataracts
　　d. spastic paralysis

56–23. What is the risk of cytomegalovirus seroconversion among susceptible women during pregnancy?

　　a. <1%
　　b. 1 to 4%
　　c. 10%
　　d. 20%

56–24. What is the rate of transmission to the fetus during primary cytomegalovirus infection?

　　a. 10%
　　b. 20%
　　c. 30%
　　d. 40%

56–25. Which of the following is NOT associated with cytomegalic inclusion disease?

　　a. microcephaly
　　b. chorioretinitis
　　c. hydrops
　　d. thrombocytopenic purpura

56–26. Which of the following is the most sensitive method to diagnose maternal primary cytomegalovirus infection?

    a. culture of cervix
    b. cytomegalovirus IgG titer
    c. cytomegalovirus IgM titer
    d. twofold increase in IgG titer

56–27. Which of the following techniques is best to diagnose fetal cytomegalovirus infection?

    a. amniocentesis plus cordocentesis
    b. chorionic villus sampling
    c. sonography
    d. magnetic resonance imaging

56–28. Which of the following is associated with *Streptococcus pyogenes* (group A streptococcus)?

    a. toxic shocklike syndrome
    b. scarlet fever
    c. erysipelas
    d. all of the above

56–29. What percent of pregnant women are colonized with *Strep. agalactiae* (group B streptococcus [GBS])?

    a. <1
    b. 5 to 10
    c. 15 to 20
    d. 40 to 50

56–30. What is the attack rate for group B streptococcus (per 1000 live births) in preterm babies born to colonized mothers?

    a. 1 to 2
    b. 10
    c. 20
    d. 40

56–31. Which of the following is a characteristic of early-onset group B streptococcus neonatal infection?

    a. onset at 1 to 2 weeks of age
    b. respiratory distress
    c. nearly always fatal
    d. end outcome is cerebral palsy

56–32. What is the most accurate method for detection of group B streptococcal infection?

    a. Gram stain
    b. latex agglutination test
    c. culture
    d. enzyme-linked immunosorbent assay

56–33. Which of the following are gram-positive aerobic bacilli?

    a. *Strep. pyogenes*
    b. *Listeria monocytogenes*
    c. *Salmonella typhi*
    d. *Strep. faecalis*

56–34. Which of the following is associated with fetal listeria infection?

    a. osteochondritis
    b. neuronal destruction
    c. granulomatous lesions with microabscesses
    d. myocarditis

56–35. What is the treatment of choice for listeria during the third trimester?

    a. metronidazole
    b. ampicillin plus gentamicin
    c. clindamycin
    d. tetracycline

56–36. Which of the following is generally used for the treatment for salmonella enteritis?

    a. intravenous fluids
    b. ampicillin
    c. ampicillin plus gentamicin
    d. ampicillin plus sulbactam

56–37. What is the most effective treatment for *S. typhi*?

    a. ampicillin
    b. erythromycin
    c. ciprofloxacin
    d. chloramphenicol

56–38. What is the attack rate for shigellosis?

    a. 10%
    b. 20%
    c. 40%
    d. 75%

56–39. What is the causative organism of Hansen disease?

    a. *Shigella hanseni*
    b. *Borrelia burgdorferi*
    c. *Mycobacterium leprae*
    d. *Toxoplasma gondii*

56–40. What is the causative organism for Lyme disease?

    a. *Treponoma pallidum*
    b. *B. burgdorferi*
    c. *B. ixodes*
    d. *T. gondii*

56–41. What is the treatment of choice for Lyme disease in pregnancy?

    a. amoxicillin
    b. clindamycin
    c. gentamicin
    d. tetracycline

56–42. Which of the following organisms is associated with eating undercooked meat?

    a. *B. burgdorferi*
    b. *Plasmodium vivax*
    c. *M. leprae*
    d. *T. gondii*

56–43. What is the overall risk of fetal infection from primary maternal toxoplasmosis?

    a. 5%
    b. 15%
    c. 50%
    d. 80%

56–44. What percentage of fetuses infected in the first trimester will have congenital toxoplasmosis?

    a. 3
    b. 10
    c. 40
    d. 70

56–45. Which of the following is associated with congenital toxoplasmosis infection?

    a. limb defects
    b. cardiac defects
    c. hepatosplenomegaly
    d. renal defects

56–46. Almost all infants with congenital toxoplasmosis develop which of the following?

    a. mental retardation
    b. microcephaly
    c. chorioretinitis
    d. hearing loss

56–47. How long can toxoplasmosis IgM persist?

    a. days
    b. weeks
    c. months
    d. years

56–48. Which of the following is potential treatment for toxoplasmosis in pregnancy?

    a. spectinomycin
    b. erythromycin
    c. sulfasalazine
    d. spiramycin

56–49. What is the treatment of choice for chloroquine-resistant falciparum infection?

    a. high-dose chloroquine
    b. chloramphenicol
    c. quinine
    d. mefloquine

57

Sexually Transmitted Diseases

57–1. Which of the following is true concerning syphilis in reproductive-age women?

    a. Rates peaked in 1950.
    b. Rates peaked in 1975.
    c. Rates peaked in 1990.
    d. Rates continue to rise.

57–2. Antepartum syphilis is NOT associated with which of the following?

    a. fetal death
    b. preterm labor
    c. neonatal infection
    d. abruptio placentae

57–3. What is the average incubation period for primary syphilis?

    a. 1 day
    b. 1 week
    c. 3 weeks
    d. 6 months

57–4. Which of the following best describes the lesion of primary syphilis?

    a. painless firm ulcer
    b. painful firm ulcer
    c. painless maculopapular
    d. painful maculopapular

57–5. What is the approximate time for development of secondary syphilis following healing of the primary chancre?

    a. 7 days
    b. 10 to 14 days
    c. 4 to 10 weeks
    d. 12 weeks or more

57–6. What is a characteristic presentation of secondary syphilis?

    a. condyloma lata
    b. multiple chancres
    c. genital ulcers
    d. generalized pruritis without rash

57–7. At what gestational age does the fetus first manifest clinical disease if infected by syphilis?

    a. 6 weeks
    b. 8 to 10 weeks
    c. 12 weeks
    d. 18 weeks or more

57–8. What are syphilitic changes in the liver termed?

    a. condyloma hepaticum
    b. syphilitic hepatitis
    c. portal syphilis
    d. hypertrophic cirrhosis

57–9. What is the gross appearance of the placenta in syphilitic infection?

    a. congested and small
    b. congested and large
    c. pale and small
    d. pale and large

57–10. After contracting syphilis, when will serological tests for syphilis be positive?

    a. within 7 days
    b. 10 to 14 days
    c. 28 to 42 days
    d. ~90 days

57–11. Which of the following is the most specific test for syphilis?

   a. fluorescent treponemal antibody absorption test (FTA-ABS)
   b. gram stain of lesion exudate
   c. rapid plasma reagin test (RPR)
   d. venereal disease research laboratory test (VDRL)

57–12. What is the best test for diagnosis of neonatal syphilis?

   a. cord blood VDRL
   b. motile spirochetes in amnionic fluid
   c. neonatal serum polymerase chain reaction
   d. sonographic evidence of large placenta

57–13. Which of the following is NOT typical of congenital syphilis?

   a. ascites
   b. cerebral calcifications
   c. lymphadenopathy
   d. rhinitis

57–14. What is the treatment of choice for syphilis in pregnancy?

   a. tetracycline
   b. doxycycline
   c. erythromycin
   d. penicillin

57–15. Penicillin G cures what percentage of maternal and neonatal syphilis infections?

   a. 70
   b. 80
   c. 90
   d. 98

57–16. Syphilis of more than one year's duration should be treated with which of the following?

   a. penicillin V 250 mg po qid × 10 days
   b. benzathine penicillin G 2.4 million U IM
   c. benzathine penicillin G 2.4 million U IM weekly × 3
   d. aqueous penicillin G 4 million U every 4 hr for 10 days

57–17. What is the best therapy for the treatment of syphilis in pregnant women who are allergic to penicillin?

   a. ceftriaxone
   b. erythromycin
   c. tetracycline
   d. penicillin desensitization

57–18. Which of the following antibiotics may be curative of syphilis in the mother but may not prevent congenital syphilis?

   a. penicillin
   b. erythromycin
   c. tetracycline
   d. ceftriaxone

57–19. Despite recommended treatment during pregnancy, what percentage of newborns of mothers with syphilis have obvious clinical stigmata of congenital syphilis?

   a. 2
   b. 5
   c. 20
   d. 44

57–20. Which of the following is commonly observed with the Jarisch-Herxheimer reaction in pregnancy?

   a. hypotension
   b. uterine quiescence
   c. fetal heart rate decelerations
   d. maternal rash

57–21. In pregnant women with latent syphilis of more than one year's duration, which of the following is NOT one of the criteria for recommending lumbar puncture?

   a. neurological symptoms
   b. treatment failures
   c. concomitant human immunodeficiency virus infection
   d. serological titer of 1 to 4

57–22. Which of the following treatment protocols is appropriate for the asymptomatic infant whose mother was treated with erythromycin for syphilis?

   a. penicillin G, IV or IM for 10 days
   b. erythromycin 500 mg for 4 doses
   c. treat only if stigmata are present
   d. no treatment necessary

57–23. Which of the following is a risk factor for gonorrhea?

   a. married
   b. age >35
   c. multiparous
   d. lack of prenatal care

57–24. What percentage of pregnant women with gonorrhea will also have chlamydia?

    a. <5
    b. 20
    c. 40
    d. 60

57–25. Which of the following is least commonly found in pregnant women with gonorrhea?

    a. oropharyngeal infection
    b. anal infection
    c. acute salpingitis
    d. disseminated infection

57–26. Which of the following is NOT associated with *Neisseria gonorrhoeae?*

    a. preterm labor
    b. chorioamnionitis
    c. premature rupture of membranes
    d. fetal hydrops

57–27. What is the treatment of choice for uncomplicated gonorrhea in pregnancy?

    a. ceftriaxone
    b. penicillin
    c. erythromycin
    d. azithromycin

57–28. Which of the following is NOT a manifestation or sign of disseminated gonococcal infection?

    a. blindness
    b. pustular skin lesions
    c. arthralgias
    d. endocarditis

57–29. Which of the following is used to treat gonorrhea in pregnant women allergic to β-lactam drugs?

    a. ciprofloxacin
    b. cefixime
    c. doxycycline
    d. spectinomycin

57–30. Which of the following is an obligate intracellular bacterium?

    a. *Treponema pallidum*
    b. *Borrelia burgdorferi*
    c. *Chlamydia trachomatis*
    d. *Escherichia coli*

57–31. Which of the following is the most common bacterial sexually transmitted disease in women?

    a. *N. gonorrhoeae*
    b. herpes simplex

    c. chancroid
    d. *C. trachomatis*

57–32. What is the sensitivity of polymerase chain reaction for the detection of chlamydia?

    a. 2%
    b. 50%
    c. 75%
    d. 97%

57–33. What is NOT considered a risk factor for chlamydia infection in pregnant women?

    a. age >25
    b. unmarried
    c. lower socioeconomic group
    d. multiple sex partners

57–34. Which of the following is the most common presentation of chlamydial infection in pregnancy?

    a. asymptomatic infection
    b. complaint of vaginal discharge
    c. septic abortion or chorioamnionitis
    d. fetal growth restriction

57–35. Vertical transmission of chlamydia is associated with which of the following neonatal infections?

    a. sepsis
    b. conjunctivitis
    c. urine infection
    d. skin rash

57–36. In pregnancies complicated by chlamydia, which of the following is positively associated with poor pregnancy prognosis?

    a. untreated cervical chlamydia
    b. recent infection as evidenced by elevated IgM
    c. history of treatment failure
    d. none of the above

57–37. What percentage of infants born through an infected cervix will develop chlamydial conjunctivitis?

    a. 10
    b. 33
    c. 50
    d. 75

57–38. Infants who develop *C. trachomatis* pneumonitis are least likely to demonstrate which of the following clinical features?

    a. chronic cough
    b. fever
    c. poor weight gain
    d. pulmonary infiltrates

57–39. Of the following which is the best treatment for chlamydial cervicitis in pregnancy?

   a. erythromycin estolate 250 mg po qid × 4 days
   b. tetracycline 500 mg po qid × 7 days
   c. erythromycin base 500 mg po qid × 7 days
   d. quinolones 500 mg po qid × 14 days

57–40. What is the cure rate for chlamydial infections in pregnancy treated with azithromycin?

   a. 25%
   b. 50%
   c. 75%
   d. 95%

57–41. Lymphogranuloma venereum is most difficult to differentiate from which of the following?

   a. chancroid
   b. granuloma inguinale
   c. herpes
   d. syphilis

57–42. Nongenital herpes virus infections are generally caused by which of the following?

   a. HSV 1
   b. HSV 2
   c. HSV 6
   d. HSV 11

57–43. What percentage of primary genital herpes infections in adults are due to HSV 1?

   a. 33
   b. 50
   c. 75
   d. 95

57–44. In a national serioepidemiological survey from 1976 to 1994, what percentage of women showed antibodies to HSV 2?

   a. 5
   b. 10
   c. 25
   d. 35

57–45. What percentage of newly acquired HSV 2 infections are symptomatic?

   a. 10
   b. 25
   c. 33
   d. 50

57–46. What is the average incubation time for primary herpes?

   a. 3 to 6 days
   b. 14 to 21 days
   c. 28 to 40 days
   d. 100 to 120 days

57–47. How long does it take for all signs and symptoms of primary herpes to resolve?

   a. 3 to 5 days
   b. 7 to 10 days
   c. 14 to 28 days
   d. 35 to 50 days

57–48. Which of the following is the "gold standard" for the diagnosis of genital herpes in adults?

   a. tissue culture
   b. enzyme-linked immunosorbent assay (ELISA) tests or serology
   c. deoxribonucleic acid (DNA) probes
   d. cytological examination

57–49. What is the incidence of viral shedding at delivery in women with a history of genital herpes?

   a. 1 to 2%
   b. 5 to 10%
   c. 12 to 15%
   d. 15 to 20%

57–50. What is the most common means for acquisition of neonatal herpes virus infection?

   a. transplacental
   b. across intact fetal membranes
   c. intrapartum exposure
   d. postnatally

57–51. What is the risk of neonatal infection with primary maternal infection during labor?

   a. <1%
   b. 5%
   c. 20%
   d. 50%

57–52. What is the risk of neonatal herpes infection with recurrent maternal infection during labor?

   a. 5%
   b. 15%
   c. 25%
   d. 50%

57–53. What proportion of women overall will have a positive herpes culture during labor?

   a. <0.03
   b. 0.3
   c. 3
   d. 13

57–54. What is the mortality rate of disseminated neonatal herpesvirus infection?

    a. 10%
    b. 25%
    c. 40%
    d. 60%

57–55. In disseminated neonatal herpesvirus infection, serious nervous system damage is seen in at least what percentage of survivors?

    a. 10
    b. 25
    c. 50
    d. 80

57–56. What type of virus is the human immunodeficiency virus (HIV)?

    a. ribonucleic acid (RNA) virus
    b. DNA virus
    c. RNA retrovirus
    d. DNA retrovirus

57–57. How often is HIV infection responsible for death in persons aged 25 to 44 years?

    a. tenth leading cause
    b. fifth leading cause
    c. third leading cause
    d. most common cause

57–58. In the United States, which ethnic group has a disparately increased HIV infection rate, with approximately 1 in 160 women infected?

    a. blacks
    b. Asian or Pacific Islanders
    c. white
    d. Native Americans

57–59. What is the most common mode of transmission of HIV-1?

    a. fecal-oral
    b. parenterally
    c. sexually
    d. perinatally

57–60. What percentage of HIV infections in women can be attributed to heterosexual contact?

    a. 10
    b. 33
    c. 50
    d. 75

57–61. What is the median time interval from asymptomatic viremia to the acquired immunodeficiency syndrome in HIV infection?

    a. 2 years
    b. 5 years
    c. 10 years
    d. 20 years

57–62. What CD4+ count is definitive for a diagnosis of acquired deficiency syndrome (AIDS)?

    a. $<50/\mu L$
    b. $<100/\mu L$
    c. $<200/\mu L$
    d. $<500/\mu L$

57–63. What is the risk of HIV transmission by screened blood?

    a. 1 per 20,000
    b. 1 per 500,000
    c. 1 per 2 million
    d. 1 per 10 million

57–64. What is the rate of perinatal transmission of the HIV virus in untreated women?

    a. 5 to 10%
    b. 15 to 25%
    c. 25 to 30%
    d. 50 to 60%

57–65. Which of the following increases the risk of perinatal HIV transmission?

    a. high maternal plasma HIV-RNA level
    b. premature delivery
    c. prolonged rupture of membranes
    d. all of the above

57–66. What is the rate of perinatal transmission in women given HAART (highly active antiretroviral therapy)?

    a. $<2\%$
    b. 8%
    c. 15%
    d. 25%

57–67. What is the risk of transmission of HIV to the newborn from breastfeeding?

    a. increased
    b. decreased
    c. remains the same
    d. unknown

57–68. At what CD4 count cutoff is primary prophylaxis for *Pneumocystis carinii* pneumonia recommended?

   a. <200/μL
   b. <100/μL
   c. <75/μL
   d. <50/μL

57–69. Management of health-care workers exposed significantly to HIV-contaminated fluids includes which of the following?

   a. observation and counseling
   b. serial ELISA and zidovudine for positive tests
   c. serial CD4 counts and zidovudine for CD4 count <500/μL
   d. multiple antiviral drug prophylaxis

57–70. What is the etiology of condylomata accuminata?

   a. *Treponema pallidum*
   b. human papillomavirus
   c. parvovirus
   d. *Hemophilus ducreyi*

57–71. What is a useful modality for treatment of condylomata accuminata during pregnancy?

   a. podophyllin resin
   b. interferon
   c. trichloracetic acid
   d. 5-fluorouracil

57–72. Of the following virus types, which are associated with laryngeal papillomatosis?

   a. HPV 6/11
   b. HPV 16/18
   c. HPV 31/35
   d. HPV 51/52

57–73. What is the etiology of soft chancres?

   a. *T. pallidum*
   b. *H. ducreyi*
   c. *Trichomonas vaginalis*
   d. Donovanosis

57–74. Which of the following is a recommended treatment for chancroid in pregnancy?

   a. ceftriaxone 250 mg IM once
   b. erythromycin 250 mg bid for 3 days
   c. tetracycline 500 mg qid for 7 days
   d. metronidazole 2 gm po once

57–75. How sensitive is a vaginal secretion wet mount for the detection of trichomoniasis?

   a. 20%
   b. 40%
   c. 60%
   d. 85%

57–76. Which is an alternate drug to metronidazole for the treatment of trichomoniasis?

   a. ampicillin
   b. ciprofolxacin
   c. spectinomycin
   d. none is available

XIII SECTION

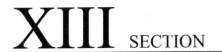

Family Planning

58

Contraception

58–1. In the absence of contraception, what percentage of fertile, sexually active women will conceive within one year?

  a. 90
  b. 75
  c. 50
  d. 40

58–2. Which of the following reliably signals the end of a woman's fertility?

  a. age >52
  b. cessation of menses for 4 months
  c. elevation of follicle-stimulating hormone (FSH)
  d. none of the above

58–3. What contraceptive method is most commonly used by women in the United States (Piccinino and Mosher, 1999)?

  a. female sterilization
  b. intrauterine device
  c. male condom
  d. oral contraceptives

58–4. With typical use, which of the following contraceptive methods has the highest failure rate within the first year of use?

  a. male condom
  b. Norplant
  c. spermicides
  d. withdrawal

58–5. What is the expected failure rate from Depo-Provera (injectable)?

  a. 0.03%
  b. 0.3%

  c. 1.0%
  d. 3.0%

58–6. What is the mechanism of action of oral contraceptives?

  a. prevent ovulation
  b. suppress gonadotropin-releasing factors
  c. impair sperm transport
  d. all of the above

58–7. Which of the following estrogens is used in oral contraceptives?

  a. estrone
  b. ethinyl estradiol
  c. estriol
  d. equilin

58–8. What is the potency of ethinyl estradiol compared to mestranol?

  a. equal potency
  b. 1.2 to 1.5 times more potent
  c. 2.1 to 2.3 times more potent
  d. 0.4 to 0.5 times weaker

58–9. What is the progestin with the least androgenic effect?

  a. norethindrone
  b. norgestrel
  c. levonorgestrel
  d. norgestimate

58–10. Which of the following drugs may decrease the effectiveness of oral contraceptives?

  a. aspirin
  b. erythromycin
  c. rifampin
  d. propranolol

58–11. Erratic use of which of the following vitamins increases the likelihood of breakthrough bleeding?

    a. A
    b. B
    c. C
    d. K

58–12. In healthy young women, which of the following activities is LEAST likely to result in a fatality?

    a. driving an automobile
    b. hysterectomy
    c. oral contraceptive use
    d. term pregnancy

58–13. Which of the following is NOT reduced with oral contraceptive use?

    a. breast milk production
    b. salpingitis
    c. endometrial cancer
    d. cervical cancer

58–14. In a patient taking oral contraceptives, which of the following is reduced?

    a. plasma thyroxine
    b. plasma cortisol
    c. T_3 resin uptake
    d. transcortin

58–15. Which progestin has the least detrimental effect on lipoproteins?

    a. desogestrel
    b. levonorgestrel
    c. norethindrone
    d. mestranol

58–16. Which of the following progestins has the greatest antagonizing effect on insulin and glucose metabolism?

    a. norgestrel
    b. norethindrone
    c. desogestrel
    d. ethynodiol diacetate

58–17. Elevated blood pressure associated with oral contraceptive use is likely related to the increased production of which of the following?

    a. angiotensin
    b. antidiuretic hormone
    c. endothelin
    d. aldosterone

58–18. Which of the following is positively associated with oral contraceptive use?

    a. ovarian cancer
    b. retinopathy
    c. malignant liver
    d. thromboembolic events

58–19. What is the effect of oral contraceptive use on the incidence of pituitary adenomas?

    a. increased
    b. decreased
    c. no change from baseline
    d. not known

58–20. The risk of cervical (preinvasive) cancer increases after how many years of oral contraceptive use?

    a. 1
    b. 3
    c. 5
    d. 10

58–21. In the evidence-based review by Speroff (2000b), what association was found between oral contraceptive use and breast cancer?

    a. increased risk with high-estrogen pills only
    b. increased risk with both high-estrogen and high-progesterone pills
    c. increased risk with duration of use >5 years
    d. no increased risk regardless of dosages or duration of use

58–22. What is the risk of venous thromboembolism with oral contraceptive use when compared with pregnancy?

    a. 5 times greater
    b. 3 times greater
    c. the same
    d. one-half as great

58–23. What is the effect of oral contraceptives on the incidence of deep venous thrombosis and embolism?

    a. decreased incidence
    b. does not effect the incidence
    c. increases the incidence
    d. increases thrombosis but not pulmonary embolism

58–24. The risk of stroke is increased with oral contraceptive use if which of the following cofactors is present?

    a. hypertension
    b. migraines
    c. smoking
    d. all of the above

58–25. What percentage of women will develop hypertension secondary to oral contraceptive use?

    a. 1
    b. 5
    c. 15
    d. 25

58–26. According to current information, what is the relation of oral contraceptive use to myocardial infarction?

    a. risk not increased in nonsmokers
    b. risk increased in both smokers and nonsmokers
    c. risk not increased in any group
    d. risk increased in nonsmokers over age 35

58–27. Oral contraceptives are currently thought to cause which of the following congenital defects?

    a. limb-reduction defects
    b. sexual ambiguity
    c. heart defects
    d. no association with any defects

58–28. Oral contraceptives have NOT been associated with which of the following?

    a. increased pigmentation of face
    b. improvement of acne
    c. depression at high doses of estrogen
    d. increased rate of HIV infection

58–29. Of the following, which is NOT an absolute contraindication to oral contraceptives?

    a. prior thromboembolism
    b. history of liver tumor while on oral contraceptives previously
    c. migraine headaches
    d. breast carcinoma with positive estrogen receptors

58–30. Regarding mechanism of action, which of the following is NOT true of progestin only contraceptive pills?

    a. inhibit ovulation reliably
    b. alter cervical mucus
    c. alter endometrial maturation
    d. impede blastocyst implantation

58–31. Which of the following is an advantage of progestin-only pills as compared with combination oral contraceptives?

    a. fewer ovarian cysts
    b. less breakthrough bleeding
    c. less effect on lactation
    d. lower incidence of ectopic pregnancy if method fails

58–32. A backup method of contraception should be considered if anticonvulsant medications or rifampin is used with which of these contraceptives?

    a. low-dose combination oral contraceptives
    b. progestin-only oral contraceptives
    c. levonorgestrel implants (Norplant)
    d. all of the above

58–33. What is a strong contraindication to oral progestin-only contraceptive use?

    a. cigarette smoking
    b. depression
    c. mild hypertension
    d. unexplained uterine bleeding

58–34. Injectable progestin contraceptives show what disadvantages?

    a. prolonged amenorrhea or irregular bleeding
    b. weight gain
    c. delayed ovulation after discontinuation
    d. all of the above

58–35. Which aspect of injectable progestin use is particularly worrisome in adolescents and young women?

    a. decreased bone mineral density
    b. increased pelvic infections
    c. worsening of acne
    d. increased risk of uterine cancer

58–36. What is the contraceptive dosage of Depo-Provera?

    a. 50 mg every 3 months
    b. 100 mg every 3 months
    c. 150 mg every 3 months
    d. 200 mg every 3 months

58–37. Which of the following is a disadvantage of progestin implants (Norplant)?

    a. low failure rate
    b. immediately effective
    c. high initial expense
    d. prompt return of fertility after removal

58–38. Which of the following has done most to limit use of Norplant by women?

    a. contraceptive failure rate
    b. expense
    c. difficulty of insertion and removal
    d. litigation

58–39. Why were the Lippes Loop and the Cu-7 intrauterine devices withdrawn from the market?

    a. unacceptable infection rate
    b. low utilization rate
    c. excessive litigation
    d. unacceptable failure rate

58–40. Which of the following is NOT a component of the Progestasert intrauterine device?

    a. barium sulfate
    b. levonorgestrel
    c. progesterone
    d. silicone

58–41. How much progesterone is supplied into the uterus daily with a Progestasert intrauterine device?

    a. 1 μg
    b. 30 μg
    c. 65 μg
    d. 100 μg

58–42. How often does the Progestasert need to be replaced?

    a. every year
    b. every 2 years
    c. every 3 years
    d. every 4 years

58–43. How often does the levonorgestrel intrauterine device need to be replaced?

    a. yearly
    b. every 2 years
    c. every 5 years
    d. every 7 years

58–44. Which of the following is NOT a mechanism of action of the intrauterine device?

    a. accelerated tubal motility
    b. prevention of ovulation
    c. local inflammatory reaction
    d. prevention of implantation

58–45. Which intrauterine device is the most effective in preventing pregnancy?

    a. Cu-T 380A
    b. levonorgestrel
    c. Progestasert
    d. all are equally effective

58–46. Which device is associated with the least menstrual blood loss?

    a. Cu-T 380A
    b. Lippes Loop

    c. Cu-7
    d. Progestasert

58–47. What percentage of women using the Cu-T 380A will have it removed due to menorrhagia?

    a. 2 to 5%
    b. 10 to 15%
    c. 20 to 25%
    d. 30 to 35%

58–48. Which of the following characterizes the risk of pelvic infection in intrauterine device users compared with nonusers?

    a. increased risk for duration of use
    b. increased risk of infection only during first 20 days after insertion
    c. increased risk of infection for first year of intrauterine device use
    d. no increased risk of infection

58–49. What is the incidence of actinomyces-like structures identified by Pap smears in women with intrauterine devices?

    a. 0.7%
    b. 1.0%
    c. 7.0%
    d. 17.0%

58–50. What is the most appropriate therapy for a woman who is 8-weeks pregnant with the string of a Cu-T 380 A visible at the cervix?

    a. antibiotics
    b. abortion
    c. removal of intrauterine device
    d. no action

58–51. Which of the following is NOT an absolute contraindication to using an intrauterine device?

    a. active or recent salpingitis
    b. pregnancy
    c. undiagnosed uterine bleeding
    d. uterine leiomyomata

58–52. How long (years) can the Copper T 380A be left in the uterus?

    a. 1
    b. 3
    c. 5
    d. 10

58–53. Use of which of the following does NOT improve the efficacy of the male condom?

    a. intravaginal spermicides
    b. oil-based lubricants
    c. reservoir tips
    d. spermicidal lubricants

58–54. What is the breakage rate of the female condom?

a. 0.6%
b. 1.0 to 2.0%
c. 3.0 to 5.0%
d. 8.0 to 10.0%

58–55. What is the duration of maximal effectiveness of spermicides?

a. 1 hr
b. 6 hr
c. 8 hr
d. 24 hr

58–56. Of the following, which is increased when spermicides are used?

a. neural tube defects
b. limb reduction defects
c. Down syndrome
d. none of the above

58–57. What is the minimum amount of time after intercourse that a diaphragm should remain in place?

a. 2 hr
b. 6 hr
c. 12 hr
d. 18 hr

58–58. The incidence of which of the following is slightly increased with use of the diaphragm?

a. cervicitis
b. cystocele
c. pelvic inflammatory disease
d. urinary tract infection

58–59. Which of the following are variations of periodic abstinence as a family planning method?

a. cervical mucous method
b. calendar rhythm
c. symptothermal
d. all of the above

58–60. Of the following, which is NOT effective for post-coital contraception?

a. ethinyl estradiol plus levonorgestrel
b. copper intrauterine devices
c. levonorgestrel alone
d. Norplant

58–61. When do adolescents typically seek contraception in relation to initiation of sexual activity?

a. a few weeks prior
b. a few months prior
c. a few weeks to months after
d. a year of more after

58–62. Postcoital hormonal contraception decreases the risk of conception by what percentage?

a. 25
b. 50
c. 75
d. 100

Sterilization

59–1. What is the most popular form of contraception in the United States?

a. condoms
b. oral contraceptives
c. intrauterine devices
d. sterilization

59–2. Which puerperal tubal sterilization procedure is least likely to fail?

a. Pomeroy
b. Irving
c. Parkland
d. fimbriectomy

59–3. The success of the Pomeroy procedure relies upon the use of what type of ligature?

    a. chromic gut
    b. plain gut
    c. synthetic polymer
    d. silk

59–4. What is the greatest failure rate for a Parkland-type tubal sterilization?

    a. 1 in 100
    b. 1 in 200
    c. 1 in 400
    d. 1 in 1000

59–5. What is the least effective sterilization procedure?

    a. fimbriectomy
    b. Madlener
    c. Parkland
    d. Irving

59–6. What is the current mortality rate directly related to female sterilization?

    a. 1.5 in 100,000
    b. 4 in 100,000
    c. 1.5 in 10,000
    d. 4 in 10,000

59–7. With laparoscopic tubal sterilization, which factors increase morbidity?

    a. obesity
    b. previous abdominal or pelvic surgery
    c. diabetes
    d. all of the above

59–8. Tubal sterilization failures are least likely due to which of the following?

    a. fistula formation
    b. mechanical devices are improperly placed
    c. inadequate coagulation with the bipolar method
    d. most are preventable

59–9. Which of the following is most likely to occur following tubal sterilization?

    a. increased psychological disorders
    b. luteal phase dysfunction

    c. menorrhagia
    d. unchanged menstrual function

59–10. What is the mortality rate from hysterectomy for benign diseases?

    a. 1 to 3 in 100,000
    b. 5 to 25 in 100,000
    c. 60 to 80 in 100,000
    d. 100 to 120 in 100,000

59–11. What is the difference with tubal sterilization when compared with vasectomy?

    a. higher complication rate
    b. higher cost
    c. higher failure rate
    d. all of the above

59–12. What is the approximate success rate of vasectomy reversal?

    a. 15%
    b. 50%
    c. 75%
    d. 90%

59–13. What are feelings of regret following male or female sterilization most strongly related to?

    a. immaturity
    b. income
    c. new partner
    d. number of children

59–14. Following a vasectomy, which statement is true?

    a. Autoimmune diseases are more common.
    b. Arteriosclerosis is accelerated.
    c. Sterility is not immediate.
    d. Testicular cancer is increased.

59–15. What method of tubal sterilization shows the highest pregnancy rate after 10 years?

    a. bipolar coagulation
    b. partial salpingectomy
    c. spring clip
    d. unipolar coagulation

ANSWERS

CHAPTER 1

1–1. **c** *(p. 4)*

1–2. **b** *(p. 4)*

1–3. **b** *(p. 4)*

1–4. **b** *(p. 4)*

1–5. **d** *(p. 5)*

1–6. **b** *(p. 5)*

1–7. **b** *(p. 5)*

1–8. **d** *(p. 5)*

1–9. **d** *(p. 5)*

1–10. **d** *(p. 5)*

1–11. **b** *(p. 5)*

1–12. **b** *(p. 5)*

1–13. **c** *(p. 6)*

1–14. **b** *(p. 6)*

1–15. **a** *(p. 6)*

1–16. **b** *(p. 6)*

1–17. **b** *(p. 6)*

1–18. **d** *(p. 6)*

1–19. **c** *(p. 6)*

1–20. **a** *(p. 6)*

1–21. **d** *(p. 8)*

1–22. **a** *(p. 8)*

1–23. **d** *(p. 9)*

1–24. **b** *(p. 10)*

1–25. **d** *(p. 12)*

CHAPTER 2

2–1. **c** *(p. 16)*

2–2. **d** *(p. 16)*

2–3. **b** *(p. 16)*

2–4. **a** *(p. 17)*

2–5. **b** *(p. 17)*

2–6. **d** *(p. 17)*

2–7. **a** *(p. 18)*

2–8. **b** *(p. 18)*

2–9. **b** *(p. 18)*

2–10. **d** *(pp. 18-19)*

2–11. **a** *(p. 19)*

2–12. **d** *(p. 19)*

2–13. **c** *(p. 20)*

2–14. **a** *(p. 20)*

2–15. **c** *(p. 20)*

2–16. **c** *(p. 20)*

2–17. c *(p. 20)*

2–18. b *(p. 20)*

2–19. d *(p. 21)*

2–20. b *(p. 21)*

2–21. a *(p. 22)*

2–22. d *(p. 22)*

2–23. c *(p. 22)*

2–24. c *(p. 22)*

2–25. c *(p. 22)*

2–26. c *(p. 22)*

2–27. c *(p. 23)*

2–28. a *(p. 23)*

2–29. b *(p. 24)*

2–30. d *(p. 24)*

2–31. a *(p. 25)*

2–32. c *(pp. 25-26)*

2–33. b *(p. 26)*

2–34. c *(p. 26)*

2–35. c *(p. 26)*

2–36. c *(p. 27)*

2–37. b *(p. 27)*

2–38. a *(p. 27)*

2–39. c *(p. 28)*

2–40. b *(p. 28)*

2–41. c *(p. 28)*

2–42. a *(p. 29)*

2–43. b *(p. 28)*

2–44. c *(p. 29)*

CHAPTER 3

3–1. a *(p. 32)*

3–2. b *(p. 32)*

3–3. d *(p. 33)*

3–4. d *(p. 34)*

3–5. a *(p. 34)*

3–6. b *(p. 34)*

3–7. d *(p. 34)*

3–8. c *(p. 35)*

3–9. d *(p. 35)*

3–10. d *(p. 36)*

3–11. c *(p. 37)*

3–12. a *(p. 37)*

3–13. b *(p. 37)*

3–14. d *(p. 37)*

3–15. b *(p. 37)*

3–16. c *(p. 38)*

3–17. d *(p. 39)*

3–18. d *(p. 39)*

3–19. b *(p. 39)*

3–20. d *(p. 40)*

3–21. c *(p. 40)*

3–22. b *(p. 40)*

3–23. a *(p. 40)*

3–24. a *(p. 42)*

3–25. d *(p. 43)*

3–26. d *(p. 43)*

3–27. b *(p. 44)*

3–28. **a** *(p. 44)*

3–29. **c** *(p. 44)*

3–30. **b** *(pp. 45-46)*

3–31. **c** *(p. 46)*

3–32. **b** *(p. 47)*

3–33. **b** *(p. 48)*

3–34. **c** *(p. 48)*

3–35. **b** *(p. 48)*

3–36. **d** *(p. 48)*

3–37. **b** *(p. 51)*

3–38. **b** *(p. 51)*

3–39. **a** *(p. 51)*

3–40. **d** *(p. 51)*

3–41. **b** *(p. 51)*

3–42. **c** *(p. 51)*

3–43. **b** *(p. 53)*

3–44. **c** *(p. 54)*

3–45. **d** *(p. 55)*

3–46. **c** *(p. 55)*

3–47. **b** *(p. 57)*

3–48. **b** *(p. 58)*

3–49. **b** *(p. 56)*

3–50. **b** *(p. 56)*

3–51. **b** *(p. 56)*

3–52. **d** *(p. 56)*

3–53. **c** *(p. 56)*

3–54. **b** *(p. 57)*

3–55. **d** *(p. 58)*

3–56. **a** *(p. 57)*

3–57. **c** *(p. 58)*

3–58. **c** *(p. 58)*

3–59. **d** *(p. 58)*

3–60. **d** *(p. 58)*

3–61. **d** *(p. 58)*

3–62. **d** *(p. 58)*

3–63. **d** *(p. 58)*

3–64. **d** *(p. 59)*

3–65. **c** *(p. 59)*

3–66. **a** *(p. 60)*

CHAPTER 4

4–1. **b** *(p. 66)*

4–2. **b** *(p. 66)*

4–3. **a** *(p. 67)*

4–4. **d** *(p. 67)*

4–5. **b** *(p. 70)*

4–6. **d** *(p. 72)*

4–7. **a** *(p. 70)*

4–8. **d** *(p. 71)*

4–9. **c** *(p. 72)*

4–10. **c** *(p. 72)*

4–11. **a** *(p. 73)*

4–12. **d** *(p. 73)*

4–13. **c** *(p. 74)*

4–14. **b** *(p. 76)*

4–15. **c** *(p. 74)*

4–16. b *(pp. 76-77)*

4–17. d *(p. 78)*

4–18. b *(p. 79)*

4–19. c *(p. 79)*

4–20. b *(p. 80)*

4–21. c *(p. 81)*

4–22. a *(p. 82)*

CHAPTER 5

5–1. b *(p. 86)*

5–2. a *(p. 86)*

5–3. c *(p. 86)*

5–4. b *(p. 86)*

5–5. c *(p. 87)*

5–6. a *(p. 87)*

5–7. b *(pp. 88-89)*

5–8. a *(p. 86)*

5–9. c *(p. 86)*

5–10. b *(p. 86)*

5–11. b *(p. 89)*

5–12. d *(p. 89)*

5–13. d *(p. 90)*

5–14. c *(p. 90)*

5–15. a *(p. 90)*

5–16. b *(p. 91)*

5–17. c *(p. 96)*

5–18. a *(p. 96)*

5–19. a *(p. 96)*

5–20. d *(p. 96)*

5–21. c *(p. 97)*

5–22. a *(p. 98)*

5–23. b *(p. 98)*

5–24. d *(p. 100)*

5–25. a *(p. 100)*

5–26. b *(p. 105)*

5–27. c *(p. 105)*

CHAPTER 6

6–1. d *(p. 110)*

6–2. c *(p. 111)*

6–3. a *(p. 111)*

6–4. b *(p. 112)*

6–5. b *(p. 112)*

6–6. d *(p. 112)*

6–7. d *(p. 112)*

6–8. d *(p. 112)*

6–9. c *(p. 113)*

6–10. a *(p. 113)*

6–11. d *(p. 113)*

6–12. b *(pp. 113-114)*

6–13. a *(p. 114)*

6–14. d *(p. 114)*

6–15. a *(p. 114)*

6–16. c *(p. 115)*

6–17. a *(p. 116)*

6–18. d *(p. 117)*

6–19. d *(p. 117)*

6–20. a *(p. 117)*

6–21. a *(p. 117)*

6–22. b *(p. 118)*

6–23. d *(p. 119)*

6–24. d *(p. 118)*

6–25. c *(p. 119)*

6–26. a *(p. 120)*

6–27. c *(p. 120)*

6–28. a *(p. 121)*

6–29. b *(p. 121)*

6–30. b *(p. 123)*

6–31. b *(p. 123)*

6–32. a *(p. 124)*

6–33. c *(p. 124)*

6–34. d *(p. 124)*

6–35. b *(p. 125)*

CHAPTER 7

7–1. c *(p. 130)*

7–2. d *(p. 130)*

7–3. b *(p. 130)*

7–4. d *(p. 130)*

7–5. c *(pp. 130-131)*

7–6. b *(p. 131)*

7–7. c *(p. 133)*

7–8. b *(p. 133)*

7–9. c *(p. 133)*

7–10. c *(p. 133)*

7–11. b *(p. 133)*

7–12. b *(p. 133)*

7–13. c *(p. 133)*

7–14. d *(p. 133)*

7–15. d *(p. 133)*

7–16. c *(p. 133)*

7–17. b *(p. 133)*

7–18. c *(p. 134)*

7–19. a *(p. 134)*

7–20. d *(p. 134)*

7–21. c *(p. 135)*

7–22. d *(p. 135)*

7–23. c *(p. 135)*

7–24. a *(p. 135)*

7–25. b *(p. 135)*

7–26. d *(p. 135)*

7–27. d *(p. 135)*

7–28. c *(p. 137)*

7–29. b *(p. 138)*

7–30. c *(p. 138)*

7–31. a *(p. 138)*

7–32. b *(p. 139)*

7–33. c *(p. 139)*

7–34. d *(p. 139)*

7–35. b *(p. 139)*

7–36. a *(p. 139)*

7–37. a *(p. 139)*

7–38. c *(p. 140)*

7–39. b *(p. 141)*

7–40. a *(p. 141)*

7–41. d *(p. 141)*

7–42. a *(p. 142)*

7–43. b *(p. 142)*

7–44. d *(p. 143)*

7–45. c *(p. 143)*

7–46. b *(p. 143)*

7–47. d *(p. 143)*

7–48. b *(p. 145)*

7–49. d *(p. 145)*

7–50. d *(p. 146)*

7–51. a *(p. 146)*

7–52. b *(p. 146)*

7–53. b *(p. 146)*

7–54. c *(p. 147)*

7–55. a *(p. 147)*

7–56. d *(p. 148)*

7–57. c *(p. 148)*

7–58. b *(p. 149)*

7–59. c *(p. 149)*

7–60. d *(p. 150)*

7–61. a *(p. 150)*

7–62. b *(p. 150)*

7–63. b *(p. 151)*

7–64. c *(p. 151)*

7–65. a *(p. 152)*

7–66. d *(p. 152)*

7–67. a *(p. 152)*

7–68. a *(p. 153)*

7–69. a *(p. 154)*

7–70. a *(p. 154)*

7–71. b *(p. 155)*

7–72. a *(p. 154)*

7–73. c *(p. 157)*

7–74. c *(p. 158)*

7–75. c *(p. 158)*

7–76. a *(p. 158)*

7–77. d *(p. 159)*

7–78. c *(p. 159)*

7–79. d *(p. 160)*

7–80. b *(p. 160)*

7–81. c *(p. 160)*

7–82. a *(p. 160)*

CHAPTER 8

8–1. d *(p. 168)*

8–2. b *(p. 168)*

8–3. b *(p. 169)*

8–4. c *(p. 169)*

8–5. d *(p. 170)*

8–6. a *(p. 170)*

8–7. a *(p. 171)*

8–8. d *(p. 171)*

8–9. c *(p. 171)*

8–10. **a** *(p. 171)*

8–11. **b** *(p. 173)*

8–12. **c** *(p. 173)*

8–13. **c** *(p. 174)*

8–14. **c** *(p. 174)*

8–15. **b** *(p. 174)*

8–16. **d** *(p. 175)*

8–17. **b** *(p. 176)*

8–18. **c** *(p. 176)*

8–19. **a** *(p. 176)*

8–20. **c** *(p. 177)*

8–21. **c** *(p. 177)*

8–22. **a** *(p. 177)*

8–23. **c** *(p. 177)*

8–24. **a** *(p. 178)*

8–25. **c** *(p. 178)*

8–26. **b** *(p. 178)*

8–27. **c** *(p. 178)*

8–28. **b** *(p. 179)*

8–29. **c** *(p. 179)*

8–30. **d** *(p. 179)*

8–31. **c** *(p. 180)*

8–32. **d** *(p. 180)*

8–33. **a** *(p. 181)*

8–34. **c** *(p. 181)*

8–35. **b** *(pp. 181-182)*

8–36. **c** *(p. 182)*

8–37. **d** *(p. 182)*

8–38. **a** *(p. 182)*

8–39. **d** *(p. 183)*

8–40. **c** *(p. 183)*

8–41. **b** *(pp. 183-184)*

8–42. **a** *(p. 185)*

8–43. **c** *(p. 185)*

8–44. **a** *(p. 185)*

8–45. **d** *(p. 186)*

8–46. **d** *(p. 186)*

8–47. **c** *(p. 188)*

8–48. **b** *(p. 188)*

8–49. **c** *(p. 190)*

8–50. **a** *(p. 190)*

8–51. **d** *(pp. 192-193)*

8–52. **b** *(p. 193)*

8–53. **b** *(p. 194)*

8–54. **b** *(p. 194)*

CHAPTER 9

9–1. **d** *(p. 204)*

9–2. **d** *(p. 204)*

9–3. **d** *(p. 205)*

9–4. **a** *(p. 205)*

9–5. **b** *(p. 205)*

9–6. **a** *(p. 206)*

9–7. **c** *(p. 206)*

9–8. **d** *(p. 206)*

9–9. **c** *(p. 206)*

9–10. c *(p. 206)*

9–11. d *(p. 206)*

9–12. c *(pp. 206-207)*

9–13. a *(p. 208)*

9–14. b *(p. 208)*

9–15. d *(p. 208)*

9–16. b *(p. 209)*

9–17. d *(p. 209)*

9–18. b *(p. 210)*

9–19. c *(p. 210)*

9–20. d *(p. 211)*

9–21. c *(p. 212)*

9–22. a *(p. 211)*

9–23. b *(p. 211)*

9–24. a *(pp. 212-213)*

9–25. a *(p. 212)*

9–26. c *(p. 213)*

9–27. d *(p. 213)*

9–28. d *(p. 213)*

9–29. d *(p. 213)*

9–30. c *(p. 214)*

9–31. a *(p. 214)*

9–32. b *(p. 215)*

9–33. b *(p. 215)*

9–34. d *(pp. 215-216)*

9–35. b *(p. 216)*

9–36. b *(p. 216)*

9–37. a *(p. 213)*

9–38. b *(p. 216)*

9–39. d *(p. 216)*

CHAPTER 10

10–1. d *(p. 222)*

10–2. a *(p. 222)*

10–3. b *(p. 225)*

10–4. d *(p. 225)*

10–5. c *(p. 226)*

10–6. c *(p. 226)*

10–7. d *(p. 226)*

10–8. a *(p. 226)*

10–9. d *(p. 226)*

10–10. a *(p. 226)*

10–11. a *(pp. 226-227)*

10–12. b *(p. 227)*

10–13. d *(p. 227)*

10–14. c *(pp. 227-228)*

10–15. c *(p. 227)*

10–16. c *(p. 228)*

10–17. d *(p. 228)*

10–18. c *(pp. 228-229)*

10–19. c *(p. 229)*

10–20. a *(p. 229)*

10–21. a *(p. 229)*

10–22. d *(p. 230)*

10–23. b *(p. 230)*

10–24. c *(p. 230)*

10–25. b *(p. 232)*

10–26. b *(p. 232)*

10–27. a *(p. 232)*

10–28. c *(p. 234)*

10–29. b *(p. 234)*

10–30. d *(p. 235)*

10–31. a *(p. 236)*

10–32. c *(p. 236)*

10–33. a *(p. 236)*

10–34. d *(p. 236)*

10–35. c *(p. 236)*

10–36. c *(p. 236)*

10–37. c *(p. 236)*

10–38. d *(pp. 236-237)*

10–39. a *(p. 237)*

10–40. a *(p. 237)*

10–41. d *(p. 237)*

10–42. d *(p. 237)*

10–43. c *(p. 237)*

10–44. c *(p. 238)*

10–45. b *(p. 238)*

10–46. c *(p. 238)*

10–47. d *(p. 238)*

10–48. a *(p. 239)*

10–49. a *(p. 239)*

10–50. d *(p. 239)*

10–51. b *(p. 240)*

10–52. b *(p. 241)*

10–53. c *(p. 241)*

10–54. b *(p. 241)*

10–55. a *(p. 241)*

10–56. b *(p. 241)*

10–57. a *(p. 241)*

10–58. d *(p. 241)*

10–59. d *(p. 241)*

10–60. d *(p. 242)*

10–61. d *(p. 242)*

10–62. a *(p. 242)*

10–63. d *(p. 243)*

10–64. c *(p. 244)*

CHAPTER 11

11–1. d *(p. 252)*

11–2. b *(p. 252)*

11–3. b *(p. 252)*

11–4. d *(p. 252)*

11–5. a. *(p. 252)*

11–6. c *(p. 253)*

11–7. d *(p. 253)*

11–8. c *(p. 253)*

11–9. a *(p. 255)*

11–10. c *(pp. 255-256)*

11–11. b *(p. 256)*

11–12. d *(p. 257)*

11–13. a *(p. 258)*

11–14. b *(p. 259)*

11–15. a *(p. 37)*

11–16. c *(p. 260)*

11–17. b *(p. 262)*

11–18. d *(p. 262)*

11–19. b *(p. 263)*

11–20. d *(p. 264)*

11–21. a *(p. 265)*

11–22. b *(p. 265)*

11–23. d *(p. 266)*

11–24. a *(pp. 266-267)*

11–25. d *(p. 267)*

11–26. c *(p. 267)*

11–27. c *(p. 269)*

11–28. a *(p. 269)*

11–29. b *(pp. 270-271)*

11–30. b *(p. 272)*

11–31. a *(p. 272)*

11–32. a *(p. 273)*

11–33. d *(p. 273)*

11–34. d *(p. 273)*

11–35. c *(p. 273)*

11–36. a *(p. 273)*

11–37. c *(pp. 275-277)*

11–38. a *(p. 277)*

11–39. b *(p. 277)*

11–40. a *(p. 277)*

11–41. b *(p. 278)*

11–42. d *(p. 279)*

11–43. d *(p. 279)*

11–44. a *(p. 280)*

11–45. a *(p. 284-85)*

11–46. c *(p. 284)*

11–47. d *(p. 284)*

11–48. d *(p. 285)*

11–49. c *(pp. 285-286)*

CHAPTER 12

12–1. b *(p. 293)*

12–2. c *(p. 293)*

12–3. d *(p. 293)*

12–4. b *(p. 293)*

12–5. a *(p. 293)*

12–6. b *(p. 293)*

12–7. d *(p. 293)*

12–8. a *(p. 293)*

12–9. a *(p. 294)*

12–10. c *(p. 295)*

12–11. d *(p. 296)*

12–12. b *(p. 296)*

12–13. c *(p. 296)*

12–14. a *(p. 298-299)*

12–15. c *(p. 298-299)*

12–16. b *(p. 298-299)*

12–17. d *(p. 299)*

12–18. a *(p. 300)*

12–19. d *(p. 300)*

12–20. d *(p. 301)*

12–21. a *(p. 301)*

12–22. c *(p. 301)*

12–23. b *(p. 301)*

12–24. c *(p. 301)*

12–25. c *(p. 301)*

12–26. c *(p. 303)*

12–27. a *(p. 303)*

12–28. b *(p. 305)*

12–29. c *(p. 305)*

12–30. a *(p. 305)*

12–31. c *(p. 305)*

12.32. a *(p. 306)*

12–33. b *(p. 306)*

12–34. d *(p. 306)*

CHAPTER 13

13–1. c *(p. 310)*

13–2. c *(p. 310)*

13–3. a *(p. 311)*

13–4. c *(p. 311)*

13–5. d *(p. 311)*

13–6. d *(p. 311)*

13–7. a *(p. 312)*

13–8. c *(p. 312)*

13–9. b *(p. 312)*

13–10. b *(p. 313)*

13–11. a *(p. 313)*

13–12. d *(p. 314)*

13–13. b *(p. 314)*

13–14. c *(p. 314)*

13–15. c *(p. 314)*

13–16. d *(p. 315)*

13–17. c *(p. 315)*

13–18. c *(p. 315)*

13–19. b *(p. 316)*

13–20. b *(p. 316)*

13–21. b *(p. 317)*

13–22. c *(p. 317)*

13–23. d *(p. 319)*

13–24. d *(p. 319)*

13–25. d *(p. 321)*

13–26. d *(p. 321)*

13–27. d *(p. 323)*

13–28. b *(p. 323)*

13–29. a *(p. 323)*

13–30. b *(p. 323)*

13–31. b *(p. 323)*

13–32. b *(p. 324)*

13–33. b *(p. 324)*

13–34. d *(pp. 325, 328)*

13–35. a *(p.325)*

13–36. c *(p. 325)*

13–37. d *(p. 326)*

CHAPTER 14

14–1. c *(p. 332)*

14–2. c *(p. 332)*

14–3. b *(p. 332)*

14–4. c *(p. 334)*

14–5. b *(p. 334)*

14–6. b *(p. 335)*

14–7. c *(p. 335)*

14–8. a *(p. 335)*

14–9. c *(p. 335)*

14–10. d *(p. 335)*

14–11. d *(p. 335)*

14–12. b *(p. 336)*

14–13. b *(p. 336)*

14–14. c *(p. 337)*

14–15. c *(p. 338)*

14–16. b *(p. 339)*

14–17. c *(p. 339)*

14–18. d *(p. 340)*

14–19. a *(p. 340)*

14–20. b *(p. 341)*

14–21. c *(p. 341)*

14–22. c *(p. 341)*

14–23. d *(pp. 343-344)*

14–24. a *(p. 344)*

14–25. d *(pp. 343-344)*

14–26. c *(p. 345)*

14–27. a *(p. 345)*

14–28. d *(p. 346)*

14–29. c *(p. 348)*

14–30. b *(p. 349)*

14–31. b *(p. 353)*

14–32. c *(p. 354)*

14–33. d *(p. 354)*

14–34. a *(p. 355)*

14–35. b *(p. 355)*

14–36. c *(p. 355)*

14.37. d *(p. 356)*

14–38. c *(p. 356)*

14–39. c *(p. 356)*

CHAPTER 15

15–1. b *(p. 362)*

15–2. d *(p. 363)*

15–3. d *(p. 363)*

15–4. c *(p. 364)*

15–5. a *(p. 364)*

15–6. d *(p. 364)*

15–7. c *(p. 364)*

15–8. b *(p. 364)*

15–9. b *(p. 364)*

15–10. b *(p. 364)*

15–11. d *(p. 365)*

15–12. a *(p. 365)*

15–13. a *(p. 365)*

15–14. a *(p. 365)*

15–15. c *(p. 366)*

15–16. c *(p. 366)*

15–17. b *(p. 366)*

15–18. a *(p. 367)*

15–19. d *(p. 367)*

15–20. c *(p. 367)*

15–21. b *(p. 368)*

15–22. d *(p. 368)*

15–23. d *(p. 368)*

15–24. b *(p. 369)*

15–25. c *(p. 369)*

15–26. c *(p. 371)*

15–27. a *(p. 372)*

15–28. b *(pp. 373, 378)*

15–29. b *(p. 374)*

15–30. b *(p. 375)*

15–31. c *(p. 375)*

15–32. c *(p. 379)*

15–33. c *(p. 379)*

CHAPTER 16

16–1. b *(p. 386)*

16–2. a *(p. 386)*

16–3. d *(p. 386)*

16–4. c *(p. 386)*

16–5. d *(p. 386)*

16–6. a *(p. 387)*

16–7. b *(p. 388)*

16–8. d *(p. 388)*

16–9. b *(p. 388)*

16–10. b *(p. 388)*

16–11. d *(p. 389)*

16–12. d *(p. 388)*

16–13. d *(p. 389)*

16–14. b *(p. 389)*

16–15. d *(p. 389)*

16–16. d *(p. 389)*

16–17. b *(p. 389)*

16–18. c *(p. 390)*

16–19. b *(p. 390)*

16–20. a *(p. 390)*

16–21. c *(p. 391)*

16–22. d *(p. 393)*

16–23. c *(p. 395)*

16–24. d *(p. 395)*

16–25. c *(p. 396)*

16–26. d *(p. 396)*

16–27. b *(p. 398)*

16–28. c *(p. 399)*

CHAPTER 17

17–1. c *(p. 404)*

17–2. b *(p. 404)*

17–3. b *(p. 404)*

17–4. b *(p. 404)*

17–5. c *(p. 405)*

17–6. c *(p. 406)*

17–7. d *(p. 406)*

17–8. d *(p. 406)*

17–9. d *(p. 407)*

17–10. d *(p. 406)*

17–11. d *(p. 407)*

17–12. a *(p. 408)*

17–13. c *(p. 408)*

17–14. b *(p. 408)*

17–15. c *(p. 409)*

17–16. d *(p. 409)*

17–17. d *(p. 409)*

17–18. a *(p. 410)*

17–19. c *(p. 410)*

17–20. b *(p. 412)*

17–21. d *(p. 412)*

17–22. c *(p. 412)*

17–23. a *(p. 413)*

17–24. c *(p. 413)*

17–25. a *(p. 413)*

17–26. b *(p. 413)*

17–27. c *(p. 413)*

17–28. a *(p. 414)*

17–29. c *(p. 414)*

17–30. d *(p. 415)*

17–31. d *(p. 416)*

17–32. d *(p. 417)*

17–33. c *(p. 418)*

CHAPTER 18

18–1. d *(p. 426)*

18–2. d *(p. 426)*

18–3. c *(p. 427)*

18–4. b *(p. 428)*

18–5. b *(p. 427)*

18–6. a *(p. 428)*

18–7. c *(p. 428)*

18–8. b *(p. 430)*

18–9. b *(p. 429)*

18–10. b *(p. 429)*

18–11. d *(p. 429)*

18–12. c *(p. 429)*

18–13. b *(p. 429)*

18–14. b *(p. 430)*

18–15. d *(p. 430)*

18–16. c *(p. 432)*

18–17. a *(p. 434)*

18–18. b *(p. 434)*

18–19. b *(p. 431)*

18–20. c *(p. 436)*

18–21. c *(p. 436)*

18–22. c *(p. 436)*

18–23. b *(p. 437)*

18–24. d *(p. 437)*

18–25. b *(p. 437)*

18–26. d *(p. 437)*

18–27. c *(p. 438)*

18–28. b *(p. 438)*

18–29. b *(p. 438)*

18–30. b *(p. 441)*

18–31. d *(p. 442)*

18–32. b *(p. 441)*

18–33. b *(p. 441)*

18–34. c *(p. 431)*

18–35. a *(p. 445)*

18–36. d *(p. 447)*

18–37. a *(p. 447)*

CHAPTER 19

19–1. b *(p. 452)*

19–2. c *(p. 452)*

19–3. b *(p. 452)*

19–4. a *(p. 452)*

19–5. c *(p. 452)*

19–6. b *(p. 454)*

19–7. a *(p. 454)*

19–8. a *(p. 455)*

19–9. c *(p. 455)*

19–10. d *(p. 455)*

19–11. b *(pp. 456-457)*

19–12. c *(p. 457)*

19–13. d *(p. 457)*

19–14. b *(p. 459)*

19–15. c *(p. 459)*

19–16. c *(p. 460)*

19–17. b *(p. 460)*

19–18. d *(p. 461)*

19–19. b *(p. 461)*

19–20. c *(p. 462)*

CHAPTER 20

20–1. c *(p. 470)*

20–2. d *(p. 470)*

20–3. c *(p. 470)*

20–4. d *(p. 470)*

20–5. a *(p. 470)*

20–6. d *(p. 471)*

20–7. c *(p. 471)*

20–8. b *(p. 471)*

20–9. a *(p. 471)*

20–10. c *(p. 472)*

20–11. d *(p. 472)*

20–12. a *(p. 472)*

20–13. c *(p. 473)*

20–14. d *(p. 474)*

20–15. d *(p. 474)*

20–16. a *(p. 475)*

20–17. d *(p. 475)*

20–18. b *(p. 476)*

20–19. d *(p. 477)*

20–20. b *(p. 476)*

20–21. b *(p. 477)*

20–22. c *(p. 478)*

CHAPTER 21

21–1. **d** *(p. 486)*

21–2. **a** *(p. 486)*

21–3. **c** *(p. 486)*

21–4. **a** *(p. 487)*

21–5. **b** *(p. 487)*

21–6. **c** *(p. 487)*

21–7. **a** *(p. 487)*

21–8. **c** *(p. 487)*

21–9. **d** *(p. 488)*

21–10. **a** *(p. 489)*

21–11. **b** *(p. 489)*

21–12. **d** *(p. 489)*

21–13. **d** *(p. 489)*

21–14. **a** *(p. 490)*

21–15. **c** *(p. 490)*

21–16. **a** *(p. 490)*

21–17. **c** *(p. 490)*

21–18. **d** *(p. 490)*

21–19. **b** *(p. 490)*

21–20. **a** *(p. 490)*

21–21. **d** *(p. 494)*

21–22. **b** *(p. 495)*

21–23. **d** *(p. 497)*

21–24. **b** *(p. 497)*

21–25. **b** *(p. 497)*

21–26. **b** *(p. 498)*

21–27. **d** *(p. 498)*

21–28. **c** *(p. 499)*

21–29. **d** *(p. 503)*

21–30. **a** *(p. 503)*

21–31. **a** *(p. 504)*

21–32. **d** *(p. 505)*

CHAPTER 22

22–1. **b** *(p. 510)*

22–2. **d** *(p. 510)*

22–3. **b** *(p. 510)*

22–4. **a** *(p. 510)*

22–5. **c** *(p. 510)*

22–6. **b** *(p. 510)*

22–7. **c** *(p. 510)*

22–8. **d** *(p. 512)*

22–9. **c** *(p. 513)*

22–10. **d** *(p. 514)*

22–11. **b** *(p. 514)*

22–12. **d** *(p. 517)*

22–13. **b** *(p. 518)*

22–14. **b** *(p. 518)*

22–15. **c** *(p. 519)*

22–16. **b** *(p. 520)*

22–17. **c** *(p. 524)*

22–18. **a** *(p. 524)*

22–19. **b** *(p. 524)*

22–20. **c** *(p. 520)*

22–21. **d** *(p. 518)*

22–22. c *(p. 528)*

22–23. c *(p. 520)*

22–24. b *(p. 525)*

22–25. c *(p. 528)*

22–26. a *(p. 530)*

22–27. d *(p. 530)*

22–28. a *(p. 531)*

22–29. c *(p. 531)*

22–30. a *(p. 530)*

22–31. d *(p. 530)*

CHAPTER 23

23–1. b *(p. 538)*

23–2. c *(p. 539)*

23–3. c *(p. 543)*

23–4. d *(p. 539)*

23–5. b *(p. 542)*

23–6. c *(p. 542)*

23–7. c *(p. 542)*

23–8. c *(p. 542)*

23–9. a *(p. 543)*

23–10. c *(p. 543)*

23–11. c *(p. 546)*

23–12. d *(p. 546)*

23–13. a *(p. 546)*

23–14. d *(p. 546)*

23–15. c *(p. 548)*

23–16. b *(p. 550)*

23–17. d *(p. 551)*

23–18. b *(p. 551)*

23–19. d *(p. 552)*

23–20. c *(p. 553)*

23–21. c *(p. 557)*

23–22. b *(p. 559)*

23–23. b *(p. 538)*

CHAPTER 24

24–1. b *(p. 568)*

24–2. b *(p. 568)*

24–3. a *(p. 572)*

24–4. c *(p. 568)*

24–5. c *(p. 569)*

24–6. c *(p. 569)*

24–7. b *(p. 569)*

24–8. c *(p. 570)*

24–9. c *(p. 570)*

24–10. d *(p. 571)*

24–11. b *(p. 569)*

24–12. c *(p. 572)*

24–13. b *(p. 572)*

24–14. b *(p. 573)*

24–15. c *(p. 574)*

24–16. c *(p. 579)*

24–17. d *(p. 576)*

24–18. a *(p. 577)*

24–19. d *(p. 577)*

24–20. b *(p. 577)*

24–21. a *(p. 578)*

24–22. c *(p. 578)*

24–23. a *(p. 579)*

24–24. d *(p. 579)*

24–25. d *(p. 579)*

24–26. b *(p. 582)*

24–27. a *(p. 581)*

24–28. c *(p. 582)*

24–29. d *(p. 582)*

24–30. d *(p. 584)*

24–31. a *(p. 585)*

24–32. c *(p. 586)*

24–33. a *(p. 590)*

24–34. a *(p. 586)*

24–35. d *(p. 585)*

24–36. b *(p. 590)*

24–37. c *(p. 592)*

24–38. a *(p. 592)*

24–39. c *(p. 593)*

24–40. d *(p. 596)*

24–41. b *(p. 597)*

24–42. c *(p. 599)*

24–43. b *(p. 599)*

24–44. c *(p. 599)*

24–45. c *(p. 599)*

24–46. c *(p. 600)*

24–47. c *(p. 604)*

24–48. b *(p. 604)*

24–49. a *(p. 605)*

24–50. b *(p. 609)*

24–51. d *(pp. 587, 609)*

24–52. b *(p. 609)*

CHAPTER 25

25–1. c *(p. 620)*

25–2. c *(p. 621)*

25–3. d *(p. 622)*

25–4. d *(p. 623)*

25–5. c *(p. 623)*

25–6. d *(p. 624)*

25–7. d *(p. 623)*

25–8. b *(p. 624)*

25–9. a *(p. 624)*

25–10. b *(p. 625)*

25–11. d *(p. 626)*

25–12. d *(p. 626)*

25–13. b *(p. 627)*

25–14. b *(p. 627)*

25–15. b *(p. 627)*

25–16. a *(p. 628)*

25–17. c *(p. 629)*

25–18. b *(p. 631)*

25–19. a *(pp. 631-632)*

25–20. d *(p. 632)*

25–21. c *(p. 632)*

25–22. c *(p. 632)*

25–23. c *(pp. 632, 633)*

25–24. d *(p. 635)*

25–25. d *(p. 636)*

25–26. a *(p. 637)*

25–27. d *(p. 637)*

25–28. c *(p. 638)*

25–29. b *(p. 638)*

25–30. c *(p. 639)*

25–31. a *(p. 639)*

25–32. b *(p. 639)*

25–33. b *(p. 639)*

25–34. a *(p. 640)*

25–35. b *(p. 640)*

25–36. d *(p. 640)*

25–37. c *(p. 642)*

25–38. d *(p. 643)*

25–39. b *(p. 645)*

25–40. d *(p. 645)*

25–41. a *(p. 645)*

25–42. d *(p. 649)*

25–43. d *(p. 646)*

25–44. c *(p. 647)*

25–45. c *(p. 648)*

25–46. d *(p. 649)*

25–47. d *(p. 650)*

25–48. c *(p. 650)*

25–49. c *(p. 651)*

25–50. b *(p. 652)*

25–51. c *(p. 652)*

25–52. d *(p. 653)*

25–53. b *(p. 653)*

25–54. b *(p. 653)*

25–55. d *(p. 654)*

25–56. b *(p. 654)*

25–57. b *(p. 654)*

25–58. a *(p. 654)*

25–59. a *(p. 654)*

25–60. c *(p. 655)*

25–61. c *(p. 655)*

25–62. c *(p. 655)*

25–63. b *(p. 656)*

25–64. c *(p. 656)*

25–65. c *(p. 656)*

25–66. a *(p. 656)*

25–67. c *(p. 657)*

25–68. d *(p. 657)*

25–69. a *(p. 657)*

25–70. a *(p. 660)*

25–71. d *(p. 660)*

25–72. d *(p. 661)*

25–73. a *(p. 663)*

CHAPTER 26

26–1. c *(p. 672)*

26–2. a *(p. 672)*

26–3. a *(p. 672)*

26–4. a *(p. 672)*

26–5. b *(p. 672)*

26–6. d *(p. 673)*

26–7. c *(p. 673)*

26–8. d *(p. 673)*

26–9. a *(p. 674)*

26–10. a *(p. 673)*

26–11. c *(p. 674)*

26–12. d *(p. 674)*

26–13. d *(p. 674)*

26–14. b *(p. 674)*

26–15. b *(p. 674)*

26–16. d *(p. 675)*

26–17. d *(p. 676)*

26–18. d *(p. 676)*

26–19. a *(p. 676)*

26–20. b *(p. 677)*

26–21. a *(p. 677)*

26–22. c *(p. 677)*

26–23. b *(p. 677)*

26–24. d *(p. 677)*

26–25. b *(p. 678)*

26–26. d *(p. 678)*

26–27. b *(p. 678)*

26–28. d *(p. 678)*

26–29. b *(p. 678)*

26–30. b *(p. 678)*

26–31. d *(p. 679)*

26–32. a *(p. 679)*

26–33. a *(p. 679)*

26–34. d *(p. 680)*

26–35. b *(p. 681)*

26–36. a *(p. 681)*

26–37. b *(p. 681)*

26–38. c *(p. 681)*

26–39. b *(p. 683)*

26–40. d *(p. 683)*

26–41. b *(p. 683)*

26–42. d *(p. 683)*

26–43. d *(p. 683)*

26–44. b *(p. 684)*

26–45. c *(p. 684)*

26–46. a *(p. 685)*

26–47. d *(p. 685)*

CHAPTER 27

27–1. c *(p. 690)*

27–2. c *(p. 690)*

27–3. c *(p. 690)*

27–4. d *(p. 692)*

27–5. a *(p. 694)*

27–6. d *(p. 695)*

27–7. b *(p. 695)*

27–8. a *(p. 697)*

27–9. d *(p. 699)*

27–10. b *(p. 699)*

27–11. a *(p. 699)*

27–12. d *(p. 700)*

27–13. d *(p. 701)*

27–14. a *(p. 702)*

27–15. b *(p. 702)*

27–16. a *(p. 703)*

27–17. d *(p. 704)*

27–18. d *(p. 704)*

27–19. b *(p. 704)*

27–20. d *(p. 705)*

27–21. c *(p. 706)*

27–22. d *(p. 706)*

27–23. d *(p. 709)*

27–24. c *(p. 708)*

27–25. b *(p. 715)*

27–26. b *(p. 714)*

27–27. b *(p. 715)*

27–28. c *(p. 716)*

27–29. d *(p. 716)*

27–30. a *(p. 717)*

27–31. c *(p. 717)*

27–32. b *(p. 717)*

CHAPTER 28

28–1. c *(p. 730)*

28–2. c *(p. 730)*

28–3. b *(p. 730)*

28–4. d *(p. 732)*

28–5. d *(p. 732)*

28–6. c *(p. 732)*

28–7. a *(p. 732)*

28–8. c *(p. 733)*

28–9. d *(p. 733)*

28–10. b *(p. 734)*

28–11. a *(p. 737)*

28–12. d *(p. 737)*

28–13. a *(p. 737)*

CHAPTER 29

29–1. c *(p. 744)*

29–2. c *(p. 744)*

29–3. c *(p. 744)*

29–4. b *(p. 744)*

29–5. d *(p. 744)*

29–6. c *(p. 744)*

29–7. c *(p. 744)*

29–8. b *(p. 745)*

29–9. c *(p. 746)*

29–10. d *(p. 746)*

29–11. b *(p. 748)*

29–12. b *(p. 748)*

29–13. b *(p. 748)*

29–14. c *(p. 749)*

29–15. d *(p. 749)*

29–16. c *(pp. 750-751)*

29–17. d *(pp. 750-751)*

29–18. a *(p. 751)*

29–19. b *(p. 751)*

29–20. c *(p. 752)*

29–21. b *(p. 753)*

29–22. d *(p. 755)*

29–23. d *(p. 756)*

29–24. c *(p. 758)*

29–25. b *(pp. 758-759)*

29–26. d *(p. 759)*

29–27. a *(p. 760)*

29–28. b *(p. 760)*

CHAPTER 30

30–1. b *(p. 766)*

30–2. c *(p. 767)*

30–3. a *(p. 767)*

30–4. b *(p. 767)*

30–5. b *(p. 767)*

30–6. d *(pp. 768-769)*

30–7. a *(p. 769)*

30–8. c *(p. 769)*

30–9. a *(p. 769)*

30–10. d *(p. 780)*

30–11. b *(p. 770)*

30–12. a *(pp. 773-774)*

30–13. d *(p. 771)*

30–14. c *(p. 773)*

30–15. b *(p. 773)*

30–16. d *(p. 774)*

30–17. c *(p. 777)*

30–18. d *(p. 777)*

30–19. b *(p. 777)*

30–20. d *(p. 778)*

30–21. c *(p. 780)*

30–22. d *(pp. 766, 777, 786)*

30–23. c *(p. 792)*

30–24. d *(pp. 781-782, 789)*

30–25. a *(p. 782)*

30–26. b *(p. 786)*

30–27. c *(p. 787)*

30–28. a *(p. 788)*

30–29. b *(p. 790)*

30–30. d *(p. 790)*

30–31. b *(p. 792)*

30–32. c *(p. 793)*

30–33. a *(p. 794)*

30–34. d *(p. 795)*

30–35. d *(p. 796)*

30–36. a *(pp. 797-798)*

30–37. d *(p. 799)*

30–38. d *(p. 802)*

CHAPTER 31

31–1. c *(p. 812)*

31–2. b *(p. 812)*

31–3. d *(p. 812)*

31–4. a *(p. 812)*

31–5. c *(p. 812)*

31–6. a *(p. 813)*

31–7. d *(p. 813)*

31–8. c *(p. 813)*

31–9. c *(p. 813)*

31–10. b *(p. 814)*

31–11. d *(p. 814)*

31–12. b *(p. 815)*

31–13. b *(p. 816)*

31–14. d *(p. 816)*

31–15. b *(pp. 816-817)*

31–16. d *(p. 817)*

31–17. b *(p. 817)*

31–18. b *(pp. 817-818)*

31–19. c *(p. 817)*

31–20. c *(p. 818)*

31–21. c *(p. 819)*

31–22. d *(p. 819)*

31–23. c *(p. 819)*

31–24. b *(p. 819)*

31–25. a *(pp. 819-820)*

31–26. a *(p. 819)*

31–27. c *(p. 820)*

31–28. c *(p. 821)*

31–29. c *(p. 822)*

CHAPTER 32

32–1. a *(p. 828)*

32–2. c *(p. 828)*

32–3. b *(p. 828)*

32–4. c *(pp. 828-829)*

32–5. d *(p. 828)*

32–6. c *(p. 829)*

32–7. c *(p. 829)*

32–8. b *(p. 829)*

32–9. d *(p. 829)*

32–10. d *(pp. 829-830)*

32–11. d *(p. 830)*

32–12. a *(p. 830)*

32–13. b *(p. 830)*

32–14. a *(p. 831)*

32–15. d *(p. 831)*

32–16. c *(p. 831)*

32–17. c *(p. 832)*

32–18. a *(p. 833)*

32–19. c *(p. 833)*

32–20. a *(p. 833)*

32–21. d *(pp. 833-834)*

32–22. c *(p. 834)*

32–23. b *(p. 834)*

32–24. d *(p. 834)*

32–25. d *(p. 834)*

32–26. a *(p. 835)*

32–27. b *(p. 835)*

32–28. c *(p. 835)*

32–29. c *(p. 835)*

32–30. a *(p. 836)*

32–31. a *(p. 836)*

32–32. c *(p. 837)*

32–33. c *(p. 837)*

32–34. d *(p. 839)*

32–35. b *(p. 838)*

32–36. d *(p. 839)*

32–37. a *(p. 839)*

32–38. c *(p. 839)*

32–39. d *(p. 839)*

32–40. c *(p. 839)*

32–41. c *(p. 840)*

32–42. b *(p. 841)*

32–43. c *(p. 842)*

32–44. b *(p. 842)*

32–45. b *(p. 843)*

32–46. b *(p. 843)*

32–47. c *(p. 843)*

32–48. a *(p. 845)*

32–49. c *(p. 846)*

32–50. a *(p. 846)*

32–51. a *(p. 847)*

32–52. a *(p. 847)*

32–53. b *(p. 847)*

32–54. b *(p. 847)*

CHAPTER 33

33–1. c *(p. 856)*

33–2. b *(p. 856)*

33–3. a *(p. 856)*

33–4. d *(p. 856)*

33–5. d *(p. 856)*

33–6. b *(p. 857)*

33–7. a *(p. 857)*

33–8. a *(p. 858)*

33–9. c *(p. 858)*

33–10. d *(p. 858)*

33–11. a *(p. 858)*

33–12. b *(p. 859)*

33–13. c *(p. 859)*

33–14. b *(p. 859)*

33–15. a *(p. 859)*

33–16. a *(p. 860)*

33–17. c *(p. 861)*

33–18. b *(p. 862)*

33–19. c *(p. 862)*

33–20. d *(p. 863)*

33–21. c *(p. 866)*

33–22. d *(pp. 866-868)*

33–23. d *(p. 866)*

33–24. d *(pp. 866-867)*

33–25. b *(p. 868)*

33–26. c *(p. 868)*

33–27. c *(p. 869)*

33–28. b *(p. 870)*

33–29. d *(p. 872)*

33–30. b *(p. 876)*

CHAPTER 34

34–1. a *(p. 884)*

34–2. d *(p. 884)*

34–3. b *(p. 884)*

34–4. a *(p. 884)*

34–5. c *(pp. 884-885)*

34–6. b *(p. 886)*

34–7. b *(p. 886)*

34–8. b *(p. 887)*

34–9. d *(p. 888)*

34–10. b *(p. 890)*

34–11. a *(p. 889)*

34–12. d *(p. 890)*

34–13. c *(p. 891)*

34–14. d *(p. 891)*

34–15. c *(p. 891)*

34–16. b *(p. 892)*

34–17. b *(p. 892)*

34–18. c *(p. 892)*

34–19. b *(p. 893)*

34–20. d *(p. 893)*

34–21. c *(p. 894)*

34–22. d *(p. 892)*

34–23. d *(p. 896)*

34–24. d *(pp. 895-896)*

34–25. c *(p. 896)*

34–26. b *(p. 898)*

34–27. d *(pp. 896-897)*

34–28. a *(p. 898)*

34–29. d *(p. 899)*

34–30. c *(p. 899)*

34–31. a *(p. 902)*

34–32. d *(p. 902)*

34–33. b *(p. 903)*

34–34. d *(p. 904)*

CHAPTER 35

35–1. b *(p. 912)*

35–2. b *(p. 912)*

35–3. d *(p. 912)*

35–4. c *(p. 912)*

35–5. d *(p. 912)*

35–6. a *(p. 913)*

35–7. c *(p. 914)*

35–8. c *(p. 915)*

35–9. d *(p. 915)*

35–10. c *(p. 915)*

35–11. c *(p. 916)*

35–12. d *(p. 917)*

35–13. a *(p. 918)*

35–14. b *(p. 918)*

35–15. b *(p. 918)*

35–16. c *(p. 920)*

35–17. b *(p. 921)*

35–18. d *(pp. 918-919)*

35–19. a *(p. 922)*

35–20. d *(p. 922)*

35–21. c *(p. 922)*

35–22. d *(pp. 923-924)*

35–23. c *(p. 924)*

35–24. d *(p. 924)*

35–25. c *(p. 924)*

35–26. b *(p. 927)*

35–27. b *(p. 927)*

35–28. c *(p. 930)*

35–29. c *(p. 931)*

35–30. a *(p. 931)*

35–31. c *(p. 931)*

35–32. c *(p. 932)*

35–33. c *(p. 931)*

CHAPTER 36

36–1. b *(p. 940)*

36–2. c *(p. 940)*

36–3. d *(p. 940)*

36–4. c *(p. 941)*

36–5. c *(p. 941)*

30–6. a *(p. 941)*

36–7. d *(p. 944)*

36–8. a *(p. 944)*

36–9. d *(p. 944)*

36–10. a *(p. 944)*

36–11. a *(p. 944)*

36–12. c *(pp. 943-944)*

36–13. a *(pp. 943-944)*

36–14. c *(p. 943)*

36–15. b *(p. 944)*

36–16. d *(p. 944)*

36–17. c *(p. 945)*

36–18. c *(p. 946)*

36–19. d *(p. 946)*

36–20. d *(p. 946)*

36–21. b *(p. 947)*

36–22. b *(p. 947)*

36–23. a *(p. 948)*

36–24. a *(p. 949)*

36–25. a *(p. 949)*

36–26. a *(p. 949)*

36–27. b *(p. 949)*

36–28. a *(p. 950)*

36–29. b *(pp. 951-952)*

36–30. d *(p. 952)*

36–31. d *(p. 951)*

36–32. c *(p. 951)*

36–33. c *(p. 951)*

36–34. d *(p. 953)*

36–35. c *(p. 953)*

36–36. d *(p. 953)*

36–37. a *(p. 953)*

36–38. a *(p. 954)*

36–39. c *(p. 954)*

36–40. d *(p. 954)*

36–41. d *(p. 954)*

36–42. a *(p. 954)*

36–43. c *(p. 954)*

36–44. b *(p. 955)*

36–45. c *(p. 955)*

36–46. c *(p. 955)*

36–47. a *(p. 957)*

36–48. d *(p. 960)*

36–49. b *(pp. 958-959)*

36–50. d *(p. 961)*

36–51. b *(p. 962)*

36–52. a *(p. 962)*

36–53. d *(p. 963)*

36–54. b *(p. 963)*

36–55. c *(p. 965)*

36–56. b *(p. 966)*

36–57. d *(p. 968)*

36–58. c *(p. 966)*

CHAPTER 37

37–1. d *(p. 974)*

37–2. c *(p. 974)*

37–3. d *(p. 974)*

37–4. b *(p. 974)*

37–5. b *(p. 974)*

37–6. b *(p. 974)*

37–7. c *(p. 975)*

37–8. a *(p. 975)*

37–9. c *(pp. 975-976)*

37–10. c *(p. 976)*

37–11. c *(p. 977)*

37–12. d *(p. 977)*

37–13. d *(pp. 977-978)*

37–14. d *(p. 979)*

37–15. d *(p. 979)*

37–16. d *(p. 979)*

37–17. a *(p. 979)*

37–18. c *(p. 979)*

37–19. c *(p. 980)*

37–20. d *(p. 980)*

37–21. b *(p. 980)*

37–22. a *(p. 980)*

37–23. a *(p. 980)*

37–24. b *(p. 980)*

37–25. d *(pp. 980-982)*

37–26. b *(p. 982)*

37–27. a *(p. 982)*

37–28. c *(p. 982)*

37–29. b *(p. 982-983)*

37–30. a *(p. 983)*

37–31. a *(p. 983)*

37–32. d *(p. 984)*

37–33. d *(p. 984)*

37–34. b *(p. 984)*

37–35. b *(p. 984)*

37–36. a *(p. 984)*

37–37. d *(p. 986)*

37–38. b *(p. 986)*

37–39. b *(p. 986)*

37–40. d *(p. 986)*

37–41. a *(p. 987)*

37–42. a *(p. 987)*

37–43. c *(p. 987)*

37–44. c *(p. 989)*

37–45. d *(p. 989)*

37–46. b *(p. 990)*

37–47. c *(p. 990)*

37–48. d *(p. 991)*

37–49. c *(p. 991)*

37–50. c *(p. 993)*

37–51. a *(p. 993)*

37–52. d *(pp. 993-994)*

37–53. d *(p. 994)*

CHAPTER 38

38–1. b *(p. 1006)*

38–2. a *(p. 1006)*

38–3. b *(p. 1006)*

38–4. c *(p. 1006)*

38–5. b *(p. 1007)*

38–6. c *(p. 1007)*

38–7. c *(p. 1007)*

38–8. b *(p. 1007)*

38–9. c *(p. 1007)*

38–10. a *(p. 1007)*

38–11. c *(p. 1007)*

38–12. a *(p. 1009)*

38–13. b *(p. 1009)*

38–14. b *(p. 1009)*

38–15. d *(p. 1009)*

38–16. d *(p. 1009)*

38–17. d *(p. 1009)*

38–18. a *(p. 1009)*

38–19. c *(p. 1009)*

38–20. d *(p. 1009)*

38–21. b *(p. 1010)*

38–22. c *(p. 1010)*

38–23. a *(p. 1011)*

38–24. b *(p. 1011)*

38–25. d *(p. 1011)*

38–26. b *(p. 1012)*

38–27. b *(p. 1012)*

38–28. a *(p. 1012)*

38–29. b *(p. 1013)*

38–30. a *(p. 1013)*

38–31. c *(p. 1014)*

38–32. b *(p. 1015)*

38–33. b *(p. 1016)*

38–34. a *(p. 1016)*

38–35. c *(p. 1016)*

38–36. b *(pp. 1016-1017)*

38–37. a *(p. 1017)*

38–38. b *(p. 1017)*

38–39. b *(p. 1017)*

38–40. c *(p. 1018)*

38–41. b *(p. 1018)*

38–42. c *(p. 1018)*

38–43. b *(p. 1018)*

38–44. c *(pp. 1018-1019)*

38–45. d *(p. 1019)*

38–46. a *(p. 1019)*

38–47. d *(p. 1019)*

38–48. d *(p. 1019)*

38–49. b *(p. 1019)*

38–50. b *(p. 1019)*

38–51. c *(p. 1019)*

38–52. c *(p. 1019)*

38–53. b *(p. 1020)*

38–54. b *(p. 1020)*

38–55. a *(p. 1020)*

38–56. b *(p. 1021)*

38–57. a *(p. 1021)*

38–58. d *(p. 1021)*

38–59. b *(p. 1022)*

38–60. d *(p. 1022)*

38–61. a *(p. 1022)*

38–62. b *(p. 1023)*

38–63. c *(p. 1023)*

38–64. a *(p. 1024)*

38–65. b *(p. 1024)*

38–66. b *(p. 1024)*

38–67. c *(p. 1024)*

38–68. a *(p. 1024)*

38–69. b *(p. 1025)*

38–70. d *(p. 1025)*

38–71. c *(p. 1025)*

38–72. d *(p. 1026)*

38–73. d *(p. 1025)*

38–74. d *(p. 1026)*

38–75. c *(p. 1027)*

38–76. b *(p. 1027)*

38–77. c *(p. 1027)*

38–78. b *(p. 1027)*

38–79. d *(p. 1027)*

38–80. a *(p. 1028)*

38–81. c *(p. 1028)*

38–82. c *(p. 1029)*

38–83. d *(pp. 1029-1030)*

38–84. d *(p. 1030)*

38–85. d *(p. 1030)*

38–86. d *(p. 1031)*

CHAPTER 39

39–1. **d** *(p. 1040)*

39–2. **a** *(p. 1040)*

39–3. **d** *(p. 1041)*

39–4. **a** *(p. 1041)*

39–5. **b** *(p. 1041)*

39–6. **c** *(p. 1042)*

39–7. **c** *(p. 1042)*

39–8. **b** *(p. 1043)*

39–9. **d** *(p. 1043)*

39–10. **d** *(p. 1043)*

39–11. **c** *(pp. 1043-1044)*

39–12. **d** *(p. 1044)*

39–13. **c** *(p. 1044)*

39–14. **d** *(p. 1045)*

39–15. **b** *(p. 1045)*

39–16. **d** *(p. 1044)*

39–17. **c** *(p. 1046)*

39–18. **a** *(pp. 1046-1047)*

39–19. **d** *(p. 1046)*

39–20. **b** *(p. 1046)*

39–21. **c** *(p. 1047)*

39–22. **d** *(p. 1047)*

39–23. **a** *(p. 1049)*

39–24. **c** *(p. 1049)*

39–25. **b** *(p. 1049)*

39–26. **b** *(p. 1049)*

39–27. **d** *(p. 1049)*

39–28. **a** *(p. 1049)*

39–29. **a** *(p. 1049)*

39–30. **d** *(p. 1050)*

39–31. **c** *(p. 1052)*

39–32. **c** *(p. 1052)*

39–33. **d** *(pp. 1054-1055)*

39–34. **a** *(p. 1055)*

39–35. **d** *(p. 1055)*

39–36. **d** *(pp. 1054-1055)*

39–37. **c** *(p. 1055)*

39–38. **c** *(p. 1056)*

39–39. **a** *(p. 1057)*

39–40. **a** *(p. 1057)*

39–41. **a** *(p. 1058)*

39–42. **c** *(p. 1058)*

39–43. **c** *(p. 1058)*

39–44. **a** *(p. 1059)*

39–45. **d** *(p. 1059)*

39–46. **c** *(p. 1058)*

39–47. **d** *(p. 1059)*

39–48. **a** *(p. 1059)*

39–49. **a** *(p. 1059)*

39–50. **b** *(p. 1062)*

39–51. **c** *(p. 1054)*

39–52. **b** *(p. 1061)*

39–53. **d** *(pp. 1063-1064)*

39–54. **d** *(pp. 1064-1065)*

39–55. **a** *(p. 1066)*

39–56. b *(p. 1066)*

39–57. b *(p. 1067)*

39–58. d *(p. 1068)*

39–59. b *(p. 1068)*

39–60. c *(p. 1068)*

39–61. b *(p. 1068)*

39–62. b *(p. 1068)*

39–63. a *(p. 1069)*

39–64. c *(p. 1071)*

39–65. a *(p. 1071)*

39–66. d *(p. 1072)*

39–67. c *(pp. 1072-1073)*

39–68. c *(p. 1073)*

39–69. b *(p. 1073)*

39–70. a *(p. 1078)*

39–71. a *(p. 1078)*

39–72. b *(p. 1079)*

39–73. c *(p. 1080)*

39–74. b *(p. 1080)*

39–75. d *(p. 1081)*

39–76. c *(p. 1081)*

39–77. b *(p. 1082)*

CHAPTER 40

40–1. c *(p. 1096)*

40–2. d *(p. 1096)*

40–3. b *(p. 1096)*

40–4. b *(p. 1096)*

40–5. c *(p. 1096)*

40–6. b *(p. 1097)*

40–7. a *(p. 1097)*

40–8. d *(p. 1097)*

40–9. c *(p. 1099)*

40–10. c *(p. 1098)*

40–11. d *(p. 1098)*

40–12. a *(p. 1100)*

40–13. b *(p. 1101)*

40–14. d *(p. 1101)*

40–15. a *(p. 1101)*

40–16. d *(p. 1102)*

40–17. b *(p. 1104)*

40–18. d *(p. 1104)*

40–19. c *(p. 1104)*

40–20. b *(p. 1104)*

40–21. a *(p. 1106)*

40–22. d *(p. 1107)*

40–23. c *(p. 1108)*

CHAPTER 41

41–1. c *(p. 1112)*

41–2. a *(p. 1112)*

41–3. d *(p. 1113)*

41–4. d *(p. 1114)*

41–5. a *(p. 1114)*

41–6. c *(p. 1114)*

41–7. b *(p. 1114)*

41–8. b *(pp. 1114–1115)*

41–9. b *(p. 1116)*

41–10. b *(p. 1116)*

41–11. b *(p. 1118)*

41–12. a *(p. 1118)*

41–13. b *(p. 1119)*

41–14. c *(p. 1120)*

41–15. a *(p. 1120)*

41–16. d *(p. 1120)*

41–17. b *(p. 1120)*

41–18. d *(p. 1120)*

41–19. a *(p. 1120)*

41–20. a *(p. 1121)*

41–21. a *(pp. 1121–1122)*

41–22. c *(p. 1121)*

41–23. c *(p. 1122)*

41–24. c *(p. 1123)*

41–25. d *(p. 1123)*

41–26. c *(p. 1123)*

41–27. b *(p. 1123)*

41–28. d *(p. 1123)*

41–29. b *(p. 1123)*

41–30. b *(p. 1125)*

41–31. d *(p. 1125)*

41–32. d *(p. 1127)*

41–33. a *(p. 1127)*

41–34. c *(p. 1128)*

41–35. c *(p. 1128)*

41–36. c *(p. 1128)*

41–37. d *(p. 1129)*

41–38. c *(p. 1131)*

41–39. b *(p. 1131)*

41–40. a *(p. 1133)*

41–41. b *(p. 1133)*

41–42. b *(p. 1133)*

41–43. d *(p. 1133)*

CHAPTER 42

42–1. a *(p. 1144)*

42–2. c *(p. 1144)*

42–3. b *(p. 1145)*

42–4. c *(p. 1145)*

42–5. b *(pp. 1145–1146)*

42–6. d *(p. 1146)*

42–7. c *(p. 1147)*

42–8. a *(p. 1147)*

42–9. a *(p. 1149)*

42–10. b *(p. 1149)*

42–11. d *(p. 1150)*

42–12. a *(p. 1149)*

42–13. b *(p. 1150)*

42–14. c *(p. 1150)*

42–15. a *(p. 1150)*

42–16. c *(p. 1150)*

42–17. d *(p. 1150)*

42–18. c *(p. 1152)*

42–19. a *(p. 1153)*

42–20. b *(p. 1154)*

42–21. c *(p. 1155)*

CHAPTER 43

43–1. d *(p. 1161)*

43–2. a *(p. 1161)*

43–3. b *(p. 1161)*

43–4. b *(p. 1162)*

43–5. b *(p. 1162)*

43–6. a *(p. 1162)*

43–7. b *(p. 1162)*

43–8. b *(p. 1162)*

43–9. c *(p. 1163)*

43–10. d *(p. 1163)*

43–11. b *(p. 1163)*

43–12. c *(p. 1164)*

43–13. d *(p. 1164)*

43–14. b *(p. 1165)*

43–15. a *(p. 1165)*

43–16. d *(p. 1165)*

43–17. c *(p. 1166)*

43–18. c *(p. 1166)*

43–19. d *(p. 1166)*

43–20. a *(p. 1167)*

43–21. d *(p. 1167)*

43–22. c *(p. 1167)*

43–23. c *(p. 1170)*

43–24. b *(p. 1171)*

43–25. a *(p. 1173)*

43–26. a *(p. 1173)*

43–27. b *(p. 1173)*

43–28. c *(pp. 1176-1177)*

43–29. c *(p. 1177)*

CHAPTER 44

44–1. b *(p. 1182)*

44–2. d *(p. 1182)*

44–3. d *(p. 1182)*

44–4. d *(p. 1183)*

44–5. a *(p. 1183)*

44–6. c *(p. 1183)*

44–7. d *(p. 1184)*

44–8. b *(p. 1184)*

44–9. a *(p. 1184)*

44–10. b *(p. 1184)*

44–11. c *(p. 1184)*

44–12. b *(p. 1185)*

44–13. a *(p. 1185)*

44–14. a *(p. 1185)*

44–15. c *(p. 1185)*

44–16. b *(p. 1186)*

44–17. a *(p. 1186)*

44–18. c *(p. 1186)*

44–19. c *(p. 1186)*

44–20. d *(p. 1186)*

44–21. **c** *(p. 1187)*

44–22. **c** *(p. 1188)*

44–23. **b** *(p. 1188)*

44–24. **c** *(p. 1188)*

44–25. **b** *(p. 1188)*

44–26. **b** *(p. 1188)*

44–27. **d** *(p. 1188)*

44–28. **b** *(p. 1189)*

44–29. **d** *(p. 1189)*

44–30. **c** *(p. 1189)*

44–31. **b** *(p. 1189)*

44–32. **d** *(p. 1190)*

44–33. **d** *(p. 1190)*

44–34. **a** *(p. 1190)*

44–35. **c** *(p. 1191)*

44–36. **a** *(p. 1191)*

44–37. **d** *(pp. 1191-1192)*

44–38. **c** *(p. 1192)*

44–39. **b** *(p. 1192)*

44–40. **c** *(p. 1192)*

44–41. **a** *(p. 1192)*

44–42. **b** *(pp. 1192-1193)*

44–43. **d** *(p. 1193)*

44–44. **a** *(p. 1193)*

44–45. **d** *(p. 1193)*

44–46. **a** *(p. 1193)*

44–47. **c** *(p. 1193)*

44–48. **d** *(p. 1193)*

44–49. **b** *(p. 1194)*

44–50. **a** *(p. 1195)*

44–51. **b** *(p. 1195)*

44–52. **a** *(p. 1195)*

44–53. **d** *(p. 1195)*

44–54. **c** *(p. 1197)*

44–55. **d** *(p. 1197)*

44–56. **c** *(p. 1198)*

44–57. **c** *(p. 1197)*

44–58. **b** *(p. 1199)*

44–59. **a** *(p. 1198)*

44–60. **d** *(p. 1199)*

44–61. **c** *(p. 1199)*

44–62. **b** *(p. 1200)*

44–63. **d** *(p. 1200)*

44–64. **d** *(p. 1200)*

44–65. **b** *(p. 1201)*

44–66. **b** *(p. 1201)*

44–67. **c** *(p. 1201)*

44–68. **c** *(p. 1201)*

44–69. **d** *(p. 1201)*

44–70. **b** *(p. 1202)*

44–71. **c** *(p. 1202)*

CHAPTER 45

45–1. **c** *(p. 1211)*

45–2. **d** *(p. 1211)*

45–3. **c** *(p. 1211)*

45–4. b *(p. 1211)*

45–5. a *(p. 1212)*

45–6. b *(p. 1212)*

45–7. a *(p. 1213)*

45–8. c *(p. 1213)*

45–9. a *(p. 1214)*

45–10. d *(p. 1214)*

45–11. b *(p. 1214)*

45–12. c *(p. 1214)*

45–13. d *(p. 1214)*

45–14. d *(p. 1214)*

45–15. a *(p. 1214)*

45–16. c *(p. 1214)*

45–17. b *(p. 1215)*

45–18. d *(p. 1218)*

45–19. b *(p. 1218)*

45–20. c *(p. 1219)*

CHAPTER 46

46–1. b *(p. 1224)*

46–2. b *(p. 1224)*

46–3. a *(p. 1224)*

46–4. c *(p. 1224)*

46–5. d *(p. 1224)*

46–6. a *(p. 1224)*

46–7. d *(p. 1225)*

46–8. a *(p. 1225)*

46–9. c *(p. 1225)*

46–10. d *(p. 1225)*

46–11. b *(p. 1226)*

46–12. d *(p. 1226)*

46–13. c *(p. 1226)*

46–14. a *(p. 1226)*

46–15. b *(p. 1226)*

46–16. c *(p. 1227)*

46–17. d *(p. 1227)*

46–18. b *(p. 1227)*

46–19. a *(p. 1228)*

46–20. d *(p. 1228)*

46–21. a *(pp. 1228-1229)*

46–22. b *(p. 1229)*

46–23. c *(p. 1229)*

46–24. c *(p. 1229)*

46–25. a *(p. 1229)*

46–26. a *(p. 1229)*

46–27. c *(p. 1229)*

46–28. b *(p. 1230)*

46–29. d *(p. 1230)*

46–30. c *(pp. 1230-1231)*

46–31. d *(p. 1231)*

46–32. c *(p. 1230)*

46–33. a *(p. 1232)*

46–34. b *(p. 1230)*

46–35. d *(p. 1231)*

46–36. c *(p. 1232)*

46–37. b *(p. 1232)*

46–38. b *(p. 1233)*

46–39. c *(p. 1234)*

46–40. a *(p. 1234)*

46–41. a *(p. 1234)*

46–42. a *(p. 1235)*

46–43. b *(p. 1235)*

46–44. a *(p. 1235)*

46–45. c *(p. 1236)*

46–46. c *(p. 1236)*

46–47. c *(p. 1236)*

46–48. b *(p. 1237)*

46–49. c *(p. 1238)*

46–50. d *(p. 1239)*

46–51. d *(p. 1239)*

46–52. a *(p. 1239)*

46–53. b *(p. 1240)*

46–54. b *(p. 1240)*

46–55. a *(p. 1239)*

46–56. a *(p. 1240)*

46–57. d *(p. 1241)*

46–58. c *(p. 1241)*

46–59. a *(p. 1242)*

46–60. d *(p. 1242)*

46–61. c *(p. 1242)*

46–62. c *(p. 1243)*

46–63. d *(p. 1243)*

46–64. a *(p. 1244)*

46–65. d *(p. 1244)*

CHAPTER 47

47–1. c *(p. 1252)*

47–2. c *(p. 1252)*

47–3. d *(p. 1252)*

47–4. a *(p. 1252)*

47–5. a *(p. 1253)*

47–6. b *(p. 1253)*

47–7. b *(p. 1253)*

47–8. c *(p. 1253)*

47–9. d *(p. 1254)*

47–10. c *(p. 1255)*

47–11. d *(p. 1255)*

47–12. d *(p. 1255)*

47–13. b *(p. 1255)*

47–14. b *(p. 1255)*

47–15. c *(p. 1255)*

47–16. a *(p. 1255)*

47–17. d *(pp. 1255-1256)*

47–18. a *(p. 1256)*

47–19. b *(p. 1256)*

47–20. d *(p. 1258)*

47–21. c *(p. 1258)*

47–22. c *(p. 1258)*

47–23. b *(p. 1258)*

47–24. a *(p. 1259)*

47–25. b *(pp. 1259-1260)*

47–26. a *(p. 1260)*

47–27. d *(p. 1260)*

47–28. c *(p. 1260)*

47–29. c *(p. 1260)*

47–30. c *(p. 1260)*

47–31. c *(p. 1261)*

47–32. c *(p. 1261)*

47–33. a *(p. 1261)*

47–34. a *(p. 1262)*

47–35. b *(p. 1262)*

47–36. d *(p. 1262)*

47–37. c *(p. 1262)*

47–38. d *(p. 1262)*

47–39. a *(p. 1262)*

47–40. d *(p. 1262)*

47–41. d *(p. 1263)*

47–42. c *(p. 1263)*

47–43. b *(p. 1263)*

47–44. c *(pp. 1263-1264)*

47–45. b *(p. 1265)*

47–46. d *(p. 1265)*

47–47. c *(pp. 1265-1266)*

47–48. a *(p. 1266)*

47–49. d *(p. 1266)*

47–50. c *(p. 1267)*

47–51. d *(p. 1267)*

CHAPTER 48

48–1. b *(p. 1274)*

48–2. c *(p. 1274)*

48–3. b *(p. 1274)*

48–4. d *(p. 1275)*

48–5. c *(p. 1275)*

48–6. a *(pp. 1275-1276)*

48–7. d *(p. 1276)*

48–8. a *(p. 1276)*

48–9. d *(p. 1276)*

48–10. d *(p. 1276)*

48–11. b *(p. 1276)*

48–12. c *(p. 1277)*

48–13. c *(p. 1277)*

48–14. a *(p. 1277)*

48–15. a *(p. 1278)*

48–16. d *(pp. 1277-1278)*

48–17. b *(p. 1279)*

48–18. a *(p. 1280)*

48–19. b *(p. 1280)*

48–20. c *(p. 1280)*

48–21. c *(p. 1281)*

48–22. d *(p. 1281)*

48–23. d *(pp. 1282-1283)*

48–24. a *(pp. 1283-1284)*

48–25. c *(p. 1284)*

48–26. b *(p. 1284)*

48–27. a *(pp. 1284-1285)*

48–28. b *(p. 1285)*

48–29. b *(p. 1285)*

48–30. d *(p. 1286)*

48–31. b *(p. 1287)*

48–32. c *(p. 1287)*

48–33. c *(p. 1287)*

48–34. c *(p. 1288)*

48–35. b *(p. 1289)*

48–36. b *(p. 1289)*

48–37. b *(p. 1289)*

48–38. c *(pp. 1289-1290)*

48–39. a *(p. 1290)*

48–40. b *(p. 1290)*

48–41. d *(p. 1290)*

48–42. c *(p. 1290)*

48–43. b *(p. 1290)*

48–44. d *(p. 1291)*

48–45. c *(p. 1291)*

48–46. c *(p. 1291)*

48–47. c *(p. 1292)*

48–48. b *(p. 1293)*

48–49. b *(p. 1293)*

48–50. c *(p. 1293)*

48–51. a *(p. 1294)*

48–52. c *(p. 1294)*

48–53. a *(p. 1295)*

48–54. b *(p. 1295)*

48–55. b *(p. 1296)*

48–56. d *(p. 1296)*

48–57. b *(p. 1296)*

48–58. c *(pp. 1296-1297)*

48–59. b *(p. 1296)*

48–60. c *(p. 1298)*

48–61. a *(p. 1298)*

48–62. d *(p. 1298)*

48–63. c *(p. 1298)*

48–64. d *(p. 1299)*

CHAPTER 49

49–1. c *(p. 1308)*

49–2. a *(p. 1309)*

49–3. c *(p. 1309)*

49–4. a *(p. 1309)*

49–5. c *(p. 1309)*

49–6. b *(p. 1310)*

49–7. d *(p. 1310)*

49–8. c *(p. 1310)*

49–9. b *(p. 1310)*

49–10. b *(p. 1310)*

49–11. c *(p. 1310)*

49–12. c *(p. 1310-1311)*

49–13. b *(p. 1311)*

49–14. c *(p. 1311)*

49–15. a *(p. 1311)*

49–16. a *(p. 1311)*

49–17. d *(p. 1311)*

49–18. d *(p. 1312)*

49–19. d *(p. 1312)*

49–20. b *(p. 1312)*

49–21. c *(p. 1312)*

49–22. d *(p. 1312)*

49–23. a *(p. 1312)*

49–24. c *(pp. 1312-1313)*

49–25. b *(p. 1313)*

49–26. d *(p. 1313)*

49–27. b *(p. 1313)*

49–28. d *(p. 1313)*

49–29. b *(p. 1314)*

49–30. c *(p. 1314)*

49–31. c *(pp. 1314-1315)*

49–32. d *(p. 1315)*

49–33. a *(p. 1315)*

49–34. c *(p. 1315)*

49–35. a *(p. 1316)*

49–36. c *(p. 1316)*

49–37. b *(p. 1316)*

49–38. c *(p. 1317)*

49–39. c *(p. 1318)*

49–40. d *(p. 1318)*

49–41. b *(p. 1318)*

49–42. b *(p. 1319)*

49–43. d *(p. 1320)*

49–44. c *(p. 1320)*

49–45. d *(p. 1320)*

49–46. a *(p. 1321)*

49–47. c *(p. 1321)*

49–48. d *(p. 1322)*

49–49. b *(p. 1322)*

49–50. b *(p. 1323)*

49–51. a *(p. 1323)*

49–52. b *(p. 1323)*

49–53. d *(p. 1323)*

49–54. b *(p. 1323)*

49–55. a *(p. 1323)*

49–56. b *(p. 1324)*

49–57. c *(p. 1324)*

49–58. a *(p. 1325)*

49–59. b *(p. 1325)*

49–60. d *(pp. 1325-1326)*

49–61. c *(p. 1326)*

49–62. d *(p. 1327)*

49–63. c *(p. 1327)*

49–64. d *(p. 1327)*

49–65. b *(p. 1327)*

49–66. d *(p. 1327)*

49–67. b *(p. 1327)*

49–68. d *(p. 1327)*

49–69. d *(p. 1328)*

49–70. c *(p. 1328)*

49–71. c *(p. 1329)*

49–72. a *(p. 1329)*

49–73. b *(p. 1329)*

49–74. d *(p. 1329)*

49–75. d *(p. 1332)*

49–76. c *(p. 1331)*

49–77. c *(p. 1332)*

49–78. c *(p. 1332)*

49–79. d *(p. 1332)*

CHAPTER 50

50–1. d *(p. 1340)*

50–2. c *(p. 1340)*

50–3. a *(p. 1340)*

50–4. c *(p. 1340)*

50–5. b *(p. 1340)*

50–6. b *(p. 1340)*

50–7. d *(pp. 1340-1341)*

50–8. c *(p. 1341)*

50–9. a *(p. 1341)*

50–10. a *(p. 1341)*

50–11. b *(p. 1341)*

50–12. a *(p. 1341)*

50–13. c *(p. 1342)*

50–14. b *(p. 1342)*

50–15. c *(p. 1342)*

50–16. b *(p. 1342)*

50–17. b *(pp. 1342-1343)*

50–18. c *(p. 1343)*

50–19. a *(p. 1343)*

50–20. d *(p. 1343)*

50–21. b *(p. 1344)*

50–22. a *(p. 1344)*

50–23. c *(p. 1344)*

50–24. d *(p. 1344)*

50–25. d *(p. 1344)*

50–26. d *(p. 1345)*

50–27. b *(p. 1345)*

50–28. d *(p. 1346)*

50–29. c *(p. 1346)*

50–30. b *(p. 1346)*

50–31. b *(p. 1346)*

50–32. b *(p. 1346)*

50–33. d *(p. 1347)*

50–34. b *(p. 1348)*

50–35. b *(p. 1348)*

50–36. d *(p. 1349)*

50–37. d *(p. 1349)*

50–38. a *(p. 1349)*

50–39. d *(p. 1350)*

50–40. b *(p. 1350)*

50–41. a *(p. 1350)*

50–42. b *(p. 1351)*

50–43. a *(p. 1351)*

50–44. d *(p. 1352)*

50–45. b *(p. 1352)*

50–46. d *(p. 1353)*

50–47. b *(p. 1353)*

50–48. d *(p. 1353)*

50–49. a *(p. 1353)*

50–50. a *(p. 1354)*

50–51. c *(p. 1354)*

CHAPTER 51

51–1. b *(p. 1360)*

51–2. d *(p. 1360)*

51–3. b *(p. 1360)*

51–4. d *(p. 1360)*

51–5. a *(p. 1360)*

51–6. c *(p. 1360)*

51–7. b *(p. 1360)*

51–8. c *(p. 1361)*

51–9. a *(p. 1361)*

51–10. d *(p. 1362)*

51–11. a *(p. 1362)*

51–12. d *(p. 1363)*

51–13. d *(p. 1363)*

51–14. a *(p. 1363)*

51–15. d *(p. 1364)*

51–16. d *(pp. 1360, 1362-1363)*

51–17. d *(p. 1364)*

51–18. b *(p. 1365)*

51–19. d *(p. 1365)*

51–20. c *(p. 1367)*

51–21. c *(p. 1369)*

51–22. d *(p. 1368)*

51–23. b *(p. 1368)*

51–24. d *(pp. 1368-1369)*

51–25. d *(p. 1369)*

51–26. b *(p. 1373)*

51–27. c *(p. 1376)*

51–28. d *(p. 1377)*

51–29. a *(p. 1373)*

CHAPTER 52

52–1. c *(p. 1384)*

52–2. b *(p. 1384)*

52–3. a *(p. 1384)*

52–4. a *(p. 1385)*

52–5. c *(p. 1385)*

52–6. d *(p. 1385)*

52–7. c *(p. 1385)*

52–8. b *(p. 1385)*

52–9. c *(p. 1385)*

52–10. c *(p. 1386)*

52–11. a *(p. 1386)*

52–12. d *(p. 1386)*

52–13. c *(p. 1386)*

52–14. b *(p. 1386)*

52–15. d *(p. 1386)*

52–16. d *(p. 1386)*

52–17. b *(p. 1387)*

52–18. a *(p. 1388)*

52–19. b *(p. 1388)*

52–20. c *(p. 1389)*

52–21. b *(p. 1389)*

52–22. a *(p. 1389)*

52–23. a *(pp. 1389-1390)*

52–24. d *(p. 1390)*

52–25. c *(p. 1390)*

52–26. d *(p. 1390)*

52–27. d *(p. 1390)*

52–28. d *(p. 1391)*

52–29. c *(p. 1391)*

52–30. b *(p. 1391)*

52–31. b *(p. 1392)*

52–32. a *(p. 1392)*

52–33. c *(p. 1392)*

52–34. c *(p. 1394)*

52–35. b *(p. 1394)*

52–36. a *(p. 1394)*

52–37. d *(p. 1395)*

52–38. c *(p. 1395)*

52–39. d *(p. 1395)*

52–40. b *(p. 1396)*

52–41. d *(p. 1396)*

52–42. c *(p. 1396)*

52–43. c *(p. 1396)*

52–44. d *(p. 1396)*

52–45. a *(p. 1397)*

52–46. b *(p. 1398)*

52–47. c *(p. 1399)*

52–48. d *(p. 1399)*

52–49. a *(p. 1399)*

CHAPTER 53

53–1. a *(p. 1406)*

53–2. c *(p. 1407)*

53–3. b *(p. 1407)*

53–4. c *(p. 1407)*

53–5. d *(p. 1407)*

53–6. a *(p. 1407)*

53–7. a *(p. 1408)*

53–8. b *(p. 1408)*

53–9. a *(p. 1409)*

53–10. b *(p. 1409)*

53–11. b *(p. 1410)*

53–12. d *(p. 1410)*

53–13. c *(p. 1410)*

53–14. b *(p. 1410)*

53–15. d *(p. 1410)*

53–16. c *(p. 1411)*

53–17. a *(p. 1411)*

53–18. d *(p. 1411)*

53–19. d *(p. 1411)*

53–20. d *(pp. 1411-1412)*

53–21. d *(p. 1412)*

53–22. d *(p. 1412)*

53–23. b *(p. 1412)*

53–24. a *(p. 1413)*

53–25. b *(p. 1414)*

53–26. a *(p. 1414)*

53–27. a *(p. 1415)*

53–28. b *(p. 1415)*

53–29. c *(p. 1415)*

53–30. b *(p. 1415)*

53–31. c *(p. 1416)*

53–32. c *(p. 1416)*

53–33. c *(p. 1416)*

53–34. d *(p. 1416)*

53–35. d *(p. 1417)*

53–36. d *(p. 1417)*

53–37. d *(p. 1417)*

53–38. a *(p. 1417)*

53–39. d *(p. 1417)*

53–40. d *(p. 1417)*

53–41. c *(p. 1418)*

53–42. c *(p. 1418)*

53–43. a *(p. 1418)*

53–44. b *(p. 1418)*

53–45. b *(p. 1418)*

53–46. d *(p. 1419)*

53–47. a *(p. 1419)*

53–48. d *(p. 1420)*

53–49. b *(p. 1420)*

53–50. c *(p. 1420)*

53–51. b *(p. 1420)*

53–52. b *(p. 1421)*

53–53. c *(p. 1421)*

53–54. d *(p. 1421)*

53–55. a *(p. 1421)*

53–56. c *(p. 1421)*

53–57. b *(p. 1421)*

53–58. c *(p. 1422)*

53–59. b *(p. 1422)*

53–60. b *(p. 1422)*

53–61. c *(p. 1422)*

53–62. c *(p. 1423)*

53–63. a *(p. 1424)*

CHAPTER 54

54–1. d *(p. 1430)*

54–2. d *(p. 1430)*

54–3. c *(p. 1430)*

54–4. c *(p. 1430)*

54–5. c *(p. 1430)*

54–6. d *(p. 1430)*

54–7. b *(p. 1430)*

54–8. a *(p. 1431)*

54–9. a *(p. 1432)*

54–10. b *(p. 1431)*

54–11. a *(p. 1431)*

54–12. d *(p. 1431)*

54–13. d *(p. 1433)*

54–14. d *(p. 1433)*

54–15. b *(p. 1433)*

54–16. a *(p. 1433)*

54–17. b *(p. 1433)*

54–18. c *(p. 1433)*

54–19. b *(p. 1434)*

54–20. c *(p. 1434)*

54–21. b *(p. 1435)*

54–22. c *(p. 1436)*

CHAPTER 55

55–1. b *(p. 1440)*

55–2. a *(p. 1440)*

55–3. c *(p. 1440)*

55–4. c *(p. 1440)*

55–5. a *(p. 1440)*

55–6. c *(p. 1440)*

55–7. a *(p. 1441)*

55–8. a *(p. 1441)*

55–9. b *(p. 1442)*

55–10. c *(p. 1443)*

55–11. d *(p. 1443)*

55–12. c *(p. 1443)*

55–13. a *(p. 1444)*

55–14. b *(p. 1444)*

55–15. d *(p. 1444)*

55–16. b *(p. 1445)*

55–17. b *(p. 1445)*

55–18. a *(p. 1446)*

55–19. c *(p. 1446)*

55–20. b *(p. 1446)*

55–21. c *(p. 1446)*

55–22. d *(p. 1446)*

55–23. c *(p. 1446)*

55–24. d *(p. 1447)*

55–25. b *(p. 1448)*

55–26. d *(p. 1448)*

55–27. d *(p. 1449)*

55–28. d *(p. 1450)*

55–29. c *(p. 1450)*

55–30. d *(pp. 1450-1451)*

55–31. b *(p. 1452)*

55–32. a *(p. 1452)*

55–33. c *(p. 1453)*

55–34. d *(p. 1454)*

CHAPTER 56

56–1. b *(p. 1462)*

56–2. d *(p. 1462)*

56–3. b *(p. 1463)*

56–4. b *(p. 1463)*

56–5. b *(p. 1463)*

56–6. b *(p. 1463)*

56–7. c *(p. 1464)*

56–8. a *(p. 1464)*

56–9. a *(p. 1464)*

56–10. b *(p. 1465)*

56–11. b *(p. 1465)*

56–12. d *(p. 1465)*

56–13. d *(p. 1465)*

56–14. d *(p. 1466)*

56–15. b *(p. 1466)*

56–16. d *(p. 1466)*

56–17. b *(p. 1466)*

56–18. c *(p. 1466)*

56–19. c *(p. 1467)*

56–20. b *(p. 1467)*

56–21. a *(p. 1467)*

56–22. a *(p. 1468)*

56–23. b *(p. 1468)*

56–24. d *(p. 1468)*

56–25. c *(p. 1469)*

56–26. c *(p. 1470)*

56–27. a *(pp. 1470-1471)*

56–28. d *(p. 1471)*

56–29. c *(p. 1471)*

56–30. a *(p. 1471)*

56–31. b *(p. 1471)*

56–32. c *(p. 1471)*

56–33. b *(p. 1473)*

56–34. c *(p. 1474)*

56–35. b *(p. 1474)*

56–36. a *(p. 1474)*

56–37. d *(p. 1474)*

56–38. d *(p. 1475)*

56–39. c *(p. 1475)*

56–40. b *(p. 1475)*

56–41. a *(p. 1475)*

56–42. d *(p. 1475)*

56–43. c *(p. 1476)*

56–44. b *(p. 1476)*

56–45. c *(p. 1476)*

56–46. c *(p. 1476)*

56–47. d *(p. 1476)*

56–48. d *(p. 1476)*

56–49. d *(p. 1477)*

CHAPTER 57

57–1. c *(p. 1486)*

57–2. d *(p. 1486)*

57–3. c *(p. 1486)*

57–4. a *(p. 1486)*

57–5. c *(pp. 1486-1487)*

57–6. a *(p. 1487)*

57–7. d *(p. 1487)*

57–8. d *(p. 1487)*

57–9. d *(p. 1487)*

57–10. c *(p. 1488)*

57–11. a *(p. 1488)*

57–12. c *(p. 1488)*

57–13. b *(p. 1488)*

57–14. d *(p. 1489)*

57–15. d *(p. 1489)*

57–16. c *(p. 1489)*

57–17. d *(p. 1489)*

57–18. b *(p. 1489)*

57–19. c *(p. 1489)*

57–20. c *(p. 1490)*

57–21. d *(p. 1490)*

57–22. a *(p. 1490)*

57–23. d *(p. 1490)*

57–24. c *(p. 1491)*

57–25. c *(p. 1491)*

57–26. d *(p. 1491)*

57–27. a *(p. 1491)*

57–28. a *(p. 1491)*

57–29. d *(p. 1491)*

57–30. c *(p. 1492)*

57–31. d *(p. 1492)*

57–32. d *(p. 1492)*

57–33. a *(p. 1492)*

57–34. a *(p. 1492)*

57–35. b *(p. 1493)*

57–36. b *(p. 1493)*

57–37. b *(p. 1493)*

57–38. b *(p. 1493)*

57–39. c *(pp. 1493-1494)*

57–40. d *(p. 1494)*

57–41. a *(p. 1494)*

57–42. a *(p. 1494)*

57–43. a *(p. 1494)*

57–44. c *(p. 1495)*

57–45. c *(p. 1495)*

57–46. a *(p. 1495)*

57–47. c *(p. 1495)*

57–48. a *(p. 1496)*

57–49. a *(p. 1497)*

57–50. c *(p. 1497)*

57–51. d *(p. 1497)*

57–52. a *(p. 1497)*

57–53. b *(p. 1497)*

57–54. d *(p. 1497)*

57–55. c *(p. 1497)*

57–56. d *(p. 1499)*

57–57. d *(p. 1498)*

57–58. a *(p. 1498)*

57–59. c *(p. 1499)*

57–60. b *(p. 1499)*

57–61. c *(p. 1499)*

57–62. c *(p. 1499)*

57–63. b *(p. 1500)*

57–64. b *(p. 1500)*

57–65. d *(pp. 1500-1501)*

57–66. a *(p. 1504)*

57–67. a *(p. 1504)*

57–68. a *(p. 1503)*

57–69. d *(p. 1503)*

57–70. b *(p. 1504)*

57–71. c *(p. 1505)*

57–72. a *(p. 1506)*

57–73. b *(p. 1506)*

57–74. a *(p. 1506)*

57–75. d *(p. 1506)*

57–76. d *(p. 1506)*

CHAPTER 58

58–1. a *(p. 1519)*

58–2. d *(p. 1519)*

58–3. a *(p. 1519)*

58–4. c *(p. 1520)*

58–5. b *(p. 1520)*

58–6. d *(p. 1521)*

58–7. b *(p. 1521)*

58–8. b *(p. 1521)*

58–9. d *(p. 1521)*

58–10. c *(p. 1525)*

58–11. c *(p. 1525)*

58–12. c *(p. 1525)*

58–13. d *(p. 1525)*

58–14. c *(p. 1526)*

58–15. a *(p. 1526)*

58–16. a *(p. 1527)*

58–17. a *(p. 1527)*

58–18. d *(p. 1527)*

58–19. c *(p. 1527)*

58–20. c *(p. 1527)*

58–21. d *(p. 1528)*

58–22. d *(p. 1528)*

58–23. c *(p. 1528)*

58–24. d *(p. 1528)*

58–25. b *(p. 1529)*

58–26. a *(p. 1529)*

58–27. d *(p. 1529)*

58–28. d *(p. 1530)*

58–29. c *(p. 1533)*

58–30. a *(p. 1531)*

58–31. c *(p. 1531)*

58–32. d *(p. 1531)*

58–33. d *(p. 1531)*

58–34. d *(pp. 1533-1534)*

58–35. a *(p. 1533)*

58–36. c *(p. 1533)*

58–37. c *(p. 1534)*

58–38. d *(p. 1534)*

58–39. c *(p. 1536)*

58–40. b *(pp. 1536-1537)*

58–41. c *(pp. 1536-1537)*

58–42. a *(p. 1537)*

58–43. c *(p. 1537)*

58–44. b *(p. 1537)*

58–45. b *(p. 1538)*

58–46. d *(p. 1538)*

58–47. b *(p. 1538)*

58–48. b *(p. 1538)*

58–49. c *(p. 1539)*

58–50. c *(p. 1539)*

58–51. d *(p. 1540)*

58–52. **d** *(p. 1541)*

58–53. **b** *(p. 1542)*

58–54. **a** *(p. 1542)*

58–55. **a** *(p. 1544)*

58–56. **d** *(p. 1544)*

58–57. **b** *(p. 1544)*

58–58. **d** *(pp. 1544-1545)*

58–59. **d** *(p. 1545)*

58–60. **d** *(pp. 1546-1547)*

58–61. **d** *(p. 1546)*

58–62. **c** *(p. 1547)*

CHAPTER 59

59–1. **d** *(p. 1556)*

59–2. **b** *(p. 1557)*

59–3. **b** *(p. 1557)*

59–4. **c** *(p. 1557)*

59–5. **b** *(p. 1557)*

59–6. **a** *(p. 1559)*

59–7. **d** *(p. 1559)*

59–8. **d** *(p. 1559)*

59–9. **d** *(p. 1559)*

59–10. **b** *(p. 1560)*

59–11. **d** *(p. 1561)*

59–12. **b** *(p. 1561)*

59–13. **a** *(p. 1561)*

59–14. **c** *(p. 1561)*

59–15. **c** *(p. 1560)*

Index

The numbers following each entry indicate chapter and question numbers.

Instructions for Obtaining CME

On the following pages are 50 test questions. Please indicate your answers to these questions on the blue answer grid that appears at the end of the book. ANSWERS MUST BE RECORDED IN PENCIL. Complete the CME evaluation form printed on the reverse side. Enclose the completed answer grid and CME evaluation form in the preaddressed envelope along with a check for $25 payable to The University of Texas Southwestern Medical Center at Dallas.

Statement of Educational Need

This study guide was designed to give the reader an understanding of the management of normal and abnormal pregnancies based on sound obstetrical practice, which is presented in detail in *Williams Obstetrics, 21st Edition.* The purpose of this study guide is to assess comprehension and retention of materials covered in the textbook.

In recent years, new data have added substantially to our knowledge of obstetrics and have changed many management schemes and practice patterns. This updated information needs to be disseminated to physicians in order to help improve recognition and management of common obstetrical problems.

Target Audience and Suggested Use of Materials

The said educational material is comprised of the study guide for the 21st edition of *Williams Obstetrics.* It is suggested that, prior to taking the examination, the participants review the 21st edition of *Williams*, complete the questions contained in the study guide, and finally complete the test evaluation.

Educational Objectives

After reviewing the above materials, individuals will be able to:
1. Determine their fund of knowledge with regard to basic obstetrics.
2. Determine their fund of knowledge with regard to high-risk pregnancies and a variety of medical complications of pregnancy.
3. Be able to assess their knowledge base of common labor problems as well as complications at the time of delivery and postpartum.

Continuing Medical Education Questions

1. For pregnancy, the National Research Council (1989) recommends a daily caloric increase of how much?

   a. 100 kcal
   b. 300 kcal
   c. 500 kcal
   d. 1000 kcal

2. Which of the following is essential for the generation of smooth muscle contractions?

   a. prostaglandins
   b. intracellular free calcium
   c. extracellular free calcium
   d. oxytocin

3. For the purpose of administering antimicrobial prophylaxis for group B streptococcus, prolonged membrane rupture is defined as duration greater than

   a. 10 hr
   b. 12 hr
   c. 18 hr
   d. 24 hr

4. What term indicates that fetal heart rate has regularity whereas noise is random?

   a. autoregulation
   b. automation
   c. autocorrelation
   d. randomization

5. What is the mechanism of action of naloxone hydrochloride?

   a. stimulates acetylcholinesterase
   b. displaces narcotic from specific receptors
   c. inhibits muscarinic receptors
   d. blocks beta receptors

6. What physiologic process is associated with closure of the ductus arteriosus?

   a. increased systemic blood pressure
   b. decreased systemic blood pressure
   c. increased pulmonary arterial pressure
   d. decreased pulmonary arterial pressure

7. Which of the following neurologic deficits is most clearly related to perinatal asphyxia?

   a. mental retardation
   b. epilepsy
   c. hypotonia
   d. cerebral palsy

8. Placental site exfoliation is brought about by what process?

   a. hypertrophic repair
   b. decrease in myometrial cell size
   c. proliferation of new endometrial glands
   d. necrotic sloughing

9. Which of the following organisms has been associated with toxic shock-like syndrome?

   a. *Staphylococcus epidermidis*
   b. *Escherichia coli*
   c. group A β-hemolytic streptococcus
   d. *Klebsiella pneumoniae*

10. What is the most common cause of indicated preterm birth?

    a. fetal distress
    b. preeclampsia
    c. fetal growth restriction
    d. abruptio placenta

11. What is the mechanism by which betamethasone reduces RDS?

  a. increased cytokine production
  b. increased prostaglandin production
  c. increased surfactant production
  d. increased latency period

12. Which of the following is the principle reason for increased fetal risks in the postterm pregnancy?

  a. placental insufficiency
  b. cord compression with oligohydramnios
  c. decreased umbilical cord diameter
  d. meconium-stained amniotic fluid

13. Which of the following compounds are elevated in the plasma of growth restricted fetuses?

  a. prostacyclin
  b. adenosine
  c. interleukin-1
  d. epidermal growth factor

14. Modulation of expression of major HLA antigens by trophoblasts facilitates

  a. decidualization of endometrium
  b. degradation of extracellular proteins
  c. immunologic acceptance of fetal tissues
  d. maintenance of corpus luteum

15. Which of the following is increased in pregnancies with long umbilical cords?

  a. abruptio placenta
  b. uterine inversion
  c. true knots
  d. funisitis

16. A transverse vaginal septum is thought to result from which of the following?

  a. defective canalization of the vagina
  b. lack of fusion of the müllerian ducts
  c. unilateral müllerian duct atresia
  d. in utero infection

17. What is the form of female genital mutilation which causes the most serious medical and obstetrical complications?

  a. complete clitoridectomy
  b. hymenectomy
  c. infibulation
  d. partial vulvectomy

18. With laparoscopic tubal sterilization, which factors increase morbidity?

  a. obesity
  b. previous abdominal or pelvic surgery
  c. diabetes
  d. all of the above

19. Erratic use of which of the following vitamins increases the likelihood of breakthrough bleeding in women using oral contraceptives?

  a. A
  b. B
  c. C
  d. K

20. Which of the following is the most specific test for syphilis?

  a. fluorescent treponemal antibody absorption test (FTA-ABS)
  b. gram stain of lesion exudate
  c. rapid plasma reagin test (RPR)
  d. venereal disease research laboratory test (VDRL)

21. In varicella-exposed susceptible immunocompromised individuals, the Centers for Disease Control and Prevention recommends prophylaxis with which of the following?

  a. varicella vaccine
  b. varicella-zoster immunoglobulin
  c. immunoglobulin
  d. gamma globulin

22. What is the most common presenting finding of Hodgkin disease in pregnancy?

  a. mediastinal adenopathy
  b. peripheral adenopathy
  c. rash
  d. fever

23. The pathophysiology of PUPP is best described as which of the following?

  a. allergic
  b. autoimmune
  c. infectious
  d. uncertain

24. What type of seizures involve a very brief loss of consciousness without muscle activity and immediate recovery of consciousness?

  a. absence or petit mal
  b. temporal lobe
  c. complex partial
  d. simple

25. Which of the following hepatitis panels is associated with acute hepatitis A and chronic hepatitis B?

	HBsAg	Anti-HAV IgM	Anti-HBc IgM
a.	−	+	−
b.	+	+	+
c.	+	+	−
d.	+	−	+

26. In the management of lupus, azathioprine should be used in the presence of which of the following?

a. seizures
b. steroid-resistant nephropathy
c. lupus activation
d. thrombocytopenia

27. Which of the following symptoms in pregnancy is most suggestive of heart disease?

a. tachycardia
b. tachypnea
c. syncope with exertion
d. peripheral edema

28. What is the caloric requirement per ideal body weight of a woman with gestational diabetes?

a. 20 to 25 kcal/kg
b. 30 to 35 kcal/kg
c. 40 to 45 kcal/kg
d. 50 to 55 kcal/kg

29. Hemoglobin S is owing to a substitution of which of the following?

a. valine for glutamic acid at position 6
b. glutamic acid for valine at position 6
c. lysine for glutamic acid at position 6
d. glutamic acid for leucine at position 6

30. Serum levels of which marker are monitored to assess thyroxine therapy of maternal hypothyroidism?

a. thyrotropin (TSH)
b. thyroid-releasing hormone
c. total T_4 plus total T_3
d. thyroid antibodies

31. In women exposed to general anesthesia during early gestation (4–5 weeks), what congenital anomaly is significantly increased?

a. congenital heart defects
b. hydrocephaly
c. limb defects
d. gastroschisis

32. Where in the myometrium do uterine contractions of normal labor begin?

a. laterally in the cornual region
b. lower uterine segment
c. cervix
d. fundus

33. Fever owing to breast engorgement is self-limited and generally, at the most, lasts how long?

a. 4 to 16 hr
b. 24 hr
c. 48 hr
d. 72 hr

34. Which of the following is associated etiologically with a face presentation?

a. contracted pelvic inlet
b. oxytocin induction
c. small for gestational age infant
d. tight abdominal musculature

35. How are Montevideo units calculated?

a. number of contractions in 10 min × peak amplitude
b. number of contractions in 20 min × peak amplitude
c. number of contractions in 30 min × peak amplitude
d. add the peak amplitude minus the baseline for each contraction in a 10-min period

36. Which of the following analgesia/anesthesia techniques is least adequate for low-forceps or midpelvic procedures?

a. pudendal block
b. spinal block
c. epidural block
d. ketamine

37. Which of the following describes a frank breech presentation?

a. flexion of the hips and extension of the knees
b. flexion of the hips and flexion of the knees
c. extension of the hips and flexion of the knees
d. extension of the hips and extension of the knees

38. Which of the following is a benefit of not reapproximating the visceral and peritoneal peritoneum?

a. decreased blood loss
b. decreased return of bowel function
c. decreased dehiscence
d. decreased analgesia postoperatively

39. Which Korotkoff phase sound is used to diagnose pregnancy-induced hypertension?

    a. phase III
    b. phase IV
    c. phase V
    d. phase VI

40. Which of the following is contraindicated in the treatment of chronic hypertension and pregnancy?

    a. methyldopa
    b. hydralazine
    c. angiotensin-converting enzyme inhibitors
    d. labetolol

41. Which of the following is characteristic of Sheehan syndrome?

    a. profuse lactation
    b. amenorrhea
    c. hyperthyroidism
    d. renal insufficiency

42. Which of the following puerperal infections is associated with scant, odorless lochia?

    a. *Chlamydia trachomatis*
    b. *Neisseria gonorrhoeae*
    c. Enterococcus sp.
    d. group A beta-hemolytic streptococci

43. Which of the following is the most specific test of amniotic fluid to exclude intraamniotic infection?

    a. glucose
    b. interleukin-6
    c. white blood cell count
    d. gram stain

44. What happens to placental apoptosis (programmed cell death) after 41 weeks gestation?

    a. no change
    b. decreases
    c. increases
    d. unknown

45. How is symmetrical growth restriction characterized?

    a. reduction in head size
    b. reduction in body size
    c. reduction in both body and head size
    d. reduction in body and femur length

46. Which of the following ultrasound characteristics is an indication of monochorionic twins?

    a. same gender
    b. dividing membrane thickness 1 mm
    c. two placentas
    d. concordancy

47. After the first trimester, amniotic fluid volume correlates most strongly with which of the following?

    a. fetal cardiac output
    b. maternal fluid status
    c. maternal rest in left lateral recumbent position
    d. fetal urine production and excretion

48. What is the etiology of true cysts of the umbilical cord?

    a. intra-amniotic infection
    b. remnants of the allantois
    c. liquefaction of Wharton's jelly
    d. associated with congenital anomalies

49. What is the mechanism of pregnancy loss in women with antiphospholipid antibodies?

    a. placental thrombosis and infarction
    b. increased vascularization of decidual basalis
    c. stimulates prosatcyclin release
    d. protein C activation

50. Which of the following would make methotrexate therapy for ectopic pregnancy less likely to succeed?

    a. pregnancy of 5 weeks' duration
    b. tubal mass 3.5 cm
    c. fetal heart motion
    d. primigravid patient